Advance Praise for *Public and Community Psychiatry*

"*Public and Community Psychiatry* creatively uses Socratic questioning, evidence-based practices, case presentations, art, and literature to describe the many complex roles of the 'contemporary public psychiatrist.' The authors skillfully paint a picture of the psychiatrist as team member, leader, and advocate across the diverse systems of care in which public psychiatrists work. No matter your style of learning or stage of career in psychiatry, there is much to be learned from this book."

Stephanie Le Melle, MD
Associate Professor of Psychiatry
Director of Public Psychiatry Education
Columbia University/NYS Psychiatric Institute

"This amazing father–daughter public psychiatrist pair has teamed up to co-edit an informative textbook on public sector work in psychiatry. This textbook will inspire young professionals considering entry into this field and provide direction to more experienced psychiatrists already serving in the public sector. The authors of this textbook interweave wisdom from existing literature with real-life illustrations from their extensive professional experience. This text will be highly informative for a variety of programs educating public sector practitioners."

Carol S. North, MD, MPE, DLFAPA
The Nancy and Ray L. Hunt Chair in Crisis Psychiatry and Professor of Psychiatry
Director, Division of Trauma & Disaster
The University of Texas Southwestern Medical Center

"Working effectively in a public psychiatry setting is not easy. The work involves so much more than seeing patients and writing prescriptions. What else does it involve? Read this primer to learn more. It does an excellent job of introducing us to public psychiatry's past and, more importantly, teaches us how to work well in the present."

Curtis N. Adams, Jr., MD
Assistant Professor of Psychiatry
University of Maryland School of Medicine

"*Public and Community Psychiatry* is a beautifully written, organized, and comprehensive must-read for every mental health care provider, including those beginning their careers and those who may feel stuck in the middle of systems of care that need tuning up. This is NOT your typical academic textbook on public psychiatry. Each chapter begins by using art and literature to reflect general themes, and in-depth literature reviews on salient topics and wise finely told stories of lived experiences to illuminate core issues. The references are timely and complete. Between a chapter on the history of public psychiatry and a final chapter which discusses overarching community psychiatry values, a broad spectrum of chapters comment on the various roles a community psychiatrist can play: clinician, team member, leader, educator, researcher, and roles in integrated health and with those living with intellectual disabilities (ID). Each chapter can be read independently of others, but each is so packed with clinical insights and evidence-based recommendations that none should be skipped. This Primer is extraordinary in its breadth, its readability, and its clinical wisdom; it is a remarkable educational opportunity for anyone associated with public psychiatry."

Jacqueline Maus Feldman, MD
Professor Emerita
University of Alabama, Birmingham

Primers on Psychiatry

Stephen M. Strakowski, MD, Series Editor

Published and Forthcoming Titles:

Anxiety Disorders
edited by Kerry Ressler, Daniel Pine, and Barbara Rothbaum

Autism Spectrum Disorders
edited by Christopher McDougle

Schizoprehnia and Psychotic Spectrum Disorders
edited by S. Charles Schulz, Michael F. Green, and Katharine J. Nelson

Mental Health Practice and the Law
edited by Ronald Schouten

Borderline Personality Disorder
edited by Barbara Stanley and Antonia New

Trauma and Stressor-Related Disorders
edited by Frederick J. Stoddard, Jr., David M. Benedek, Mohammed R. Milad, and Robert J. Ursano

Depression
edited by Madhukar H. Trivedi

Bipolar Disorder
edited by Stephen M. Strakowski, Melissa P. Del Bello, Caleb M. Adler, and David E. Fleck

Public and Community Psychiatry
edited by James G. Baker and Sarah E. Baker

Substance Use Disorders
edited by F. Gerard Moeller and Mishka Terplan

PUBLIC AND COMMUNITY PSYCHIATRY

Edited by

James G. Baker, MD, MBA

University of Texas Dell Medical School

Austin, Texas

Sarah E. Baker, MD, MA

University of Texas Southwestern Medical School

Dallas, Texas

OXFORD
UNIVERSITY PRESS

Oxford University Press is a department of the University of Oxford. It furthers
the University's objective of excellence in research, scholarship, and education
by publishing worldwide. Oxford is a registered trade mark of Oxford University
Press in the UK and certain other countries.

Published in the United States of America by Oxford University Press
198 Madison Avenue, New York, NY 10016, United States of America.

Library of Congress Cataloging-in-Publication Data
Names: Baker, James G., editor. | Baker, Sarah E., editor.
Title: Public and community psychiatry / [edited by] James G. Baker, Sarah E. Baker.
Other titles: Primer on.
Description: New York, NY : Oxford University Press, [2020] |
Series: Primer on |
Includes bibliographical references.
Identifiers: LCCN 2019036459 (print) | LCCN 2019036460 (ebook) |
ISBN 9780190907914 (paperback) | ISBN 9780190907921 (updf) | ISBN 9780190907938 (epub) |
ISBN 9780190907945 (online) | ISBN 9780190907952 (online)
Subjects: MESH: Community Psychiatry | Community Mental Health Services | United States
Classification: LCC RA790.55 (print) | LCC RA790.55 (ebook) |
NLM WM 30.6 | DDC 362.2/2—dc23
LC record available at https://lccn.loc.gov/2019036459
LC ebook record available at https://lccn.loc.gov/2019036460

9 8 7 6 5 4 3 2 1

Printed by Marquis, Canada

CONTENTS

Foreword   vii
   Steve Strakowski

Contributors   ix

Introduction   1

1. The Public Psychiatrist in History   3
   Sarah E. Baker and Erica Hua Fletcher

2. The Public Psychiatrist as Clinician   31
   James G. Baker and Sarah E. Baker

3. The Public Psychiatrist as Clinical Team Member   55
   Ashley Trust and James G. Baker

4. The Public Psychiatrist and the Patient with Intellectual Disability   75
   Emily Morse, Kelly Vinquist, and Jodi Tate

5. The Public Psychiatrist and Integrated Health   103
   Helena Winston and Elizabeth Lowdermilk

6. The Public Psychiatrist as a Leader   127
   Michael D. Ross and Octavio N. Martinez, Jr.

7. The Public Psychiatrist as Educator   149
   Sarah E. Baker and Adam Brenner

8. The Public Psychiatrist as Researcher   169
   Gopalkumar Rakesh and Marvin Swartz

9. The Public Psychiatrist as Advocate 193
   Ebony Dix and Ayana Jordan

10. Back to the Future of Community Psychiatry 221
    David Saunders and Kenneth Minkoff

Index 253

FOREWORD

Dear Reader,

Thank you for purchasing *Public and Community Psychiatry*. In this volume, Drs. Sarah and James Baker recruited leading experts in public psychiatry from throughout the United States, as well as provided material directly themselves, to create an engaging and highly informative description of the entire breadth of modern public psychiatry. Each chapter is, typically, written with a resident or early career psychiatrist paired with a senior expert to ensure that it is relevant to our target audience of early career practitioners. Indeed, the Drs. Baker are a father–daughter team! The role of a public psychiatrist is often highly misunderstood (so often I have heard it completely misrepresented as a "prescriber"), and this volume highlights the wide range of responsibility—advocate, educator, epidemiologist, and clinician. For those of you pursuing a public psychiatry career, we believe you will find this book an invaluable guide. For the rest of you, this book provides an outstanding overview of public psychiatry to allow better collaboration and care coordination, regardless of your practice (because all clinicians eventually need to refer to or work with public mental health resources).

This volume is part of the Oxford University Press *Primer On* series; I am honored to lead this series since 2016 and was particularly pleased to join an already successful venture. The *Primer On* series has been designed specifically to support psychiatry residents, early stage practicing psychiatrists, psychology graduate students, and other interested medical trainees and practitioners. Specifically, in this series we have asked international experts to create books that focus on a specific set of conditions to provide the basic science and clinical tools to diagnose, treat, and manage these major psychiatric disorders. We have also expanded the scope of the series to provide this audience information and guidance to major aspects of mental health care practices. With these considerations in mind, each volume is written with an eye toward early stage practitioners to present current evidence and recommendation in a format that is user-friendly and informative.

These texts compliment other resources, such as the Oxford American Psychiatry Library, by offering more comprehensive basic and clinical knowledge so that psychiatric and other trainees are better prepared for clinical practice and fellowships (and to take board exams). As they are released, each volume will be available in print, e-book, and Oxford Medicine Online (http://oxfordmedicine.com). We have aimed to make these affordable books that bridge handbooks and more lengthy and expensive highly specialized textbooks. I hope you enjoy this text!

Best wishes

Steve Strakowski, MD
Associate Vice President, Regional Mental Health
Dell Medical School, University of Texas at Austin
Series Editor

CONTRIBUTORS

James G. Baker, MD, MBA
University of Texas Dell Medical School
Austin, TX

Sarah E. Baker, MD, MA
University of Texas Southwestern
  Medical School
Dallas, TX

Adam Brenner, MD
University of Texas Southwestern
  Medical School
Dallas, TX

Ebony Dix, MD
Department of Psychiatry
Yale University School of Medicine
New Haven, CT

Erica Hua Fletcher, PhD
Hope and Healing Center & Institute
Houston, TX

Ayana Jordan, MD, PhD
Department of Psychiatry
Yale University School of Medicine
New Haven, CT

Elizabeth Lowdermilk, MD
Department of Psychiatry
University of Colorado School of
  Medicine
Aurora, CO

**Octavio N. Martinez, Jr., MD, MPH,
  MBA, FAPA**
Division of Diversity and Community
  Engagement
Hogg Foundation for Mental Health
University of Texas
Austin, TX

Kenneth Minkoff, MD
Harvard University
Cambridge, MA
ZiaPartners
Catalina, AZ

Emily Morse, DO
University of Iowa Carver College of
  Medicine
Iowa City, IA

Gopalkumar Rakesh, MD
Duke University School of Medicine
Durham, NC

Michael D. Ross, MD
University of Texas Dell Medical School
Austin, TX

David Saunders, MD, PhD
Yale Child Study Center
Yale University School of Medicine
New Haven, CT

Marvin Swartz, MD
Duke University School of Medicine
Durham, NC

Jodi Tate, MD
University of Iowa Carver College of
    Medicine
Iowa City, IA

Ashley Trust, MD
Department of Psychiatry
University of Texas Dell Medical School
Austin, TX

Kelly Vinquist, PhD
University of Iowa Carver College of
    Medicine
Iowa City, IA

Helena Winston, MD
Department of Psychiatry
University of Colorado School of
    Medicine
Aurora, CO

INTRODUCTION

Since the beginning of the deinstitutionalization movement, the American public has turned to public psychiatrists to care for those in the community who are challenged by a mental illness and who otherwise would go without care. Public psychiatry, the subspecialty within psychiatry that typically focuses on care in publicly funded systems (whether in public or nonprofit organizations), has historically been referred to as *community psychiatry*. Yet in contemporary practice, the terms *public psychiatry* and *public mental health* seem preferential because the work of the public psychiatrist has much in common with the discipline of public health, generally.

The term *community psychiatrist* reflects the subspecialty's roots in the deinstitutionalization movement in the 1960s, when psychiatrists began to treat people with serious mental illness in the community instead of in state-sponsored hospitals. And, indeed, much of the discussion that follows will reference care in community-based settings.

However, changes in models of mental health care, new treatments, and evolution in financing have meant that the roles and responsibilities of the public psychiatrist have changed significantly during the subspecialty's 50-plus year history. Likewise, evolving models of public health care, including the integration of psychiatry into primary and specialty care settings, are harbingers of more change ahead for the public psychiatrist in contemporary health care.

Taken together, it is clear that the contemporary practice of public psychiatry is no longer based in place but, rather, in the subspecialty's tenets. These tenets include:

- addressing mental health from a population perspective;
- using a wide array of community-based services and supports;
- offering person-directed, recovery-oriented treatment planning focused on the goals and strengths of individual patients;

- insisting upon use of evidence-based care; and
- practicing advocacy as a patient-centered health care strategy.

That is, the contemporary public psychiatrist is called upon to do much more than provide individual patient care in a public sector setting. Recognizing that the community should not view mental health problems as solely individual problems, the contemporary community psychiatrist insists that systems of care pay attention to social, cultural, and political influences on the health and well-being of people who live with neuropsychiatric disorders, as well as their families.

Today, the public psychiatrist may find herself testifying in a commitment hearing in the morning and then in a state legislative hearing in the afternoon, evaluating a clinic's new quality initiative, helping develop treatment plans for repeat mentally ill jail offenders, seeing patients at a school-based clinic one day and at the jail the next day, or facilitating translational research in a community mental health center. These are all common roles of the contemporary public psychiatrist.

However, physicians who choose to serve in public sector settings and physicians-in-training assigned to public sector clinics may not be fully prepared for many of these important roles. Therefore, the chapters in this volume offer practical information and guidance to the psychiatrist called upon to serve in the roles of public sector clinician, team member, advocate, administrator, and academician. They include concise descriptions of each of these roles and responsibilities and offer engaging examples of the public psychiatrist at work. They also ask readers to thoughtfully consider case-based problems typically faced by the public psychiatrist.

Each chapter also features works of art and literature, usually from the public domain. Medical humanities help physicians keep sight of the lived experiences of public sector patients; this includes not only the pain and suffering endured by them due to both the medical disorders with which they live and the disparities they endure in health, educational, and occupational outcomes but also their resilience while facing so many challenges. Medical humanities also serve to reinforce the physician's individual and collective will to address the disparities endured by our patients.

There are several excellent and very comprehensive textbooks available that examine community psychiatry broadly. By contrast, this work is a concise guide for the resident and early career psychiatrist to the many roles he or she might be asked to provide in a public sector mental health setting. Our hope for this primer is that it provides a level of support to psychiatrists that fosters their desire, individually and collectively, to serve the poor and the marginalized with grit and determination and to broadly consider their potential to improve not only patient well-being but also these patients' incorporation into their communities.

/// 1 /// THE PUBLIC PSYCHIATRIST IN HISTORY

SARAH E. BAKER AND ERICA HUA FLETCHER

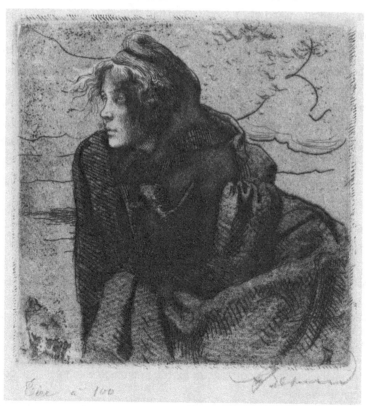

FIGURE 1.1 Paul-Albert Besnard, *Melancholy* (*Mélancolie*), 1888, etching on paper.

Paul-Albert Besnard was born in 1849 in Paris. His parents were both accomplished artists, and his wife was an accomplished sculptor. Besnard is known primarily for his paintings, and particularly for his attention to the illumination of the subjects of his portraits, primarily women (Figure 1.1). His etchings frequently were of women as well, including his series of 12 etchings titled *La Femme*, portraying various emotions of the woman as mistress, wife, and mother (Van Vorst, 1904).

CASE STUDY: INITIAL PRESENTATION

Mr. T is a 58-year-old male who is a new admission to the state psychiatric hospital where you are an attending psychiatrist. Concerned about his welfare, his sister brought Mr. T to the hospital for a psychiatric evaluation. His sister tells you that he spends the majority of time in the trailer in which he lives. She had been dropping off meals for him once a week, and during her last visit, she noticed that he had left the food uneaten for several days. When she went to his home to check on him this morning, she overheard him say, "It is all over . . . life is over." She noted that he seemed to mumble to himself at times. After she learned that he had purchased a gun recently and had also been collecting old medications, she was concerned that he might be planning to kill himself.

Mr. T's chief complaint is "I'm dead. I can't bear this anymore." He tells you that he has felt particularly bad for the past 8 months, beginning when the local manufacturing warehouse laid him off. Although he had episodes of depression in the past, none had been so severe as this one. Two months ago, Mr. T lost his unemployment benefits, and he has little savings left to sustain himself. He says to you, "I just can't get ahead. There is no point in living anymore. . . . I plan to shoot myself." He also reports that he has been hearing voices telling him that he would be better off dead. He looks unkempt, as though he has not changed his clothes or showered in several days. Because he is unwilling to sign himself into the hospital, you determine that Mr. T should be admitted involuntarily.

QUESTIONS
1. How did perceptions and fears about mental illness shape psychiatric treatment in the 19th century? Are these still issues today?
2. What causal factors would you attribute Mr. T's poor mental state if you had been his attending physician at an asylum in the 1850s compared to now?
3. How do the somatic and nonsomatic therapies that you are able to offer Mr. T compare with what you would have been able to offer in a mid-19th-century asylum?
4. How does the inpatient length of stay for Mr. T compare with treatment durations in 19th-century asylums?
5. What contemporary community organizations may be helpful for Mr. T and/or his family?

PSYCHIATRY AND LITERATURE

Memorial to the Legislature of Massachusetts

I found, near Boston, in the jails and asylums for the poor, a numerous class brought into unsuitable connection with criminals and the general mass of paupers. I refer to idiots and insane persons, dwelling in circumstances not only adverse to their own physical and moral improvement, but productive of extreme disadvantages to all other persons brought into association with them. . . .

I come as the advocate of helpless, forgotten, insane, and idiotic men and women; of beings sunk to a condition from which the most unconcerned would start with real horror; of beings wretched in our prisons, and more wretched in our almshouses. . . . I proceed, gentlemen, briefly to call your attention to the *present* state of insane persons confined within this Commonwealth, in *cages, closets, cellars, stalls, pens! Chained, naked, beaten with rods*, and *lashed into obedience*. . . .

Prisons are not constructed in view of being converted into county hospitals, and almshouses are not founded as receptacles for the insane. And yet, in the face of justice and common sense, wardens are by law compelled to receive, and the masters of almshouses not to refuse, insane and idiotic subjects in all stages of mental disease and privation. . . .

Gentlemen, I commit to you this sacred cause. Your action upon this subject will affect the present and future condition of hundreds and of thousands. . . .

Respectfully submitted,

D. L. Dix

January 1843 (Dix, 1843)

Advocate Dorothea Dix began to champion the construction of asylums in 1841, when she volunteered to teach Sunday school classes to women housed at a jail in East Cambridge, Massachusetts. When she arrived at the jail, Dix found people neglected—naked, undernourished, often in chains—because they were suffering from mental illness. Dix sought to increase the number of asylum beds available to those living with a mental illness. As Dix describes in her legislative letter excerpted here, jails and almshouses were required to accept people who suffered from acute mental illness even though they had no treatment to offer, a problem related to the incarceration of those with mentally ill that persists to this day (Parry, 2006).

INTRODUCTION

Public psychiatrists today work across a patchwork of public mental health services, physical health services, public health efforts, criminal justice systems, and social welfare programs in order to improve the lives of the people they serve. It is important for public psychiatrists to know the history of the field's shifting understandings of the causes and treatments of mental illness and the relationship of these understandings to the development of state and local mental health systems in the United States. Accordingly, this chapter describes psychiatry's search to understand mental illness and the evolution of models of mental health service delivery that have been based on that understanding.

SHIFTING PARADIGMS IN PSYCHIATRY'S SEARCH FOR A CURE

Before outlining the mental health system's evolution, however, it is important to note briefly the historic divide between treatments of the mind and the body that parallel the relatively separate development of medicine and psychiatry in the 17th and 18th centuries. The origins of this divide can be traced as far back as Cartesian dualism in the Western intellectual era of Enlightenment, as Western scholars sought to classify and order disease processes (Taylor, 1995). Such dualistic categorizations that historically separated diseases of the mind from diseases of the body now hold less sway in psychiatry. Nevertheless, the effects of these divisive categorizations separating mental health from physical health are still reflected in community psychiatry's challenges working across fragmented health and social services system in the Unites States.

Relatively indistinct from each other until the 19th century, the disciplines of the mind—psychiatry, neurology, and psychoanalysis—developed from nonempirical theories generated by elite men educated in Western intellectual tradition. In this vein, theoretical concepts of what it meant to be "sane" or "insane" and the causes of mental illness often reflected early scholars' views on what they believed to be rational, orderly behavior within strict social, cultural, and religious practices. Whereas mental illness had been variously attributed throughout the centuries to vengeful gods or to imbalanced humors, scholars in the Enlightenment era and onward searched for visible, physical sources of mental illness and created classification systems for those considered to be "inferior"—due to their behavior, skull shape or other physical attribute, or perceived intelligence (Gould, 1981; Scull, 2015).

In the early 18th century, new theories attributing mental illness to a disease of the body took hold, in part due to the teachings of Herman Boerhaave, a medical anatomist at Leiden in the Netherlands. Boerhaave taught that mental illness was caused by beliefs, mistaken for reality, but with a physical source (Porter, 2002). However, his belief system was problematic. Applied broadly, it led over time to the problematic diagnosis and psychiatric treatment of those living in poverty (Pick, 1989), women (Showalter, 1988; Chesler, 2005; Tomes, 1994), ethnic and racial minorities (Metzl, 2009; Gould, 1981), those with intellectual or developmental disabilities (Lombardo, 2008; Sheffer, 2018), and those with nonconforming gender identities and non-heteronormative sexualities (Drescher, 2015; Plant, 1988).

In the early 19th century, and in response to his belief in psychological and sociological etiologies of mental illness, the descriptive psychopathologist Philippe Pinel popularized the idea of improved morale as contributing to good mental health (Charland, 2010). Likewise, Pinel also subscribed to the notion that "the passions" were major causes of mental illness. These "passions" were viewed as personal attributes that could improve with appropriate care. Affective states "irritated" the nervous, muscular, cardiovascular, and other systems and thereby caused physiological effects, including mental illness (Charland, 2008). Intensity and disorder of emotions were believed to be due to behavior, poor self-esteem, and a patient's psychological sensitivity to her environment. Therefore, Pinel proposed a cure for mental illness that involved creating an orderly, structured environment for patients—a therapeutic approach that became known as moral treatment, which greatly influenced the design and operation of early American asylums.

During the early 20th century, there was an increased interest in Freudian and Jungian psychoanalytic theories, which emphasized the role of talk therapy in uncovering subconscious desires that often stemmed from early childhood experiences and resulted in deviant behavior in adulthood. This form of psychiatric treatment often spanned several years as rapport developed and as transference and countertransference could be observed between psychiatrist and patient. Although psychoanalysis most frequently catered to the needs of the elite, efforts to bring such treatments into public psychiatry resulted, for example, in the widespread recognition of post-traumatic stress disorder for both veterans and other populations that experience extreme duress (Dayan & Olliac, 2010). The impact of psychoanalysis in public psychiatry can also be seen in the growth of the art therapy movement, first popularized by Brazilian psychiatrist Nise da Silveira (Amendoeira & Tavares Cavalcanti, 2006).

The early 20th century also brought the first wave of new somatic therapies for psychiatric disorders, such as insulin shock therapy and electroconvulsive therapy. These new treatments were followed by the discovery and introduction of psychotropic medications (Turner, 2007; Brown & Rosdolsky, 2015; Shorter, 2009). This new wave of treatments catalyzed a new focus on biological understandings of mental illness as brain disorders and ushered in psychopharmacology as the mainstay of public sector psychiatric treatment. Although the search for biological underpinnings of mental illness continues, most contemporary public psychiatrists recognize that biological interventions are just one component of a strategy for mental health recovery. Patients who are able to access psychosocial rehabilitation services, have stable housing, enjoy financial stability, experience close social ties, and able to participate in meaningful work have much better mental health outcomes than those without these structural supports within their communities (McAllister et al., 2018). For these reasons, community psychiatrists increasingly recognize the need to advocate for supporting the social, political, and economic drivers of community mental well-being.

SYSTEMS CREATION AND EVOLUTION

Given the previously presented chronology of evolving ideas on the cause and treatment of mental illness, this section describes the development of mental health systems from the rise of the asylum movement to its decline and later transition into primarily community-based outpatient services. Throughout these shifts, we note the changing role of public psychiatry and its leaders as that role evolved from service not only as care providers but also as community liaisons and advocates for the expansion and reformation of mental health services.

Mental Illness in Colonial America

Before the prevalence of asylums, which arose in the late 18th century and lasted into the mid-20th century, historian David Rothman (1971) notes that in colonial America the responsibility for those unable to care for themselves fell upon local communities. Gerald Grob (1994) describes ways in which rural communities in pre-asylum America assimilated, and cared for, the mentally ill—ways that offer lessons for contemporary practice as well. In 17th-century America, communities rallied to support a local family in caring for a "distracted" relative at home. In keeping with Puritan beliefs on social duty, locals from small colonial towns often pooled money and provided food and shelter for poor villagers, vagabonds, orphaned, and those deemed mad or otherwise unfit for traditional participation in society. The community residents might agree, for example, to provide the family a subsidy to pay for room and board for a relative, an acknowledgment not only of the family burden for providing the care but also of the lost productivity when a family member was unable to work on the family farm (Grob, 1994).

In larger cities, almshouses and workhouses became centers to support those in need, including those with mental illness, as well as strangers unable to find lodging and work.

In exchange for labor, people were able to live with their families in these facilities and come and go at their leisure. Flexibility for handling people on a case-by-case basis was necessary during a time when small communities held great power in determining the fate of their most vulnerable members.

The Asylum Movement

As the United States became more urban, alternatives to home-based care evolved that were based on the almshouse concept. From an urban community's perspective, it was simply more cost-effective to manage patients in a single setting, especially because there were more people needing care. Furthermore, increased immigration into the United States meant that many people with mental illness could no longer rely on extended families or strong ties to the community for support and so were less likely to be welcomed into homes to be cared for individually.

The history of public psychiatry as a distinct profession in the United States arguably starts with one such urban strategy. The Public Hospital of Williamsburg (also known as Eastern State Hospital or Eastern Lunatic Asylum) in Virginia was built in an attempt to address a familiar problem to public psychiatrists even today: a large number of people in jail primarily due to behaviors associated with a mental illness and as a last resort for their own families or other families in town who could not take care of them. In November 1766, Governor Francis Fauquier asked the legislature to fund a hospital, describing "a poor unhappy set of people who are deprived of their senses and wander about the countryside, terrifying the rest of their fellow creatures" (p. 5). One community strategy for dealing with the "terror" was to confine those with mental illness to the local jail, where people were often whipped, chained, or restrained (Rothman, 1971). Recognizing that this population was not dangerous and therefore did not warrant these measures, leaders still felt the need to be responsive to community misunderstanding of mental illness. Therefore, Fauquier proposed a hospital staffed by doctors who would "endeavour to restore to (patients) their lost reason" using contemporary care such as restraint, medication, and bleeding (Zwelling, 1985, p. 5).

Virginia was not the only state seeking alternatives for the mentally ill. Not many years after the Williamsburg hospital was started, Benjamin Rush, a physician who is often considered the father of American psychiatry, also took up the pursuit of new treatments for the mentally ill. A signer of the *Declaration of Independence* who also wrote the first American textbook on mental illness, Rush was distraught at the dismal conditions for the mentally ill in Pennsylvania Hospital and advocated for the construction of a separate ward for the mentally ill. He was also an advocate of less violent and coercive ways of caring for the mentally ill (Osborn, 2009).

Nonphysicians also served as early advocates for the mentally ill. William Tuke was moved by the story of a widow who had died at the York Lunatic Asylum and advocated for the construction of a new type of asylum. Tuke's hospital, the New York Retreat, became an influential model for hospitals in the early 19th century. His hospital advocated gentler methods for caring for the mentally ill, emphasizing the importance of proper diet and exercise and limited use of physical restraints (Osborn, 2009).

In addition to the need for an efficient way to house people with mental illness in urban settings, as psychological and social etiologies of mental illness gained traction, the rise of the asylum movements stemmed from beliefs that cures could come from institutionalization—through Pinel's moral treatment—and the related desire to create a disciplined society. Describing the power of this institution as a cure for mental illness in the public imagination, Rothman (1971) states,

> The asylum was to fulfill a dual purpose for its innovators. It would rehabilitate inmates and then, by virtue of its success, set an example of right action of the larger society. There was a utopian flavor to this first venture, one that looked to reform the deviant and dependent and to serve as a model for others. The well-ordered asylum would exemplify the proper principles of social organization and thus ensure the safety of the republic and promote its glory. (p. xix)

This promise to "reform the deviant" provided a powerful impetus to support their construction and implementation throughout the Jacksonian era (1820–1845). The institutions themselves—through their orderly design and construction, their placement in rural areas outside of large chaotic cities, and their set routines for patients—were thought to have a wholesome effect, and the prevalent, optimistic view of the day was that the asylum would cure mental illness and return patients to productive lives.

The first public psychiatrists were employed by these early asylums, and their role would not be unfamiliar to contemporary physicians. John de Sequeyra, a Dutch-university-trained physician, arrived at the Public Hospital in Williamsburg in 1745 and served as the first visiting physician. He examined each patient at admission and then once weekly. It was a part-time position—the census at the hospital typically ran between 6 and 15 patients—for which he was paid 50 pounds per year. Dr. de Sequeyra spent the rest of his time in general practice in Williamsburg, one of five physicians in the area (Shosteck, 1971).

The admission process for the Public Hospital likewise would be familiar to the contemporary public psychiatrist. It was derived from British legal practice, and medical historian Joel Braslow (2013) notes, "Hospital admission resembled a criminal procedure as much as a medical one" (p. 789). Usually a family member would petition the local magistrate on behalf of the patient. A warrant was issued, and a sheriff deputy would bring the proposed patient before a court of three justices. If a majority of the three justices determined that the person was "insane," he or she would be sent to the hospital. In order to distinguish the hospital from an almshouse for the poor, proposed patients had to be judged either curable or dangerous so that, just as today, even patients with serious and persistent mental illness were not appropriate for admission unless they were deemed dangerous (Zwelling, 1985).

By the mid-1800s, the standard of care was that the superintendent of an asylum would be a psychiatrist serving in his asylum as both physician and chief executive officer. The superintendent not only prescribed treatment for each patient but also oversaw everyday business operations of the asylums, including hiring attendants, purchasing supplies, and construction projects. He (because few women were allowed to practice psychiatry at that time) was also the face of the asylum in its interactions with the community and government. In addition to moral therapies, medical treatments administered in the asylums included bloodletting, which dominated in the early 1800s, and opium and cathartics, which were the treatments of choice by the mid-1800s (Zwelling, 1985).

Early public psychiatrists became strong proponents for institutional care. For example, Thomas Kirkbride, whose model for the physical structure of an insane asylum and the treatment it provided was emulated throughout the United States, served as superintendent of the Pennsylvania Hospital for the Insane starting in the 1840s (Kirkbride, 1854; see also Grob, 1994). Kirkbride's asylum design was believed to promote mental stability and patients' transformation into virtuous citizens. In a time marked by optimism and idealism in the triumph of science and medicine in eradicating disease, the asylum served as a site for medical superintendents of asylums, their staff, and their staff's families who lived there to model virtuous behavior and to demonstrate "proper" family dynamics as a way to facilitate their patients' improvement. Indeed, social isolation from the outside world was thought to improve a patient's mental well-being because the family unit was often suspected of contributing to the onset of mental illness. Families were allowed to make the trip to rural areas where asylums were built to visit their loved one 3–6 months after a patient's admission. Patients often spent their time farming, cooking, cleaning, or otherwise contributing to the asylum's operations (Rothman, 1971).

In the spirit of reformation, moral treatment infused asylum life for at least 150 years and is arguably a precursor of contemporary psychosocial rehabilitation (Lilleleht, 2002). According to Piney Earle, an early asylum superintendent (as cited in Bockoven, 1963), moral treatment intended to return patients to their previous functioning so far as their condition will possibly admit, as if they were still in enjoyment of the healthy exercise of their mental faculties. School-like exercise, work, much of it intended to distract attention from symptoms of pathology and normalize day-to-day life. (p. 69)

Another early superintendent, Amariah Brigham, explained (as cited in Bockoven, 1963),

The melancholy and despairing, and all those that are uneasy and nervous, that are constantly restless and disposed to find fault and to annoy the attendants and quarrel with all about them, because they had nothing else to occupy their minds, are frequently cured by mental occupation and the exercise of a school. . . . Various are the methods that may be adopted to awaken into activity the dormant faculties of the mind and to dispel delusions and melancholy trains of thought. (p. 74)

Despite the evolving understanding of mental illness as attributable to physical and/ or psychological sources, successful treatment remained elusive. Aiming to be treatment facilities, 18th-century asylums in reality were little different from their contemporary almshouses. Their primary function was to provide physical support for the insane, not treatment. Their goal was to provide relief, not cure. In addition, although the development of hospitals stemmed from the desire of enlightened leaders to treat the sick rather than simply warehouse them, their development also served to marginalize and stigmatize the people with mental illness who they treated, setting up the problem of balancing access to cost-effective care with social integration—a problem familiar to the contemporary public psychiatrist. Women and people of color were especially vulnerable to that stigma, as described in Box 1.1.

Asylum Alternatives

The asylum model of care predominated into the early 20th century when prominent psychiatrists began to advocate for the alternative of providing care in academic institutes and outpatient settings. Adolf Meyer played a key role in this transition (Lamb, 2012). Meyer, a pathologist with special interest in the brain who trained with the pioneer German psychiatrist Emil Kraepelin, emphasized the importance of scientific principles and academic engagement in the treatment of patients. He also developed university-affiliated research institutes in psychiatry and "psychopathic" hospitals focused on diagnosis and short-term treatment, rather than custodial care, for long-term patients. Meyer recognized the issues referred to today as "social determinants of mental health,"

BOX 1.1
RACE AND GENDER IN EARLY PUBLIC PSYCHIATRY

Early public psychiatry has faced criticism for its treatment of women and African Americans. Scholars have noted that reformers such as Benjamin Rush and Dorothea Dix were largely uncritical of slavery and that psychiatric practice of the time labeled as psychiatric illness symptoms that were the direct result of the trauma caused by family separation, enslavement, and extreme social marginalization (Jackson, 2005, p. 6; Bankole, 1998).

In addition, African American patients faced segregation in asylums and psychiatric hospitals, even into the 20th century. Jackson (2005) notes that Thomas Kirkbride advocated for the separation of patients based on race (p. 6), and in the 1840s, Dr. Francis T. Stribling, the superintendent of the Western Lunatic Asylum in Virginia, successfully launched a campaign within the Association of Medical Superintendents of American Institutions for the Insane to promote segregation of patients by race. Stribling advocated that all patients of color from his asylum be sent to Public Hospital in Williamsburg, the first public asylum built in the United States; this asylum received fewer public funds for its patient population than asylums for White patients (p. 6). It was common throughout New England and the South for African American patients to receive treatment within segregated wards and hospitals that were even more underfunded and understaffed than facilities for White patients. The Civil Rights Act of 1964 forbade segregation of publicly funded institutions, leading to integration of public psychiatric facilities.

The treatment of women within the field of psychiatry has also faced similar criticism. Through most of the 19th century, husbands held the right to send their wives to asylums when they behaved in ways their husbands considered inappropriate. Most famously, Elizabeth Packard—who later became an activist for patient rights—was committed to the Illinois State Asylum at Jacksonville. In 1860, her husband, a devout Calvinist reverend, had her committed for 3 years for her public stance that she should have the right to interpret biblical text and doctrine and discuss her views with fellow women. After learning more about other women's stories of their commitments, she formed the Anti-Insane Asylum Society and began to advocate for state laws mandating forced commitment to allow potential asylum inmates to represent themselves in court and plead their cases to a jury (Chamberlin, 1990). Packard saw short-term wins for women patients' rights in Illinois and other states in the surrounding area, and she remains an early champion of mental patient rights (Wood, 1994).

and so patient care was based on his "psychobiological" theory of mind and mental illness. Meyer viewed the body as composed of mechanical, chemical, and mental functions that develop and function together as a unit, giving the patient her personality. For that reason, Meyer's original clinic featured treatment that sought to integrate physical and mental health through a structured daily routine for patients, as well as psychotherapy with both cognitive and psychodynamic components, occupational therapy (primarily arts and crafts), exercise, and hydrotherapy (Lamb, 2010).

During this same time period, training in psychiatry became a university function, generally teaching Meyer's models of psychopathology and treatment. Diagnostically, new psychiatrists were trained in the ability to discern the relationships between symptoms and dysfunction in social interactions (Lamb, 2015). The American Board of Psychiatry and Neurology, intended to set standards to be met in training in psychiatry and neurology, was founded in the 1930s (Scheiber, Madaan, & Wilson, 2008). As training moved into academic settings, fewer psychiatrists were associated with traditional public psychiatric hospitals and instead served in more popular academic research institutes such as that of Meyer.

While Meyer and his contemporaries were advocating for specialty institutes over traditional asylums, attacks on asylums also came from patients. Clifford Beers, a former patient who suffered from mental illness throughout his life, spent several years in private and public hospitals in Connecticut. His 1908 book, *A Mind That Found Itself*, intended to expose the injustices he believed patients endured in mental hospitals. In it, for example, Beers wrote,

> No incidents of my life have ever impressed themselves more indelibly on my memory than those of my first night in a strait-jacket. Within one hour of the time I was placed in it I was suffering pain as intense as any I ever endured, and before the night had passed it had become almost unbearable. My right hand was so held that the tip of one of my fingers was all but cut by the nail of another, and soon knifelike pains began to shoot through my right arm as far as the shoulder. After four or five hours the excess of pain rendered me partially insensible to it. But for fifteen consecutive hours I remained in that instrument of torture; and not until the twelfth hour, about breakfast time the next morning, did an attendant so much as loosen a cord. (pp. 127–128)

Beers wrote about the goal for his book, which was well-received by the public:

> "'Uncle Tom's Cabin,'" I continued, "had a very decided effect on the question of slavery of the negro race. Why cannot a book be written which will free the

helpless slaves of all creeds and colors confined today in the asylums and sanitariums throughout the world?" (p. 176)

Beers sent a manuscript of his book to Adolf Meyer, who viewed Beers' work as an opportunity to leverage new non-asylum initiatives in psychiatry with public sentiment to reform psychiatric care. Worried about knee-jerk reaction to Beers' book leading to the dismissal of experienced asylum superintendents and thereby making matters worse for patients, Meyer collaborated with Beers to initiate a new movement that focused less on the conditions in mental hospitals and more on the lack of funding for mental health care and also advocated for the creation of outpatient psychiatry clinics and population-based prevention. To address the social determinants of mental health, Meyers and Beer sought to improve family dynamics, education, sufficient living conditions, labor conditions, and economic stability (Winters, 1969). The National Committee for Mental Hygiene, initiated by Beers in 1909, was the instrument for that movement. Now known as Mental Health America, it remains one of the strongest mental health advocacy groups in the United States.

The Revolution in Somatic Treatments

The 1930s brought the first wave of new somatic therapies for psychiatric disorders—insulin shock therapy and electroconvulsive therapy, in particular. These new and effective treatments, followed by advances in medication treatment for schizophrenia, depression, and bipolar disorder starting in the 1950s, revolutionized the role of the public psychiatrist.

Shock Therapy

In 1934, Hungarian neuropsychiatrist Ladislas Meduna pioneered shock therapy in the treatment of a catatonic patient who had barely spoken or cared for himself in 4 years. Adopting a treatment used for neurosyphilis, Meduna used an injection of a camphor extract to induce a grand mal seizure in the patient. He continued to give the patient injections at 3- or 4-day intervals. With each injection, the patient remained subsequently alert for longer periods of time until, after the eighth such injection, the patient was able to go home (Fink, 2001). At approximately the same time, Austrian psychiatrist Manfred Sakel introduced insulin shock as a treatment for schizophrenia (James, 1992).

Camphor and insulin seizures caused panic and fear in patients and physicians had safety concerns about their use, so searches began for better methods to induce seizures. In 1938, Ugo Cerletti and Luigi Bini first used electrodes on the temples to induce the seizures (Fink, 2000). The technique was just as effective as camphor or insulin, and it reduced patients' fear of the treatment; an article in *The New York Times* from July 6, 1940, described the early use of electroconvulsive therapy (ECT) at the New York State Psychiatric Institute as a "less disagreeable" treatment than insulin and other shock treatments (TimesMachine, n.d.). It was not long until ECT became the dominant treatment of the severely mentally ill. The efficacy of various forms of shock therapy led to its use as the primary treatment in public psychiatric hospitals in the 1940s and 1950s, but its side effects, especially its impact on memory, fostered continued searches for different treatments.

The introduction of three medications—chlorpromazine for psychosis, imipramine for depression, and lithium for mania—ushered in psychopharmacology as the mainstay of public sector psychiatric treatment.

Chlorpromazine

In 1952, two French psychiatrists, Pierre Deniker and his assistant Jean Delay, at St. Anne Hospital in Paris treated 38 psychotic patients with daily injections of 75–150 mg of chlorpromazine. Initially developed as a surgical sedative and introduced into psychiatry for that purpose, chlorpromazine's treatment success was first reported to the Paris Medico-Psychological Society and published in the *Annales Médico-Psychologiques* that year (Turner, 2007). Patients showed significant improvement in agitation, delusions, and engagement with staff, and the psychiatrists were especially impressed with the impact that the novel medication had on these symptoms in patients with persistent mental illness who had been living on the locked wards of their hospital (Ban, 2007). These patients, previously thought to be hopeless and untreatable, frequently improved enough to be released from the hospital. In the United States, state mental hospital psychiatrists started using chlorpromazine in 1955 when, because of its successful use abroad, nearly all hospitalized patients were tried on it (Healy, 2009).

Imipramine

In 1955, Roland Kuhn, a Swiss psychiatrist, tried imipramine on patients with schizophrenia in the small hospital in which he worked. It did not seem to help with psychosis, but he noted that it made some of his patients hypomanic and also seemed to help the mood symptoms in his patients with both schizophrenia and depression. In a paper and presentation 2 years later, Kuhn describes using dosages of 75–150 mg on approximately 100 patients with predominantly depressive symptoms. Forty patients seemed to improve on clinical observation, as Kuhn did not use rating scales.

Kuhn's discovery was likely unexpected because the prevailing theory of his day was that depression was a psychological disorder that required a psychoanalytic approach to treatment. It is also interesting to consider that due to increased efforts to protect research subjects and decreased lengths of stay in state psychiatric hospitals, Kuhn's research might not even be possible today. Indeed, even if the study were to be done, it is quite likely that the research that led to his game-changing treatment of depression would not even reach publication today (Brown & Rosdolsky, 2015).

Lithium

Although lithium was first tried for mania at Bellevue Hospital in New York in the late 1800s, that early use was forgotten, and the medication was reintroduced in 1949 by John Cade in Australia. Noting historic use of lithium for gout and wondering if uric acid might play a role in mania, Cade tried 10 patients on lithium. Just like with chlorpromazine, lithium led to such remarkable improvements that some patients with very long hospital stays were able to be discharged. Open trials followed worldwide, but the widespread use of lithium did not occur until lithium blood levels were possible in the late 1950s, allowing dosages to be titrated without risking toxicity (Shorter, 2009).

BOX 1.2

THE INFLUENCE OF CULTURE ON UNDERSTANDINGS OF MENTAL ILLNESS

In the 1940s and 1950s, schizophrenia was an affliction most often diagnosed in White, middle-class women, who were thought to have experienced a "splitting" of their personalities—due to an inability to cope with the rigid demands of motherhood and highly gendered roles they held in society at the time (Metzl, 2009, p. 37). Many of these women were sent to psychiatric institutions, where they stayed for a short period—often 6–9 months—and experienced full recovery. Afterwards, most returned to their lives as mothers and wives.

However, currently the diagnosis is disproportionally made in African American men (Metzl, 2009, pp. 178–185). Metzl, a psychiatrist and anthropologist, has noted that as the civil rights movement gained traction and protests broke out across the nation in the 1960s, psychiatrists increasingly committed large numbers of young African American men to psychiatric hospitals when they expressed the anger and outrage of their time (p. 8). Moreover, he writes that schizophrenia has now become more closely associated with violent, aggressive behavior among African American men, who are then incarcerated for their behavior (pp. 96–108).

CASE STUDY: CONTINUED

Mr. T is committed to the hospital by the local probate court. Your diagnosis for him is major depressive disorder with psychotic features. Mr. T works with the treatment team to develop a person-centered treatment plan, after you have discussed with Mr. T the various options to address his depression, including medication, psychotherapy, and ECT. As part of the plan, Mr. T is agreeable to beginning an antidepressant medication (sertraline), as well as an antipsychotic (olanzapine). He also begins daily group psychotherapy and individual psychotherapy to work on his personal goals for treatment.

Although he tolerates his sertraline well, Mr. T believes that olanzapine makes him feel too tired, and so you and Mr. T agree to switch him to aripiprazole, which he tolerates well.

Deinstitutionalization

Deinstitutionalization is not solely a late 20th-century phenomenon because, as described previously, deinstitutionalization and institutional reform movements have waxed and waned throughout the history of psychiatric institutions. Yet histories of psychiatry after World War II focus on the impact of deinstitutionalization, typically described as driven by the discovery of psychotropic treatment and the concomitant social reform movement. However, there were clearly many other factors in the second half of the 20th century that led to deinstitutionalization. For example, Braslow (2013) notes that "the war [World War II] transformed American psychiatry by vastly increasing the number of psychiatrists working in non-institutional settings, strengthening psychodynamic, psychoanalytic, and sociocultural explanations for illness and emphasizing treatment outside of hospitals" (p. 794).

Another driver was a shift in government's funding of mental health systems. State-government divestiture of mental health hospitals was driven by a wave of federal reform bills in the wake of a booming economy following World War II, which in turn drove efforts to offer alternatives to hospital-based care for patients with severe mental illness. Progressive legislation in the New Deal era led to the creation of national and international organizations to support the efforts of community psychiatrists. The formation of the National Institute of Mental Health in 1949 further legitimated the field of psychiatry, and its provision of federal research grants spurred synergies between public psychiatrists, public health officials, policy analysts, and leaders in government. It also laid the groundwork for the eventual establishment of what is now known as the Substance Abuse and Mental Health Services Administration under the US Department of Health and Human Services. Under President Eisenhower's administration, Congress passed the Mental Health Study Act, which led to the creation of the Joint Commission on Mental Illness and Health. In 1961, the Commission published a report that outlined strategies for deinstitutionalization and the creation of community health centers, and its policy recommendations became known as the Community Mental Health Act of 1963 (Rochefort, 1984).

Despite Eisenhower's contributions to transfer mental health care to communities, President John Kennedy is often credited with this "bold new approach" to the transformation of public mental health (Novella, 2010). Kennedy, whose sister Rosemary suffered from mental illness, felt a very personal need to address mental health in the United States (O'Brien, 2004). Kennedy successfully passed the Community Mental Health Act of 1963, which ordered the release of patients from publicly funded facilities and the construction of a robust system of community mental health centers throughout the country as a replacement for state institutions. As one of his final acts in office before his assassination, Kennedy was unable to oversee the implementation of the act, which was left underfunded by subsequent administrations (Thomas, 1998).

Despite the lack of funding for community alternatives, the census in public psychiatric hospitals dropped 70% between the 1950s and the 1970s as service provision moved out of inpatient settings (Geller, 2000). Money saved from closing state facilities was absorbed back into state budgets rather than being allocated to community mental health centers, and patients discharged from state hospitals were not directly connected to care at community mental health centers (Brodwin, 2013, p. 32). One of the consequences for patients is described in Box 1.3.

Evolution of the Community Mental Health System

In the decades following deinstitutionalization, the effects of underfunding the Community Mental Health Act, especially the failure to create less than half of the intended community mental health centers, became very evident (Thomas, 1998). For example, the homeless population with mental health issues—which was now composed mainly of veterans suffering from post-traumatic stress disorder, youth and adults with drug addiction, and former state hospital residents who lacked stable housing and adequate mental health care—skyrocketed at an alarming rate (Grob, 1994). These individuals became a part of what is now known as the "revolving door" or the "institutional circuit," in which people experiencing homelessness move from acute hospitalization to the streets, homeless shelters, and jails and prisons, without much possibility for recovery under extreme poverty (Lurhmann, 2016). To meet these emerging needs, the public system of mental health care began to develop alternative models of care for patients in the community.

BOX 1.3
PUBLIC PSYCHIATRY AND MASS INCARCERATION

With the rise of mass incarceration in the 1960s, the growth of the public and private prison industry, and the failures of deinstitutionalization, the role of public psychiatrists in the criminal justice system has grown significantly, and according to a national survey of data from 2004 and 2005, prisons provide mental health treatment for individuals at a rate three times higher than that of hospitals (Torrey, Kennard, Eslinger, & Lamb, 2010). Psychiatrists are federally mandated to provide mental health care in juvenile detention centers, immigration detention centers, county jails, and state and federal prisons—institutions that are now the largest providers of mental health care in the United States (Slate & Johnson, 2008).

Although it is important to note that patients with mental health issues are no more likely to be violent than the general population and are much more often the victims of violence, prisoners with mental health issues often lack the necessary rehabilitation and re-entry programs needed to avoid future hospitalizations and incarcerations. In a retrospective study of the country's largest prison system in Texas, researchers noted that prisoners with major psychiatric disorders were at a much higher risk for multiple incarcerations compared to prisoners with no major psychiatric disorder over the course of 6 years (Baillargeon, Biswanger, Penn, Williams, & Murray, 2009). In addition, public policy analyst Rebecca Vallas (2016) writes that prisoners who previously did not have a mental illness diagnosis may experience poorer mental health and require psychiatric treatment as a result of their confinement and that prisoners with serious mental illness diagnoses and cognitive disabilities often experience solitary confinement and inadequate mental health treatment. Considering the current state of mental health care for prisoners, public psychiatrists working in the criminal justice system can serve as crucial advocates for creating specialty mental health courses, jail diversion programs, and better continuity of care for inmates with mental illness as they transition into the free world.

For example, as local mental health authorities found their systems of care taxed by increasing rates of psychiatric hospitalization and fewer beds to provide patient treatment, residential units for pre-emergency mental stabilization and step-down units following psychiatric hospitalization offered some form of relief to overwhelmed emergency departments and psychiatric hospitals (Stroul, 1988). Various forms of short-term crisis residential housing have provided voluntary treatment for patients who do not require hospitalization but may benefit from the presence of a psychiatrist and other mental health professionals who staff these centers.

Since the 1970s, another model of care, assertive care teams (ACTs), have brought clinical and social services into client's homes (Brodwin, 2013). The ACT model consists of a psychiatrist, mental health nurse, social worker, case manager, and occasionally a peer support specialist, who is a person with lived experience of psychiatric history trained to promote hope for improvement and empower clients. Patients visit a psychiatrist at community mental health centers for medication prescription or adjustment, and the rest of the team meets with the patient in the community or at their place of residence to provide wrap-around care, including discussing goals, delivering groceries, offering community resources, and supporting stable housing. The most studied intervention in community mental health and overwhelmingly considered a success, the ACT model is lauded for its ability to keep patients housed, maintain their adherence to medication, and reduce rates of incarceration (Brodwin, 2013, p. 44; Corrigan, 2016).

Another strategy to deal with underfunding that community mental health centers have adopted in recent years is the recovery-oriented model of care. This model seeks to align treatment recommendations with patient goals instead of, for example, maintaining a focus on psychiatric symptoms. In addition, clinicians and case managers have attempted to become more attuned to addressing the social determinants of patient health and goals (Thomas, Despeaux, Drapalski, & Bennett, 2017).

As the community mental health system developed, the role of the public psychiatrist evolved. In many states, the early community mental health centers were extensions of the state hospitals, and hospital-based psychiatrists were involved in their development. Public psychiatrists who had previously worked only in state hospitals began working in these new community mental health centers, providing care for the crisis units and ACTs. Especially in rural settings, public sector psychiatrists also served as attendings on acute care units, and even today, a psychiatrist working in a rural setting may be the only public psychiatrist for a large catchment area (Robinson, 1966). In addition to their role in community-based care movement, public psychiatrists also continued to provide leadership and clinical care in traditional state hospitals.

CASE STUDY: CONTINUED

After 2 weeks in the hospital, Mr. T's suicidal thoughts resolve and his mood shows some improvement. He becomes more future-oriented and adds the goal of finding a new job to his treatment plan. As his social worker begins to prepare for discharge, she talks to Mr. T about establishing care in his local community mental health center. Mr. T is linked with a peer support specialist to navigate the transition. His family expresses interest in learning more about community organizations that might support both the patient and the family after discharge.

The Recovery Paradigm

In the 1970s, mental health consumers discharged from state facilities began to speak out about their negative hospitalization experiences. Like Clifford Beers before them, they demonstrated that patients have a role to play not only in their own care but also in policymaking. Mental health and disability activists also premised their lived experience of psychiatric treatment and recovery over the "expertise" of psychiatrists (Benson, 1994). These activists embraced the idea that patients should be actively involved in their own care and championed the belief that recovery is possible for everyone who has suffered from mental illness. Forming what became known as the consumer/survivor/ex-patient movement, former patients fought against involuntary treatment and for their rights within psychiatric commitment orders (Sharfstein & Dickerson, 2006). The effects of their advocacy can be seen, for example, in public psychiatry's adoption of recovery-oriented mental health care, which seeks to empower patients to make their own choices about their treatment by offering them a range of options to support their mental health.

Just as Beers had done, the movement ultimately reached out to public officials, professional organizations, and family member advocates for support in their movement to improve care practices. For example, the family self-help group, the National Alliance for the Mentally Ill (NAMI), which was started by two mothers with sons who were diagnosed with schizophrenia, began lobbying policymakers for a higher quality of mental health care in 1979. Now widely inclusive of mental health professionals, family caregivers, and patients and backed by support from major pharmaceutical companies, NAMI has had success in lobbying for increased federal funding and in bringing public attention to the stigmatization of the people served by public psychiatrists (Benson, 1994).

Another precursor of the contemporary peer support movement is the work of Fountain House, an early patient empowerment group that started in the late 1940s with meetings among peers in collaboration with clinicians at Rockland State Hospital in New York. It was the idea of Michael Obolensky, a former patient, and Elizabeth Schermerhorn, a former volunteer. While hospitalized, Obolensky and five other patients routinely met in the "club room" of the hospital to share histories and social activities such as reading and painting. After leaving Rockland, the group continued to meet on the steps of the New York Public Library and later at the Third Street YMCA in Manhattan. With philanthropic support, the group bought a building in New York City and started Fountain House, intending to help other former state hospital patients reintegrate after discharge (Doyle, Lanoil, & Dudek, 2013, p. 186). This approach became known as the clubhouse model. As it evolved under the leadership of John Beard in the 1950s, the organization focused on members helping each other find jobs and places to live (Beard,

Goertzel, & Pearce, 1958). In many areas of the United States, clubhouses continue to offer day centers for people with mental illness to receive and provide social support.

Mental health activism continues to evolve away from just advocacy toward more focus on peer-led support and recovery-oriented services. Mental health activists' advocacy for the support of recovery for all people who have experienced mental illness was finally realized in the recommendations made by the Bush administration's New Freedom Commission on Mental Health of 2003, which ushered in a paradigm shift in public mental health care to integrated, consumer-driven, and recovery-oriented service provision. Critics of the recovery movement note that the commission's recommendations actually are aligned with the growth of managed care organizations and other cost-saving measures that further place the financial burden of services on consumers, family members, and local government, not the federal government (Braslow, 2013). However, patient rights' advocates and mental health activists who had firsthand experience of public mental health systems viewed the recommendations as validation of their hard-won efforts to infuse public mental health care with values such as self-empowerment and self-determination of patients and the reformation of services toward flexible, patient-centered service delivery on the part of clinicians (Jacobson, 2004; Crowley, 2000; Deegan, 1988).

In addition to the paradigm shift to recovery, the Commission recommended new funding mechanisms to further integrate peer services into community mental health care. Peer services—support services provided by people with psychiatric histories—now have meaningful employment opportunities within public psychiatry (Jacobson, Trojanowski, & Dewa, 2012). Many states have developed formal training for certified peer support specialists, and the profession now has formal job descriptions, qualifications, and duties that have allowed certified peer support workers to become eligible for Medicaid reimbursement in many states (Delaney, 2010). Peer specialists employed at community mental health centers may work with clients by staffing warmlines (talk lines for clients in need of encouragement and support) and peer-operated crisis respites—home-like environments for people who are eligible for diversion from psychiatric hospitals.

Some critics argue that peer specialists—as people with great sensitivity and empathy for mental health consumers—are unfairly placed in low-wage roles with minimal training in the public mental health system. In addition, they are often not incorporated as full members of the multidisciplinary treatment team, and their roles are viewed as upholding traditional hierarchies within public mental health (Voronka, 2017). Thus, some critics of the recovery paradigm view peers as comprising a highly vulnerable and undercompensated arm of service delivery that serves as a token gesture toward greater equality and empowerment in mental health services. However, emerging peer specialist programs do offer the opportunity to create a new face to community mental health care and establish more equitable dynamics between psychiatrists, other clinical staff, and their patients.

Mental Health Parity and the Affordable Care Act

One of the historic problems with access to mental health care has been the relatively poor coverage for psychiatric care provided by private health insurance plans. To address this barrier, Congress passed mental health parity legislation. The Paul Wellstone and Pete Domenici Mental Health Parity and Addiction Equity Act of 2008 was the first law to require US health insurance plans to use the same coverage limitations for mental health and substance use that they allow for other illnesses. A recent study shows that the law was successful in increasing, albeit modestly, the percentage of insured patients who have access to, and use, mental health and substance use services (Harwood et al., 2017).

In 2010, Congress passed the Patient Protection and Affordable Care Act (ACA), also known as Obamacare. One of the problems associated with the transition in the 1960s to a community-based system of care was an increase in the use of hospital emergency rooms as first-line treatment for mental health disorders for the uninsured. By increasing the number of people with insurance, one goal of ACA was to increase access to mental health services in non-emergent settings. Therefore, mental health and substance use services were an essential benefit of ACA health plans, and mental health parity was a plan requirement. ACA also increased the number of people with mental health insurance coverage through mandates to cover pre-existing conditions and to allow children to remain on their parents' insurance until age 26 years. Contemporary care strategies for those diagnosed with serious mental illness were incentivized as well, including supported housing services and chronic disease management programs (Mechanic, 2012).

Data on the efficacy of ACA in reaching these mental health goals are not yet robust. Emergency rooms in Los Angeles County reported a significant decrease in indigent patients after ACA was implemented, and between 2013 and 2014, the number of Los Angeles County emergency room patients with Medicaid doubled. However, it is not clear that patients have transitioned to non-emergent settings to access care. In Maryland, emergency room use for mental health services by traditionally high users did not decrease (Gingold, Pierre-Mathieu, Cole, Miller, & Khaldun, 2017). In addition, although ACA's expanded age range for dependent coverage led to a reduction in psychiatric emergency room visits by adults younger than age 26 years, it also led to a slight increase in inpatient admissions for psychiatric diagnoses in the age range (Golberstein et al., 2014).

CASE STUDY: CONCLUSION

Although the symptoms with which Mr. T presented to your hospital have been understood in different ways over time, they have been a common reason for admission to American institutions for people with mental illness for approximately 300 years. Historic and contemporary treatment approaches have much in common, as illustrated throughout this chapter. Somatic therapies, such as ECT and lithium, chlorpromazine, and imipramine, are still used today, and psychosocial rehabilitation, as popularized through Pinel's "moral treatment" approach to psychiatric care, is still a part of modern-day psychiatric care. The contemporary focus on person-centered treatment planning, as offered to Mr. T, can be compared to Meyer's early 20th-century treatment focus on the psychosocial aspects of the presentation of mental illness. Somatic therapies have evolved since the mid-20th century, including the introduction of numerous new antipsychotics, antidepressants, and anti-anxiolytics, as well as neuromodulation techniques. Furthermore, a wide variety of psychotherapy techniques, such as cognitive–behavioral therapy and dialectical behavioral therapy, have also been studied and developed. Social supports in the community in the forms of housing, rehabilitation, case management, peer support, and/or engagement with NAMI and similar organizations are also critical adjuncts to somatic treatments available today.

Although contemporary inpatient psychiatric care is usually provided by a hospitalist, the professional life of Dr. de Sequeyra at the Williamsburg Public Hospital is not dissimilar from the life of the contemporary generalist psychiatrist who might make rounds at the hospital in the morning and see patients in her office in the afternoon. Public psychiatrists serving as superintendents in the 1800s gave way to specialized health administrators in the 1900s, and there is no longer the same expectation that public psychiatrists live at the asylums and serve as "models for morality" in the way they did during the era of moral treatment. However, the recent trend toward business or health administration training among physicians, including public psychiatrists, has led many contemporary public psychiatrists into executive leadership positions in mental health organizations such as the community mental health center to which Mr. T was referred.

Finally, public psychiatrists today can learn from the examples of their predecessors in both the 1800s and 1900s about the powerful impact of advocacy for patients. This advocacy can occur not just through being a member of a comprehensive team in which patients' ideas about treatment are acknowledged and incorporated into the treatment plan but also through advocacy in the community, in state and national legislatures, and in professional organizations. Public psychiatrists now often represent their patients' needs through service in state government, by participating in public hearings at legislatures, serving on governmental commissions and task force committees, and otherwise educating lawmakers about patients' needs. The history of the profession also demonstrates the power of engaging with patients, families, and others to advocate to improve the lives of the people we serve. Many public psychiatrists are actively involved in organizations such as Mental Health America and NAMI.

As is evident in this chapter, the US government has played a crucial role in the practice of public psychiatry. As a result of its policies, public psychiatrists now serve on the front lines of the "institutional circuit"—the social systems, medical systems, and criminal justice systems that impoverished patients are forced to navigate (Luhrmann, 2016). Throughout the mental health system transformations over time, public psychiatrists have played an important role as advocates for social reform. Today, public psychiatrists can use their experience from the clinical front lines to be on the front lines of advocacy for policy changes as well, urging governments to address social determinants of mental health for their patients. In doing so, public psychiatrists can amplify the voices of their patients, peer support specialists, and family caregivers as advocacy groups continue to fight for greater access to mental health care, transparency in clinical trial outcomes, and the protection of patient's rights.

REFERENCES

Amendoeira, M. C., & Tavares Cavalcanti, M. (2006). Nise Magalhães da Silveira (1905–1999). *American Journal of Psychiatry, 163*(8), 1348–1348. https://doi.org/10.1176/ajp.2006.163.8.1348

Baillargeon, J., Biswanger, I. A., Penn, J. V., Williams, B. A., & Murray, O. J. (2009). Psychiatric disorders and repeat incarcerations: The revolving prison door. *American Journal of Psychiatry, 166*(1), 103–109.

Ban, T. A. (2007). Fifty years chlorpromazine: A historical perspective. *Neuropsychiatric Disease and Treatment, 3*(4), 495–500.

Bankole, K. (1998). The Human/Subhuman Issue and Slave Medicine in Louisiana. *Race, Gender & Class, 5*(3), 3–11.

Beard, J. H., Goertzel, V., & Pearce, A. J. (1958, January 1). The effectiveness of activity group therapy with chronically regressed adult schizophrenics. *International Journal of Group Psychotherapy, 8*(1), 123–136.

Beers, C. W. (1908). *A mind that found itself: An autobiography.* New York, NY: Longmans, Green. Retrieved from http://hdl.handle.net/2027/nyp.33433082549217

Benson, P. R. (1994, March 1). Deinstitutionalization and family caretaking of the seriously mentally ill: The policy context. *International Journal of Law & Psychiatry, 17*(2), 119–138.

Bockoven, J. S. (1963). *Moral treatment in American psychiatry.* New York, NY: Springer. Retrieved from https://babel.hathitrust.org/cgi/pt?id=mdp.39015072209912;view=1up;seq=7

Braslow, J. T. (2013). The manufacture of recovery. *Annual Review of Clinical Psychology, 9,* 781–809.

Brodwin, P. (2013). *Everyday ethics: Voices from the front line of community psychiatry.* Berkeley, CA: University of California Press.

Brown, W. A., & Rosdolsky, M. (2015). The clinical discovery of imipramine. *American Journal of Psychiatry, 172*(5), 426–429.

Chamberlin, J. (1990). The Ex-Patients' Movement: Where We've Been and Where We're Going. *The Journal of Mind and Behavior, 11*(3), 323–336.

Charland, L. C. (2008, September 1). Alexander Crichton on the psychopathology of the passions. *History of Psychiatry, 19*(3), 275–296.

Charland, L. C. (2010, March 1). Science and morals in the affective psychopathology of Philippe Pinel. *History of Psychiatry, 1,* 38–53.

Chesler, P. (2005). *Women and madness.* New York, NY: Palgrave Macmillan.

Corrigan, P. W. (2016). *Principles and practice of psychiatric rehabilitation: An empirical approach*. New York, NY: Guilford.

Crowley, K. (2000). *The power of procovery in healing mental illness*. LosAngeles: Procovery Institute.

Dayan, J., & Olliac, B. (2010). From hysteria and shell shock to posttraumatic stress disorder: Comments on psychoanalytic and neuropsychological approaches. *Journal of Physiology–Paris, 104*(6), 296–302. https://doi.org/10.1016/j.jphysparis.2010.09.003

Deegan, P. E. (1988). Recovery: The lived experience of rehabilitation. *Psychosocial Rehabilitation Journal, 9*(4), 11–19.

Delaney, K. (2010, January). The peer specialist movement: An interview with Gayle Bluebird, RN. *Issues in Mental Health Nursing, 31*(3), 232–234.

Dix, D. L. (1843). *Memorial. to the Legislature of Massachusetts* [Protesting against the confinement of insane persons and idiots in almshouses and prisons]. Boston, MA: Munroe & Francis. Retrieved from http://hdl.handle.net/2027/loc.ark:/13960/t9p281h9p

Doyle, A., Lanoil, J., & Dudek, K. J. (2013). *Fountain House: Creating community in mental health practice*. New York, NY: Columbia University Press.

Drescher, J. (2015). Out of DSM: Depathologizing homosexuality. *Behavioral Sciences, 5*, 565–575.

Fink, M. (2000). Electroshock revisited. *American Scientist, 88*(2), 162–167.

Fink, M. (2001). Convulsive therapy: A review of the first 55 years. *Journal of Affective Disorders, 63*(1), 115.

Geller, J. L. (2000, January 1). The last half-century of psychiatric services as reflected in *Psychiatric Services*. *Psychiatric Services, 51*(1), 41–67.

Gingold, D. B., Pierre-Mathieu, R., Cole, B., Miller, A. C., & Khaldun, J. S. (2017, May 1). Impact of the Affordable Care Act Medicaid expansion on emergency department high utilizers with ambulatory care sensitive conditions: A cross-sectional study. *American Journal of Emergency Medicine, 35*(5), 737–742.

Golberstein, E., Busch, S. H., Zaha, R., Greenfield, S.F., Beardslee, W.R., & Meara, E. (2014, October 31). Effect of the Affordable Care Act's young adult insurance expansions on hospital-based mental health care. *American Journal of Psychiatry, 172*(2), 182–189.

Gould, S. J. (1981). *The mismeasure of man*. New York, NY: Norton.

Grob, G. (1994). *The mad among us*. New York, NY: Free Press.

Harwood, J. M., Azocar, F., Thalmayer, A., Xu, H., Ong, M. K., Tseng, C.-H., … Ettner, S. L. (2017, February). The Mental Health Parity and Addiction Equity Act evaluation study: Impact on specialty behavioral health care utilization and spending among carve-in enrollees. *Medical Care, 55*(2), 164–172.

Healy, D. (2009). *The creation of psychopharmacology*. Boston, MA: Harvard University Press Retrieved December 7, 2017, from https://www.degruyter.com/viewbooktoc/product/463164

Jackson, V. (2005). *Separate and Unequal: The Legacy of Racially Segregated Psychiatric Hospitals, a Cultural Competence Training Tool*. Healing Circles. Retrieved from: http://www.healingcircles.org/uploads/2/1/4/8/2148953/sauweb.pdf

Jacobson, N. (2004). *In recovery: The making of mental health policy*. Nashville, TN: Vanderbilt University Press.

Jacobson, N., Trojanowski, L., & Dewa, C. S. (2012, July 19). What do peer support workers do? A job description. *BMC Health Services Research, 12*, 205.

James, F. E. (1992). Insulin treatment in psychiatry. *History of Psychiatry, 3*(10), 221–235.

Kirkbride, T. S. (1854). *On the construction, organization, and general arrangements of hospitals for the insane*. Philadelphia, PA: Lippincott. Retrieved from http://hdl.handle.net/2027/nyp.33433011466384

Lamb, S. (2010). *Pathologist of the mind: Adolf Meyer, psychobiology and the Phipps Psychiatric Clinic at the Johns Hopkins Hospital, 1908–1917*. Doctoral dissertation. Retrieved from https://search.proquest.com/docview/846615664/abstract/944B01CD880A4A4APQ/1

Lamb, S. (2012, December). "The most important professorship in the English-speaking domain": Adolf Meyer and the beginnings of clinical psychiatry in the United States. *Journal of Nervous and Mental Disorders, 200*(12), 1061–1066.

Lamb, S. (2015, July). Social skills: Adolf Meyer's revision of clinical skill for the new psychiatry of the twentieth century. *Medical History, 59*(3), 443–464.

Lilleleht, E. (2002). Progress and power: Exploring the disciplinary connections between moral treatment and psychiatric rehabilitation. *Philosophy, Psychiatry, & Psychology, 9*(2), 167–182.

Lombardo, P. A. (2008). *Three generations, no imbeciles: Eugenics, the Supreme Court, and Buck v. Bell.* Baltimore, MD: Johns Hopkins University Press.

Luhrmann, T. M. (2016). The culture of the institutional circuit in the United States. In T. M. Luhrmann & J. Marrow (Eds.), *Our most troubling madness: Case studies in schizophrenia across cultures* (pp. 153–166). Oakland, CA: University of California Press.

McAllister, A., Fritzell, S., Almroth, M., Harber-Aschan, L., Larsson, S., & Burström, B. (2018). How do macro-level structural determinants affect inequalities in mental health? A systematic review of the literature. *International Journal for Equity in Health, 17,* article 180.

Mechanic, D. (2012, February). Seizing opportunities under the Affordable Care Act for transforming the mental and behavioral health system. *Health Affairs, 31*(2), 376–382.

Metzl, J. (2009). *The protest psychosis: How schizophrenia became a Black disease.* Boston, MA: Beacon Press.

Novella, E. J. (2010, September). Mental health care in the aftermath of deinstitutionalization: A retrospective and prospective view. *Health Care Analysis, 18*(3), 222–238.

O'Brien, G. (2004). Rosemary Kennedy: The importance of a historical footnote. *Journal of Family History, 29*(3), 225–236.

Osborn, L. A. (2009, December). From beauty to despair: The rise and fall of the American state mental hospital. *Psychiatry Quarterly, 80*(4), 219–231.

Parry, M. S. (2006, April). Dorothea Dix (1802–1887). *American Journal of Public Health, 96*(4), 624–625.

Pick, D. (1989). *Faces of degeneration: A European disorder, c. 1848–1918.* New York, NY: Cambridge University Press.

Plant, R. (1988). *The pink triangle: The Nazi war against homosexuals.* New York, NY: Holt.

Porter, R. (2002). *Madness: A brief history.* Oxford, UK: Oxford University Press.

Robinson, L. D. (1966, July). The hospital psychiatrist's role in community psychiatry. *Journal of the National Medical Association, 58*(4), 271–274.

Rochefort, D. A. (1984). Origins of the "third psychiatric revolution": The Community Mental Health Centers Act of 1963. *Journal of Health Politics, Policy and Law, 9*(1), 1–30.

Rothman, D. J. (1971). *The discovery of the asylum: Social order and disorder in the new republic.* Boston, MA: Little, Brown.

Scheiber, S. C., Madaan, V., & Wilson, D. R. (2008, March 1). The American Board of Psychiatry and Neurology: Historical overview and current perspectives. *Psychiatry Clinics of North America, 31*(1), 123–135.

Scull, A. (2015). *Madness in civilization: A cultural history of insanity, from the Bible to Freud, from the madhouse to modern medicine.* Princeton, NJ: Princeton University Press.

Sharfstein, S. S., & Dickerson, F. B. (2006, June). Psychiatry and the consumer movement. *Health Affairs, 25*(3), 734–736.

Sheffer, E. (2018). *Asperger's children: The origins of autism in Nazi Vienna.* New York, NY: Norton.

Shorter, E. (2009). The history of lithium therapy. *Bipolar Disorders, 11,* 4–9.

Shosteck, R. (1971, November). Notes on an early Virginia physician. *American Jewish Archives,* 198–212.

Showalter, E. (1988). *The female malady: Women, madness, and English culture: 1830–1980.* London, UK: Virago.

Slate, R., & Johnson, W. W. (2008). *The Criminalization of Mental Illness: Crisis and Opportunity for the Justice System.* Durham, NC: Carolina Academic Press.

Stroul, B. A. (1988). Residential crisis services: A review. *Hospital and Community Psychiatry, 39,* 1095–1099.

Taylor, C. (1995). Two theories of modernity. *Hastings Center Report, 25*(2), 24–33.

Thomas, A. R. (1998). Ronald Reagan and the commitment of the mentally ill: Capital, interest groups, and the eclipse of social policy. *Electronic Journal of Sociology.* Retrieved from http://www.sociology.org/ejs-archives/vol003.004/thomas.html

Thomas, E. C., Despeaux, K. E., Drapalski, A. L., & Bennett, M. (2017). Person-oriented recovery of individuals with serious mental illnesses: A review and meta-analysis of longitudinal findings. *Psychiatric Services, 69*(3), 259–267. doi:https://doi.org/10.1176/appi.ps.201700058

TimesMachine: July 6, 1940.(n.d.). Insanity Treated by Electric Shock. *The New York Times.* Retrieved October 2, 2017, from https://timesmachine.nytimes.com/timesmachine/1940/07/06/113098496. html?pageNumber=17&login=email

Tomes, N. (1994). Feminist history of psychiatry. In M. S. Micale & R. Porter (Eds.), *Discovering the history of psychiatry* (pp. 348–383). New York, NY: Oxford University Press.

Turner, T. (2007). Chlorpromazine: Unlocking psychosis. *BMJ, 334*(Suppl. 1), s7.

Van Vorst, M. (1904, June). Paul Albert Besnard. *Pall Mall Magazine, 33*(134), 145–158.

Voronka, J. (2017). Turning mad knowledge into affective labor: The case of the peer support worker. *American Quarterly, 69*(2), 333–338.

Winters, E. E. (1969, September). Adolf Meyer and Clifford Beers, 1907–1910. *Bulletin of the History of Medicine, 43*(5), 414–443.

Wood, M. E. (1994). *The Writing on the Wall: Women's Autobiography and the Asylum.* Urbana, IL: University of Illinois Press.

Zwelling, S. (1985). *Quest for a cure.* Williamsburg, VA: Colonial Williamsburg Foundation.

///2/// THE PUBLIC PSYCHIATRIST AS CLINICIAN

JAMES G. BAKER AND SARAH E. BAKER

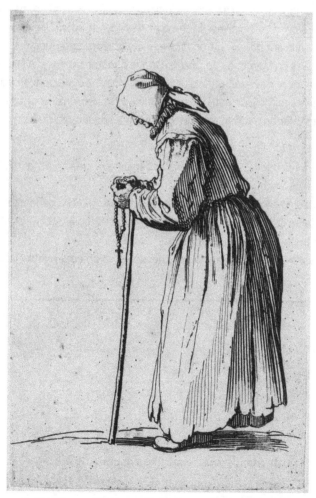

FIGURE 2.1 Jacques Callot, *Beggar Woman with Rosary*, c. 1622, etching.

Jacques Callot was born in 1592 in the northeast of France, but he traveled extensively in Europe starting at age 15 years. He made nearly 1,500 etchings and engravings that were popular in Europe in his own time, and portraits of the impoverished were common among them (Figure 2.1) (1).

CASE STUDY: INITIAL PRESENTATION

You are serving as a psychiatrist in an urban community mental health center's clinic. Your roles include clinic medical director and the clinic's only psychiatrist. The clinic cares for adults with severe and persistent mental illness, offering patient-centered treatment planning, medication management services, and psychosocial rehabilitation. Although the clinic is in a fairly large city, it is still located several blocks from the nearest bus stop.

In your role as medical director, you believe that the clinic is understaffed, thus accounting for the long wait list to access an initial psychiatric evaluation, especially because there are no other low-income clinics in the area to which to refer. The clinic's executive director is under significant pressure from community leaders to reduce the wait list, and so he asks you for ideas on how to do so. The executive director suggests a strategy: You could schedule and see more new-patient evaluations each day. You are concerned that reducing the wait list by increasing your patient load will lead to poor quality of care. You consider whether or not to offer an alternative strategy: hiring a second psychiatrist.

QUESTIONS

1. In addition to wait lists, what other access-to-care issues might public sector mental health patients encounter?
2. Although adding more psychiatrist time or scheduling more patients per physician are both viable strategies for addressing a wait-list problem, can you think of other strategies that might balance quality and access?
3. What are some strategies to address the access problems related to the clinic's location?

PSYCHIATRY AND LITERATURE

I Am!
by John Clare

I am—yet what I am none cares or knows;
My friends forsake me like a memory lost:
I am the self-consumer of my woes—
They rise and vanish in oblivious host,

Like shadows in love's frenzied stifled throes
And yet I am, and live—like vapours tossed
Into the nothingness of scorn and noise,

Into the living sea of waking dreams,
Where there is neither sense of life or joys,
But the vast shipwreck of my life's esteems;
Even the dearest that I loved the best

Are strange—nay, rather, stranger than the rest.

I long for scenes where man hath never trod
A place where woman never smiled or wept
There to abide with my Creator, God,
And sleep as I in childhood sweetly slept,
Untroubling and untroubled where I lie
The grass below—above the vaulted sky.

PUBLIC PSYCHIATRY: THE MISSION

The first experience most psychiatrists have in public sector psychiatry is providing psychiatric evaluations and medication management in an outpatient clinic, either as a resident or early in practice. The illnesses endured by the patients are often severe, and the acuity of some patients while living in the community can make it seem as if they would be better served inside of a hospital. Conversations with patients bring the realization that some rely on a fragmented system of emergency rooms and crisis residential centers while struggling with adherence to treatment recommendations due to lack of continuity of care and poor access to resources such as housing or shelters, pharmacies, or walk-in appointments. The social and financial support systems for these patients in the community offer more challenges to serving them, and the sheer volume of patients to be cared for sometimes can seem overwhelming.

Despite all these challenges, the day-in and day-out interactions with patients that are part of the public psychiatrist's role as a clinician are often the most rewarding part of the profession, and they are critical to the public psychiatrist's success at other aspects of the job (2). The mission is compelling, as well, as is the sense of professional satisfaction from caring for people whose economic and social misfortune leave them with no other place to turn for help. The sense of satisfaction is especially great when working with a team that engages the most difficult-to-treat in a manner that successfully keeps them out of hospitals, out of jails, and off the streets despite all the social challenges that patients and the treatment team collectively face.

The 19th-century poet John Clare, who composed the poem presented previously, suffered from mental illness. Clare was born in 1793 in England, the son of illiterate parents. He dropped out of school at age 12 years in order to work in various labor jobs. Despite some success related to his poetry, which described life in the English countryside, he often lived in poverty and struggled to provide for his family and continue to write his poetry. Although he always had bouts of depression, severe delusions led to his admission to a private asylum, High Beach, in 1837 and to admission to Northampton General Lunatic Asylum in 1841, where he spent the last 20 years of his life. It is believed that he wrote "I Am" while institutionalized because the superintendent, Dr. Thomas Octavius Pritchard, encouraged him to continue to write (3). Clare's poem describes the loneliness and isolation that can be a part of living with a mental illness. Fortunately, his hospital's superintendent believed in moral treatment, as described in Chapter 1, and Clare's writing was considered to be a part of his plan of care.

Today's public sector patients face struggles similar to those faced by Clare, including poverty, alienation from family, and challenges to maintaining career and educational trajectories. Along with these patient struggles, public psychiatrists face many dilemmas as they pursue their mission. This chapter discusses common clinical dilemmas and decisions that the public psychiatrist faces, including a discussion of the balance between quality versus access, concerns about productivity, medication formulary development, the oversight of physician assistants and advanced nurse practitioners, and a short consideration of the challenges of rural community psychiatry practice.

QUALITY VERSUS ACCESS

One common dilemma that public mental health providers must confront is finding the balance between access to care and quality of care, driven by limited resources in the public sector. Sometimes psychiatrists are concerned that high caseloads may hamper the ability to provide high-quality care to individual patients. However, limiting the number of patients seen by individual providers as a strategy to improve quality may mean that access to care will be limited, leaving many people without any care at all.

To find the proper balance, three aspects of access to care must be considered: front-door access, access to optimal services, and use of services (4). *Front-door access* is the ability of a patient to get into the front door of the clinic rather than being placed on a wait list. *Access to optimal services* is the ability of the clinic to provide the services that the patient actually needs. *Use of services* references the barriers, and approaches to overcoming them, that individuals face in obtaining optimal services. When trying to balance access and quality, it is important to consider barriers in all three areas, as discussed next.

Managing "Front-Door" Access

Wait lists are a significant problem in community mental health. Timely access to care can have a critical impact on outcomes of both acute and chronic mental disorders. Yet 20–50% of people with moderate to severe mental illness experience access-to-care problems (5), and a study of access to a psychiatrist for adolescents in Ohio showed an average wait of almost 2 months (6).

If demand for care is high enough that wait lists are forming, pressure on community mental health center leadership to improve access often trickles down to the clinic psychiatrist as pressure to see increasingly more patients each day. The pressure to eliminate wait lists often leads to worries about the quality of service provided to individual patients. It is not surprising, then, that physicians may experience access and quality as opposing values.

Queuing theory offers health care providers one way to understand and address the problems of meeting service demand while maintaining quality of care. Queuing theory is used to observe the relation between demand, capacity, and wait lists. It explores, for example, the variables that determine how long a wait list grows: patient demand, time per service, and the variability in both. From an administrator's perspective, hiring more psychiatrists as a strategy to ensure there is never a wait list may be wasteful of limited funding if it leads to expensive physicians with idle time. On the other hand, increasing capacity by increasing the number of patients each physician sees during a day may lead to concerns about poor outcomes (7).

To apply queuing theory to the problem of access versus quality, start by measuring how many patients need to see a psychiatrist (i.e., how many patients are asking for care in a given time period—for example, patient inquiries per month). Next, measure how many patients are receiving care—typically the number of unique patients who were actually seen by a psychiatrist in a period of time—for example, the number of unique patients who were seen in a 3-month quarter.

The next step is to determine capacity. Caseload capacity is the calculated maximum number of patients that a public psychiatrist can care for. Its measurement considers the average amount of time required per patient visit and the average frequency with which patients need to be seen. Methodologies for measuring caseload capacity have been proposed to help public mental health center leadership determine the number of psychiatrists that a center requires. In determining capacity, it is important to make allowances for historic no-show rates (which will increase capacity) and for recordkeeping and other clinical administrative demands, including vacation time (all of which will decease capacity) (8).

These data collectively can be used to calculate how many psychiatrists are required to meet patient demand—that is, to ensure the elimination of wait lists while still maintaining a desired standard of care. From there, psychiatrist and administrators can work together on strategies that would impact the second queuing variable—that is, strategies that increase capacity of the psychiatric staff primarily by reducing average time per patient. Several such strategies are presented here.

Implementation of a triage process to prioritize access to a psychiatrist is one possible strategy to increase clinic capacity. In psychiatry, a triage process can be used to determine if there is clinical need for a psychiatrist as well as the urgency for providing a psychiatric intervention. Triage was recommended by the Task Force on Community Based Systems of Care of the American Academy of Child and Adolescent Psychiatry as a strategy for responding to decreased funding availability when Medicaid managed care was implemented (9).

One possible model uses a licensed mental health clinician doing individual assessments that lead to one of three outcomes: no psychiatric intervention required, immediate referral to a psychiatrist, and wait list for psychiatric assessment. However, studies in general health care show problems with interrater reliability in triage decisions (10). Therefore, another possible strategy involves a team review of assessments and decisions, including the availability of a psychiatrist to review cases (11).

Another strategy to reduce the average time required per patient by a psychiatrist (from a queue theory perspective) is to use non-physician medical providers. Advanced nurse practitioners and physician assistants can also be used to extend the reach of limited psychiatric time. These relationships are described in more detail later in this chapter.

Individual access is not just a problem in the community. Public sector psychiatrists who work in jails and prisons often deal with understaffing as well. The following vignette presents an example in which a licensed social worker is used to do initial jail-based care assessments, which in turn are reviewed by a psychiatrist.

A VIGNETTE: CASELOAD CAPACITY AT A JAIL

Recently appointed as medical director of behavioral health for the jail in your urban city, you are quickly confronted with an average time from incarceration to psychiatric evaluation of well over a week. The consequence is that many people with known histories of severe mental illness are going more than a week without medications. As a triage strategy to address the issue, you decide to start each morning by reviewing the licensed social worker's admission assessments completed in the past 24 hours on all new referrals. Your process includes identifying patients known to the public mental health system whose medications can be continued, patients who appear to have new-onset disorders and require rapid assessment, and patients who appear to need a medical evaluation for medical etiologies of presentation or to begin detox regimens.

Public psychiatrists should advocate for eliminating wait lists as a strategy to reducing patient morbidity and societal costs of serious mental illness, and they should offer suggestions such as those presented previously for actively addressing the problem. Ensuring front-door access requires an organizational commitment to eliminating wait lists, and making that commitment is the first step to addressing the many barriers to achieving the access-to-care goal.

Access to Optimal Services

If a patient with new-onset psychosis is able to get in the front door of the clinic promptly but is still unable to access any evidence-based services other than medication management and case management, then an access problem still exists (12). Or if a patient meets criteria for, as an example, assertive community treatment (the intensive, community-based strategy intended to maintain high utilizers of acute services in the community) but cannot do so for lack of funding, then this, too, is an access problem (13). Service-array access problems such as these can have a major impact on quality of care and clinical outcomes in the public sector, especially for the difficult-to-treat patient.

Queuing theory offers at least three strategies for the public psychiatrist to employ that may help more patients obtain access to optimal care. One strategy is setting specific criteria for obtaining access to a given level of service and screening referrals to ensure that the criteria are met. This type of utilization management criteria was developed initially in the 1980s to reduce unnecessary expenses and the negative clinical impact of unnecessary hospitalizations (14). Insurance companies embraced the concept as a cost management strategy and broadened the use of utilization management to include outpatient services, especially psychotherapy. In public psychiatry, resource limitations have led to the use of similar criteria for access to other levels of service, such as assertive community treatment.

However, implementing criteria that require a patient to meet a threshold of acuity in order to access even intensive outpatient services runs the risk of driving up cost and reducing quality of care as patients go without necessary services until they become very ill. An alternative strategy to manage program access is the use of protocols to foster aggressive treatment as a way of reducing the length of time patients are served in specialty programs. Protocols should be measurement driven; that is, they should use validated treatment and screening and monitoring instruments. Goals for improvement on the measures should be set. Then, the protocols should include measurement of the instruments at decision points when changes in treatment will be made if the measures do not demonstrate progress toward treatment goals.

The same measures can be used to drive a third strategy—that is, setting thresholds at which patients are discharged from a level of care, either because treatment goals are achieved or because other criteria are met (or not met). For example, if a patient is struggling to engage with an assertive community treatment team, an argument could be made for allowing access to a second patient while motivational interviewing and other strategies are used to engage the first patient (15).

Managing Use of Services

Even when services are available, patients served by public psychiatrists often face many barriers to using them. Transportation, child care services, obtaining leave from work, and many other factors can lead to missed appointments and poor outcomes. Public psychiatrists should explore these potential barriers with patients and engage case workers/managers to help address them. For example, patients' utilization of services increases when resources are located in convenient locations and also when their basic needs for food, safe housing, and daily activity are fulfilled (16).

Adherence to treatment is another service-utilization problem in public mental health care settings generally, but patient use of psychotropic medication as prescribed is particularly poor (17). Reasons for poor adherence vary. In schizophrenia, reduced adherence has been tied to substance use, higher levels of hostility, and impaired insight (18). In depression, adherence has been tied to both the number of and the specific medications prescribed (19, 20).

Another important service-use issue is disparity in access to, and quality of, treatment by racial and ethnic minorities (21). Factors related to the disparity include lack of insurance coverage, disjointed services, unavailability of cultural-specific services, cultural insensitivity of mental health clinicians, and stigma toward mental illness (22). Treatment adherence among racial and ethnic minorities is low, as well, compared to that of non-Latino White populations (23–25). In Latinos, risk factors for nonadherence include speaking only Spanish, being poor, and lacking health insurance (26). Fear of becoming addicted to medications and the belief that medications are symbols of mental illness were factors in poor adherence among African Americans with bipolar disorder (27).

Culturally competent care—that is, consideration of treatment preferences of racial, ethnic, or cultural groups—is a critical component of improving service utilization. Unfortunately, requisite training sessions can leave clinicians with the impression that cultural competency is a series of "do's and don'ts" that define how to treat a patient of a given ethnic background (28). However, patients should not be assumed to have a core set of beliefs based on their ethnicity so that treatment planning degenerates into cultural stereotypes. Instead, treatment planning should explore and take into consideration the beliefs and choices of the individual patient.

In addition to providing care that takes into account the culture of individuals patients, most community centers in which public psychiatrists serve have developed a comprehensive array of community-based services intended to improve service accessibility. For example, case managers are usually field-based instead of office-based, and much of the rehabilitation care that they provide occurs in the homes of adults or at home and school with children. Case management can play a critical role in service utilization by connecting patients with services and helping patients ensure that their basic needs are met. In urban areas, community centers have been called upon to offer jail-based care, and case managers will often spend time in court, working with judges to develop plans to keep clients safe and out of trouble with the law. Many centers have mobile crisis units that can respond, much as an ambulance would, to the needs of law enforcement and families for crisis care.

From the perspective of the individual provider, the primary strategy for improving service utilization and adherence to treatment is to engage each patient through collaborative styles of communication, empathy, discussion of treatment specifics, and collaborative styles of communication (29). Patient perception of listening, empathy, and respectfulness influences patient satisfaction and adherence (30). Empathy varies as a function of gender and age, and it arguably also varies with professional experience, in the sense that some data suggest that empathic sensitivity seems to decrease in the last stages of medical training (31, 32). In addition, mental health workers have been shown to have more empathy for the sorts of difficulties mental health patients experience (33).

Therefore, it is important for public psychiatrists to understand how to foster and maintain clinician empathy as a strategy toward improving service utilization in patients and to advocate for applying those strategies in treatment teams. Coursework (34), simulated patients (35), and many other strategies (36) have been suggested as approaches to teaching empathy. The public psychiatrist should encourage collective exploration of evidence-based approaches to fostering empathy for implementation in the treatment team and in the clinic.

Patient education about the need for treatment, and about the need for specific treatment, is a predictor of adherence (37). Participants receiving psychoeducation have also been found to be more satisfied with mental health services and reported a better quality of life, and psychoeducation programs involving the family are more likely to produce positive results on the course of the disorder (38). Exploration with patients of the link between taking a medication and a real or imagined outcome is a key component of education. For example, a patient may believe that he will be perceived as emotionally weak for taking medication, leading to poor adherence (39). Education efforts should focus on reducing this type of harmful belief. Education should also focus on the specifics of side effects and their management, as well as helping patients understand the value of psychosocial rehabilitation and other interventions intended to help them face everyday problems associated with their disorders (40).

Poor communication can lead to a disconnect between patient and physician goals of treatment, which is another reason for poor service utilization. One strategy toward ensuring patient–physician agreement on goals of care is person-centered treatment planning, which has been shown to be associated with treatment engagement and medication adherence (41). Person-centered planning asks the public psychiatrist, as part of a treatment team, to actively collaborate with patients to identify life goals as the focus of treatment rather than, for example, simply focusing on symptom management. It strongly depends on motivational interviewing to identify goals, barriers to those goals, and strategies for overcoming those goals (42). In this model, medication adherence, for example, becomes a strategy toward attaining a life goal rather than toward attaining symptom relief or disease remission.

A VIGNETTE: PATIENT-CENTERED CARE PLANNING

John has been referred to your community mental health center by the local Federally Qualified Health Center for management of treatment-resistant depression. Your review of John's electronic health record at the community mental health center shows past poor adherence to recommendations for a combination of medication and cognitive behavioral therapy. The treatment plan cites "improved mood" and "medication compliance" as treatment goals. In exploring John's personal goals with him, you discern that he is focused on wanting a hernia repair that a surgeon has declined to do until his blood pressure, blood sugar, and depression are better controlled. In implementing a person-centered treatment plan, you recommend that the plan's treatment goals be changed to reflect his desire for the surgery and that interventions be changed to focus on how treatment of his depression fits with his plan to achieve his goal.

Self-directed care is another recent strategy intended to foster patient service utilization. Self-directed care is a model in which patients are given control of how their service delivery dollars are used. Patients are offered the opportunity to use the dollars to purchase physician and therapist services outside of the community mental health center, and even nontraditional services such as gym memberships and alternative therapies (43). The patient and the case manager develop a person-centered treatment plan together, and then the patient is assisted in deciding how to spend available dollars in a manner consistent with the recovery plan. The amount of money available to the patient to spend in this discretionary way is based on the typical average cost per patient served in the financing agency. In a Texas study of self-directed care, one-third of the discretionary dollars were spent on nontraditional goods and services, including fitness classes, massage therapy, and educational expenses (44). In a Florida study of the model, functional status improved modestly, and very few patients required hospitalization during the study period (45).

Strong engagement of individual patients in treatment planning coupled with data-driven evaluation of the three aspects of access to care—front-door access, access to optimal services, and use of services—can help public psychiatrists and clinic administrators find the balance between access to care and quality of care provided.

QUALITY VERSUS PRODUCTIVITY

Public psychiatrists often work in settings that wrestle with the financial challenge of paying adequately to recruit and retain highly trained physicians, as well as other professionals who are able to meet the community's need for high-quality care. In this environment, clinical administrators often implement productivity strategies to help make the salaries of medical professionals possible, including daily patients-served requirements, overbooking to compensate for no-shows, and straight productivity-based pay (46). Public psychiatrists may find these productivity strategies burdensome and worry about the implications of productivity requirements on quality of care.

Confronted with this fiscal pressure, the public psychiatrist can offer alternative strategies intended to help ensure that quality is a consideration in managing productivity. Offering compensation strategies to physicians that allow them to choose the number of patients served may help physicians find an individual workload that balances personal income goals and individual perception of quality of care. One possible compensation strategy mixes a base salary with per-patient augmentation (47). Although pay-for-performance strategies based on quality of care are common, studies have demonstrated only modest improvements in quality from such approaches, and an argument can also be made that the natural economic way to maintain quality is through patient demand for it (48). Indeed, compensation strategies that mix base salary with per-patient pay augmentation have been shown to maintain quality of care (49).

Team-based compensation is another alternative strategy (50).

A VIGNETTE: BALANCING PRODUCTIVITY AND QUALITY

The medical director of your community mental health clinic approaches you, a team psychiatrist, asking that you "do something" about the low volume of patients that you are seeing each day, because there are pressures on the medical director to increase the revenue to cover the costs of the medical staff. The medical director reports to you that the new chief financial officer is suggesting that the medical director move all physicians from a salary-based compensation system to a pay based entirely on billable hours. As an alternative, you suggest to the medical director that your treatment team—you as the psychiatrist, the licensed social worker doing cognitive–behavioral therapy, and five rehabilitation workers—have its productivity measured collectively and be held accountable to "paying its way." As an incentive to doing so, you suggest that all members of the team remain on salary but be given individual bonus pay if the team collectively makes its revenue target.

In this proposed compensation plan, the cost of the physician is viewed as just one part of the cost of an entire treatment team. Instead of considering each member individually and asking each to serve enough patients to cover his or her own costs, the model proposes setting productivity targets for the team as whole, with the goal that the team covers its cost as a whole. This gives the team some autonomy in how it wants to seek a balance of productivity and quality.

CASE STUDY: CONTINUED

You propose to the executive director that a second psychiatrist be hired as a way of addressing the long wait lists to access care at your clinic. The executive director, however, is worried about the high cost of a psychiatrist, especially because physician salaries seem to be rising particularly quickly, and wonders if you have other ideas. You suggest that the clinic consider adding an advanced nurse practitioner instead. When you do so, the executive director brings up another problem: the rising medication costs for patients who have no insurance. He wonders about moving to a restricted formulary. You suggest expanding the clinic's use of patient assistance programs instead.

QUESTIONS
1. What regulatory considerations would need to be considered before your clinic follows your suggestion to hire an advanced nurse practitioner?
2. What are the advantages and disadvantages, financially and clinically, of the use of formulary restrictions?
3. What clinical issues should you consider in the development of a restricted formulary?
4. What are the advantages and disadvantages of patient assistance programs?

WORKING WITH MANAGED FORMULARIES

Rising medication costs are another driver of clinical policy under which public psychiatrists must serve. One very common strategy for controlling medication costs is the use of formulary restrictions. The appeal of this simple approach is clear. A study of the impact of general medical formulary restrictions on costs at the Veterans Administration system in Oklahoma City, Oklahoma, showed an approximately 5% reduction in pharmacy budget by restricting access to just 15 medications (51).

Various formulary restriction strategies have been described (52). A popular strategy for private insurance companies uses tiered formularies, in which the patient's co-pay is higher for brand-name medications than for generics. A three-tier formulary is the most common, in which nonpreferred brand names have an even higher co-payment and may also require the physician request payment authorization before prescribing (53).

So-called "fail-first" formularies are designed so that coverage of expensive medication is not available until a patient demonstrates failed treatment with a lower cost alternative. Fail-first policies have the potential to create conflict between the goals of cost control and the ability to tailor care to the perceived needs of the individual patient, and so design criteria have been suggested to ensure that fail-first policies are based on sound ethics (54).

Both commercial insurance companies and public insurers, such as Medicaid and Medicare, have used pharmaceutical benefit management companies (PBMs) to help manage medication costs. PBMs negotiate the price to be paid by the insurance company to the drug manufacturer and also the prices to be paid to pharmacies. They also manage tiered co-pays and other formulary restrictions (55).

Rather than limiting formularies up front, alternative strategies consider the overall cost of treatment instead of the cost of the medication alone. For example, an analysis of patterns of inappropriate use of high-cost drugs might be used to develop interventions with individual physicians and/or patients that both maximize savings and minimize patient harm (56). Or, if there is evidence that a high-cost antipsychotic reduces the frequency of admission to the hospital, then that cost reduction can be taken into consideration in determining access to the medication. Indeed, caps on access to antipsychotic medications resulted in an increase in the use of emergency services that cost nearly 20 times as much as the medications would have cost (57). Similarly, Medicaid restrictions on access to antidepressant medications were not associated with lower overall spending (58).

The Clinical Antipsychotic Trials of Intervention Effectiveness ((CATIE) study lends more support for this broader view of the cost of medications. Its comparison of first- and second-generation antipsychotics left many psychiatrists concerned that the results would be used to justify formulary restrictions. However, the CATIE investigators argued that although the results of the CATIE study did not appear to justify the high utilization rate for second-generation agents because they were not significantly superior to first-generation treatment, they did suggested the need for the availability of a wide array of treatment options. In the CATIE study, almost three-fourths of patients or their clinicians wanted to switch medications, so side effects and limitations in efficacy argue for open access to allow medication changes based on side effects and individual patient/ physician preference (59).

Another strategy that has been recommended to help balance access to medications, quality, and cost management is the use of treatment-decision tools such as medication algorithms. Medical algorithms are evidence-based guidelines intended to assist physicians in the timing and choice of changes in medication and medication dosages. These algorithms incorporate relative efficacy (if there are differences), cost, and side effect profiles into the decision-making process for choosing medications (60). Although studies demonstrate the impact of physician adherence to treatment-decision tools on patient outcomes (61), research also show relatively low rates of algorithm use (62).

Finally, patient assistance programs (PAPs) are another strategy that administrators often seek to use to help manage medication costs. PAPs are used by pharmaceutical manufacturers to offset drug costs to public sector clinics and their patients by offering medications free of charge or at greatly reduced prices. However, public psychiatrists need to understand that rather than serving as philanthropy, PAPs are a marketing strategy for manufacturers. They increase demand, allow companies to charge higher prices, and provide public relations benefits. Psychiatrists and administrators who work in indigent care settings may view PAPs as a financial lifeline because they do, indeed, pay for medications that the clinic might otherwise have to finance, but commercial and public insurance programs do not favor their use because they may discourage the use of more cost-effective medication choices (63). However, no rigorous studies have been performed examining the impact of PAPs on access to medications, clinical outcomes, or cost of medications or care overall (64).

Public psychiatrists may be asked to help develop strategies to manage medication costs, including the use of restricted formularies. When so engaged, public psychiatrists should advocate for strategies that maintain the well-being of patients as the first priority but also help the institution manage its service costs. A good approach would be to advocate for evidence-based decision-making around formulary restrictions, based on the following principles (65):

1. Advocate for the use of actual data over economic modeling. In particular, formulary decisions should not be based on the relative purchase price of medications alone but, rather, when possible, on longer term studies of cost-effectiveness and relative safety.

2. When data are available, formulary decisions should be made based on how a medication helps improve overall function in the community, not just its impact on symptom rating scales. Two medications might have equal efficacy in improving symptoms on the Brief Psychiatric Rating Scale or the Positive and Negative Syndrome Scale but be markedly different when assessed by patient-centered remission criteria, such as social function and quality of life (66).

3. New medications should be added to the formulary only in the context of a thorough understanding of potential academic and economic influences on the reporting of trial outcomes (67). Academic and funding pressures and incentives may also favor publication of positive outcomes (68).

4. "First-line" restrictions should be avoided, or at least be easily overridden, because of variations in medication efficacy and side effects from patient to patient.

5. Patients who are stable on their current medications should not be required to change medications for financial reasons.

It is important that public psychiatrists help financial decision-makers in their centers recognize that medication cost is a complex problem that cannot be addressed in the absence of a broader review of the impact of medications on overall service utilization.

WORKING WITH OTHER MEDICAL PROVIDERS

The Substance Abuse and Mental Health Services Administration has described the severity of the shortage of public psychiatrists, which leads to a problem with access to care. Nearly 2,000 psychiatrists are currently needed just in Mental Health Professional Shortage Areas alone (69). Because of this shortage of public sector psychiatrists, mental health clinic leaders may ask public psychiatrists to collaborate with advanced practice nurses (APNs) and physician assistants (PAs) working as medication prescribers. In some states, the arrangement requires the psychiatrist to function in a clinical supervisory role with the APNs or PAs.

Advanced practice nurses typically have 2 years of training in an accredited nursing program beyond their registered nurse training, including hundreds of hours of supervised clinical hours. Practice requires either a Master of Science in Nursing or a Doctorate in Nursing Practice, national certification in a specialty area, and a specific state license. They are trained in psychiatric evaluation, differential diagnosis, ordering and interpreting diagnostic tests, prescribing pharmacologic agents, and psychotherapy. Similar to physicians, they are responsible for managing their scope of practice to ensure that they recognize the limits of their expertise and when to refer.

Physician assistants have at least 2 years of college coursework in basic and behavioral sciences, 3 years of classroom and clinical rotations usually ending in attaining of a master's degree, and a state license. There are few PAs in public psychiatry; most are in primary care. The American Academy of Physician Assistants found that only approximately 1% of PAs are practicing in mental health settings (70).

Many advantages of a treatment team model involving supervision by a physician of a team of APNs and PAs have been described, including more effective and efficient use of the psychiatrists and increased access to primary medical care screening (70). This model should also lead to increased access to care because having more providers (at lower cost per provider) allows for increased clinic capacity. Disadvantages of the model relate to training and "turf" issues because some psychiatrists and nursing staff may be resistant to having a PA or APN in their practice. Other disadvantages include concerns about quality and liability in this model (71). With regard to the concern about quality of care, APNs seem to provide high-quality behavioral health service, as measured by retrospective medical record review (72). Studies also suggest that patients are equally satisfied with psychiatrists and psychiatric nurse practitioners (73).

With regard to the liability concern, physicians and the public sector systems in which they serve should consider medicolegal responsibility before establishing collaboration between PAs and APNs. Courts may rule against physicians in liability cases for lack of supervision, vicarious liability, and negligent hiring of APNs and PAs (74). In public clinics, hiring is typically an organizational responsibility, and liability is generally borne by these organization broadly. However, it is still important for the physician to ensure that she knows the supervision laws in her state, including any limit on the number of nurse practitioners and/or PAs that she may supervise and the requirements (if any) for documenting adequate supervision (75). In many states, APNs can practice independently, but in others there may be a requirement for a written supervisory agreement with a psychiatrist. There also may be restrictions on the ability of PAs and APNs to prescribe stimulants, for example.

WORKING IN A RURAL PRACTICE

Access to care is an issue in rural communities, as well. Long distances to the nearest clinic and the associated travel time to get there serve as barriers. A shortage of psychiatrists willing to work in rural areas is an additional barrier. Recruitment of psychiatrists to rural practice may be hampered by fear of the prospect that one might not be able to make a living, and the presence of APNs or PAs in rural settings may fuel the fear that there is not enough to do in a rural practice (76). In addition, rural practice provides unique challenges for the physician, including feelings of professional isolation, the absence of subspecialty expertise for referrals, difficulties in recruiting psychiatrist colleagues to help with the workload, and unique boundary and confidentiality issues (77).

A VIGNETTE: WORK–LIFE BALANCE IN RURAL PSYCHIATRIC PRACTICE

As the only psychiatrist in 17 counties in Montana, Dr. Dickson reports getting two or more phone calls every night from emergency departments about psychiatric cases. She is burning out, but limits are difficult to set. She works 4½ days per week, but her medical center wants her to work 5 days per week and remain on call around the clock for psychiatric emergencies because her services are losing money: Lack of insurance means that her services are reimbursed at only 25 cents on the dollar. Dr. Dickson decides that if she is unable to come to an agreement with the medical center regarding work hours and call schedule, she will simply leave the practice (78).

For the public psychiatrist who elects to work in a rural setting, there are good strategies for addressing some of the challenges short of shuttering the practice. Web-based solutions offer some help with the professional isolation. Email, telephone, and applications such as Skype and FaceTime offer the potential for more professional peer contact than were available in the past (76). Ng et al. (77) report that after opening a practice in a rural California county serving approximately 150,000 citizens, they dealt with professional isolation and the absence of academic collaboration by maintaining contact with faculty at the academic medical center where they trained by phone, email, and in person and also by offering rural rotations for trainees. They report rural practice as ripe for academic research in the factors unique to the practice setting, including poverty, low-density population, and poor public transpiration.

Public psychiatrists working in rural communities must be especially sensitive to boundary issues with their patients due to relatively limited options for care that their friends and acquaintances may have. Psychiatrists may have dual, or even multiple, relationships with patients. Typically, these dilemmas cannot be avoided, and so it is important to address them openly and quickly, clarifying boundaries at initial appointments and reassuring patients that strict confidentiality will be maintained in social settings. Failure to clarify these concerns with new patients may negatively affect the therapeutic relationship, impair clinical judgment, or lead to poor decision-making (79).

In addition to providing the possibility of call coverage for the rural psychiatrist, telemedicine avoids some of the drawbacks for physicians about practicing in rural settings by allowing patients in these settings to be seen by public psychiatrists working from an urban location. For this reason, among others, telemedicine has rapidly become a strategy to increase access to mental health services in rural communities. Between 2004 and 2014, the number of telemedicine visits for mental health services increased almost 50% annually so that by 2014 there were more than 11 telemedicine visits per 100 rural Medicare patients with severe mental illness (80). Its cost-effectiveness has been demonstrated by its use in offering consultation to rural primary care physicians who are managing psychiatric disorders (81). Few studies have examined the relative efficacy of telemedicine versus face-to-face care, but outcomes generally appear to be the same and patients seem to accept telemedicine (82, 83).

CASE STUDY: CONCLUSION

As medical director, you and your executive director in this case face the common and unenviable task of trying to balance access, quality, and cost (84). You are attempting to do so in a system of care that is typically underfunded and for patients who face a myriad of barriers to access to quality care, including wait lists, service arrays that are not always current and evidence-based, and numerous social barriers to obtaining care. So it is important, as medical director, to take a broad perspective in engaging with your clinic leadership to develop strategies to address the clinic's challenges. Increasing the number of psychiatrists is not necessarily the first-line strategy for eliminating a wait list. Steps need to be taken, first, to ensure that current psychiatric time is being used optimally by addressing no-show rates and by reviewing medical records and other clinical–administrative work performed by psychiatrists that reduces the number of patients they are able to serve in a high-quality way.

Short of physically moving the clinic, access could be improved by outreach services, including using case managers to address social barriers such as transportation and child care. This, too, would help with no-show rates and thus would have the added benefit of addressing physician productivity issues.

Converting vacant psychiatrist positions into APN and PA positions, whether working independently or under the supervision of a clinic psychiatrist (depending on the state in which the clinic is located), has the potential to increase the medical staff without an increase in budget and so offers a cost-effective way to increase access. If your clinic decides to go this route, then the leadership and psychiatrists would need to learn the state regulatory rules on supervision, documentation of supervision, and APN/PA scope of practice.

If formulary changes are under consideration as a cost-saving strategy, then, as medical director, you can advocate for using the five principles for evidence-based decision-making on formulary restrictions. You should encourage the clinic to think broadly about cost of care, rather than focusing on the relative costs of different medications. You should encourage literature reviews that consider economically driven biases in research reports. Also, you should encourage an open formulary unless there is clear evidence of the equity of medications from the perspective of patient-centered outcomes. If you are asked to weigh in on bolstering the clinic's patient assistance program, you need to be mindful of the clear and positive impact that these programs can have on medication costs of a clinic, but also be clear with administrators of the role of PAPs in pharmaceutical industry marketing.

REFERENCES

1. Mayor AH, Baskin L. The etchings of Jacques Callot. Mass Rev. 1961;3(1):121–132.
2. Osborn L, Stein C. Mental health care providers' views of their work with consumers and their reports of recovery-orientation, job satisfaction, and personal growth. Community Ment Health J. 2016;52(7):757–766.
3. Martin F. The life of John Clare. [Internet]. London, UK: Macmillan; 1865. Available from http://hdl.handle.net/2027/uc1.b4580525
4. Wilson AB, Barrenger S, Bohrman C, Draine J. Balancing accessibility and selectivity in 21st century public mental health services: Implications for hard to engage clients. J Behav Health Serv Res. 2013 Apr 1;40(2):191–206.
5. Rowan K, McAlpine DD, Blewett LA. Access and cost barriers to mental health care, by insurance status, 1999–2010. Health Aff Chevy Chase. 2013 Oct;32(10):1723–1730.
6. Steinman KJ, Shoben AB, Dembe AE, Kelleher KJ. How long do adolescents wait for psychiatry appointments? Community Ment Health J. 2015 Oct 1;51(7):782–789.
7. Palvannan RK, Teow KL. Queueing for healthcare. J Med Syst. 2012 Apr 1;36(2):541–547.
8. Baker J. A spreadsheet method for calculating maximum caseload and intake capacity for CMHC psychiatrists. Psychiatr Serv. 1997 Dec 1;48(12):1578–1581.
9. Pumariega AJ, Nace D, England MJ, Diamond J, Fallon T, Hanson G, et al. Community-based systems approach to children's managed mental health services. J Child Fam Stud. 1997 Jun 1;6(2):149–164.
10. Harding KE, Taylor NF, Leggat SG, Wise VL. Prioritizing patients for community rehabilitation services: Do clinicians agree on triage decisions? Clin Rehabil. 2010 Oct 1;24(10):928–934.
11. Parkin A, Frake C, Davison I. A triage clinic in a child and adolescent mental health service. Child Adolesc Ment Health. 2003 Nov 1;8(4):177–183.
12. Dixon LB, Goldman HH, Bennett ME, Wang Y, McNamara KA, Mendon SJ, et al. Implementing coordinated specialty care for early psychosis: The RAISE Connection Program. Psychiatr Serv. 2015 Mar 16;66(7):691–698.
13. Phillips SD, Burns BJ, Edgar ER, Mueser KT, Linkins KW, Rosenheck RA, et al. Moving assertive community treatment into standard practice. Psychiatr Serv. 2001 Jun 1;52(6):771–779.
14. Rodriguez AR. Evolutions in utilization and quality management: A crisis for psychiatric services? Gen Hosp Psychiatry. 1989 Jul 1;11(4):256–263.
15. Lawrence P, Fulbrook P, Somerset S, Schulz P. Motivational interviewing to enhance treatment attendance in mental health settings: A systematic review and meta-analysis. J Psychiatr Ment Health Nurs. 2017 Nov 1;24(9–10):699–718.
16. Fleury M-J, Grenier G, Bamvita J-M, Caron J. Mental health service utilization among patients with severe mental disorders. Community Ment Health J. 2011 Aug 1;47(4):365–377.
17. Lacro JP, Dunn LB, Dolder CR, Jeste DV. Prevalence of and risk factors for medication nonadherence in patients with schizophrenia: A comprehensive review of recent literature. J Clin Psychiatry. 2002 Oct 1;63(10):892–909.

18. Czobor P, Van Dorn RA, Citrome L, Kahn RS, Fleischhacker WW, Volavka J. Treatment adherence in schizophrenia: A patient-level meta-analysis of combined CATIE and EUFEST studies. Eur Neuropsychopharmacol. 2015 Aug 1;25(8):1158–1166.
19. Serna MC, Real J, Cruz I, Galvan L, Martin E. Monitoring patients on chronic treatment with antidepressants between 2003 and 2011: Analysis of factors associated with compliance. BMC Public Health Lond. 2015;15:1184.
20. Sawada N, Uchida H, Suzuki T, Watanabe K, Kikuchi T, Handa T, et al. Persistence and compliance to antidepressant treatment in patients with depression: A chart review. BMC Psychiatry. 2009 Jun 16;9:38.
21. Wells K, Klap R, Koike A, Sherbourne C. Ethnic disparities in unmet need for alcoholism, drug abuse, and mental health care. Am J Psychiatry. 2001 Dec 1;158(12):2027–2032.
22. US Department of Health and Human Services. Mental health: Culture, race, and ethnicity: A supplement to Mental health: A report of the Surgeon General. [Internet]. Rockville, MD: US Department of Health and Human Services; 2001. Available from http://hdl.handle.net/2027/mdp.39015053542414
23. Dixon L, Lewis-Fernandez R, Goldman H, Interian A, Michaels A, Kiley MC. Adherence disparities in mental health: Opportunities and challenges. J Nerv Ment Dis. 2011 Oct;199(10):815–820.
24. Diaz E, Woods SW, Rosenheck RA. Effects of ethnicity on psychotropic medications adherence. Community Ment Health J. 2005 Oct 1;41(5):521–537.
25. Fleck DE, Hendricks WL, Strakowski SM. Differential prescription of maintenance antipsychotics to African American and White patients with new-onset bipolar disorder. J Clin Psychiatry. 2002 Aug 15;63(8):658–664.
26. Lanouette NM, Folsom DP, Sciolla A, Jeste DV. Psychotropic medication nonadherence among United States Latinos: A comprehensive literature review. Psychiatr Serv. 2009 Feb 1;60(2):157–174.
27. Fleck DE, Keck PE, Jr., Corey KB, Strakowski SM. Factors associated with medication adherence in African American and White patients with bipolar disorder. J Clin Psychiatry. 2005 May 15;66(5):646–652.
28. Betancourt JR. Cultural competence—Marginal or mainstream movement? N Engl J Med Boston. 2004 Sep 2;351(10):953–955.
29. Thompson L, McCabe R. The effect of clinician–patient alliance and communication on treatment adherence in mental health care: A systematic review. BMC Psychiatry. 2012 Jul 24;12:87.
30. Kim SS, Kaplowitz S, Johnston MV. The effects of physician empathy on patient satisfaction and compliance. Eval Health Prof. 2004 Sep 1;27(3):237–251.
31. Gleichgerrcht E, Decety J. Empathy in clinical practice: How individual dispositions, gender, and experience moderate empathic concern, burnout, and emotional distress in physicians. PLoS One. 2013 Apr;8(4):e61526.
32. Chen P-J, Huang C-D, Yeh S-J. Impact of a narrative medicine programme on healthcare providers' empathy scores over time. BMC Med Educ. 2017 Dec 1;17(1):108.
33. Santamaría-García H, Baez S, García AM, Flichtentrei D, Prats M, Mastandueno R, et al. Empathy for others' suffering and its mediators in mental health professionals. Sci Rep. 2017 Jul 25;7(1):6391.
34. Cheung DH, Reeves A. Can we teach empathy? Evidence from the evaluation of a course titled "Compassion in Medicine." J Altern Complement Med. 2014 May 1;20(5):A7.
35. Foster A, Chaudhary N, Kim T, Waller JL, Wong J, Borish M, et al. Using virtual patients to teach empathy: A randomized controlled study to enhance medical students' empathic communication. Simul Healthc. 2016 Jun;11(3):181–189.
36. Stepien KA, Baernstein A. Educating for empathy. J Gen Intern Med. 2006 May 1;21(5):524–530.
37. Lincoln TM, Wilhelm K, Nestoriuc Y. Effectiveness of psychoeducation for relapse, symptoms, knowledge, adherence and functioning in psychotic disorders: A meta-analysis. Schizophr Res. 2007 Nov 1;96(1):232–245.
38. Xia J, Merinder LB, Belgamwar MR. Psychoeducation for schizophrenia. Schizophr Bull. 2011;37(1):21–22.

39. Reach G. An intentionalist model of patient adherence. In: The Mental Mechanisms of Patient Adherence to Long-Term Therapies. Cham, Switzerland: Springer; 2015: pp. 55–66. Retrieved December 22, 2917, from https://link.springer.com/chapter/10.1007/978-3-319-12265-6_4

40. Petretto DR, Preti A, Zuddas C, Veltro F, Rocchi MBL, Sisti D, et al. Study on Psychoeducation Enhancing Results of Adherence in Patients with Schizophrenia (SPERA-S): Study protocol for a randomized controlled trial. Trials. 2013 Dec 1;14(1):323.

41. Stanhope V, Ingoglia C, Schmelter B, Marcus SC. Impact of person-centered planning and collaborative documentation on treatment adherence. Psychiatr Serv. 2013 Jan 1;64(1):76–79.

42. Adams N, Grieder D. Treatment planning for person-centered care: The road to mental health and addiction recovery: Mapping the journey for individuals, families, and providers. Boston, MA: Elsevier; 2005.

43. Cook JA, Russell C, Grey DD, Jonikas JA. Economic grand rounds: A self-directed care model for mental health recovery. Psychiatr Serv. 2008 Jun 1;59(6):600–602.

44. Cook JA, Shore SE, Burke-Miller JK, Jonikas JA, Ferrara M, Colegrove S, et al. Participatory action research to establish self-directed care for mental health recovery in Texas. Psychiatr Rehabil J. 2010;34(2):137–144.

45. Spaulding-Givens JC, Lacasse JR. Self-directed care: Participants' service utilization and outcomes. Psychiatr Rehabil J. 2015;38(1):74–80.

46. Tarshis TP, Langer JA, Muniz B, Nelson G, Quiterio NM. Effects of a productivity model on care delivery and financial health of a nonprofit community clinic. J Am Acad Child Adolesc Psychiatry. 2016 Oct 1;55(10, Suppl):S203–S204.

47. Barham V, Milliken O. Payment mechanisms and the composition of physician practices: Balancing cost-containment, access, and quality of care. Health Econ. 2015 Jul 1;24(7):895–906.

48. Van Herck P, De Smedt D, Annemans L, Remmen R, Rosenthal MB, Sermeus W. Systematic review: Effects, design choices, and context of pay-for-performance in health care. BMC Health Serv Res. 2010 Aug 23;10(1):247.

49. Allard M, Jelovac I, Léger PT. Treatment and referral decisions under different physician payment mechanisms. J Health Econ. 2011 Sep 1;30(5):880–893.

50. Greene J, Hibbard JH, Overton V. A case study of a team-based, quality-focused compensation model for primary care providers. Med Care Res Rev. 2014 Jun 1;71(3):207–223.

51. Moore NH. Effects of evidence-based formulary restrictions at a Veterans Affairs medical center. Formulary. 2006 Dec;41(12):657.

52. Moffic HS. Ethical principles for psychiatric administrators: The challenge of formularies. Psychiatr Q. 2006 Dec 1;77(4):319–327.

53. Motheral B, Fairman KA. Effect of a three-tier prescription copay on pharmaceutical and other medical utilization. Med Care. 2001;39(12):1293–1304.

54. Nayak RK, Pearson SD. The ethics of "fail first": Guidelines and practical scenarios for step therapy coverage policies. Health Aff Chevy Chase. 2014 Oct;33(10):1779–1785.

55. Teagarden JR. The effect of pharmacy benefit manager clinical programs and services on access to prescription drug benefit coverage. Drug Inf J. 1998 Apr 1;32(2):373–377.

56. Soumerai SB. Benefits and risks of increasing restrictions on access to costly drugs in Medicaid. Health Aff Chevy Chase. 2004 Feb;23(1):135–146.

57. Soumerai SB, McLaughlin TJ, Ross-Degnan D, Casteris CS, Bollini P. Effects of limiting Medicaid drug-reimbursement benefits on the use of psychotropic agents and acute mental health services by patients with schizophrenia. N Engl J Med. 1994 Sep 8;331(10):650–655.

58. Seabury S, Lakdawalla DN, Walter D, Hayes J, Gustafson T, Shrestha A, et al. PMH78—Medicaid formulary restrictions and expenditures for patients with major depressive disorder. Value Health. 2014 May 1;17(3):A222.

59. Lieberman JA. What the CATIE study means for clinical practice. Psychiatr Serv. 2006 Aug 1;57(8):1075.

60. Rosenheck RA, Leslie DL, Busch S, Rofman ES, Sernyak M. Rethinking antipsychotic formulary policy. Schizophr Bull. 2008 Mar 1;34(2):375–380.

61. Garg AX, Adhikari NKJ, McDonald H, Rosas-Arellano MP, Devereaux PJ, Beyene J, et al. Effects of computerized clinical decision support systems on practitioner performance and patient outcomes: A systematic review. JAMA. 2005 Mar 9;293(10):1223–1238.

62. Yeisen RAH, Joa I, Johannessen JO, Opjordsmoen S. Use of medication algorithms in first episode psychosis: A naturalistic observational study: Adherence to medical algorithms. Early Interv Psychiatry. 2016 Dec;10(6):503–510.

63. Howard DH. Drug companies' patient-assistance programs—Helping patients or profits? N Engl J Med. 2014 Jul 10;371(2):97–99.

64. Felder TM, Palmer NR, Lal LS, Mullen PD. What is the evidence for pharmaceutical patient assistance programs? A systematic review. J Health Care Poor Underserved. 2011 Feb 9;22(1):24–49.

65. Simon GE, Psaty BM, Hrachovec JB, Mora M. Principles for evidence-based drug formulary policy. J Gen Intern Med. 2005 Oct 1;20(10):964–968.

66. Mortimer AM. Symptom rating scales and outcome in schizophrenia. Br J Psychiatry. 2007 Aug 1;191(50):s7–s14.

67. Page MJ, McKenzie JE, Kirkham J, Dwan K, Kramer S, Green S, et al. Bias due to selective inclusion and reporting of outcomes and analyses in systematic reviews of randomised trials of healthcare interventions. Cochrane Database Syst Rev. 2014 Oct 1;10(10): MR000035.

68. Als-Nielsen B, Chen W, Gluud C, Kjaergard LL. Association of funding and conclusions in randomized drug trials: A reflection of treatment effect or adverse events? JAMA. 2003 Aug 20;290(7):921–928.

69. US Department of Health and Human Services. Report to Congress on the nation's substance abuse and mental health workforce issues. 2013. Available from https://www.cibhs.org/sites/main/files/file-attachments/samhsa_bhwork_0.pdf

70. Sharma TR, Nicely MD. Physician assistants in mental health: South Med J. 2011 Feb;104(2):87–88.

71. Pollack DA, Ford SM. Is there a role for physician assistants in community mental health? Community Ment Health J. 1998 Apr 1;34(2):209–217.

72. Feldman S, Bachman J, Cuffel B, Friesen B, McCabe J. Advanced practice psychiatric nurses as a treatment resource: Survey and analysis. Adm Policy Ment Health Ment Health Serv Res. 2003 Jul 1;30(6):479–494.

73. Wortans J, Happell B, Johnstone H. The role of the nurse practitioner in psychiatric/mental health nursing: Exploring consumer satisfaction. J Psychiatr Ment Health Nurs. 2006 Feb 1;13(1):78–84.

74. Moses RE, Feld AD. Physician liability for medical errors of nonphysician clinicians: Nurse practitioners and physician assistants. Am J Gastroenterol. 2007 Jan;102(1):6–9.

75. Buchbinder M, Regan J, Aldea M, Makowski D. Improving mental health services through physician assistants: Legislation in several southern states. South Med J. 2017 Apr;110(4):239–243.

76. Stevens CB. The dilemma of the rural psychiatrist: J Psychiatr Pract. 2012 Sep;18(5):369–372.

77. Ng B, Camacho A, Dimsdale J. Rural psychiatrists creating value for academic institutions. Psychiatr Serv. 2013 Nov 1;64(11):1177–1178.

78. Stress of practicing in rural area takes toll on psychiatrist. Psychiatr News. Retrieved October 27, 2017, from http://psychnews.psychiatryonline.org.ezproxy.lib.utexas.edu/doi/full/10.1176%2Fpn.41.9.0004a

79. Scopelliti J, Judd F, Grigg M, Hodgins G, Fraser C, Hulbert C, et al. Dual relationships in mental health practice: Issues for clinicians in rural settings. Aust N Z J Psychiatry. 2004 Dec 11;38(11–12):953–959.

80. Mehrotra A, Huskamp HA, Souza J, Uscher-Pines L, Rose S, Landon BE, et al. Rapid growth in mental health telemedicine use among rural medicare beneficiaries, wide variation across states. Health Aff. 2017 May 1;36(5):909–917.

81. Pyne JM, Fortney JC, Tripathi SP, Maciejewski ML, Edlund MJ, Williams DK. Cost-effectiveness analysis of a rural telemedicine collaborative care intervention for depression. Arch Gen Psychiatry. 2010 Aug 1;67(8):812–821.

82. Antonacci DJ, Bloch RM, Saeed SA, Yildirim Y, Talley J. Empirical evidence on the use and effectiveness of telepsychiatry via videoconferencing: Implications for forensic and correctional psychiatry. Behav Sci

Law. 2008;26(3):253–269. Retrieved December 25, 2017, from http://www.readcube.com/articles/10.1002/bsl.812

83. García-Lizana F, Muñoz-Mayorga I. Telemedicine for depression: A systematic review. Perspect Psychiatr Care. 2010 Apr 1;46(2):119–126.

84. Whittington JW, Nolan K, Lewis N, Torres T. Pursuing the triple aim: The first 7 years. Milbank Q. 2015 Jun 1;93(2):263–300.

///3/// THE PUBLIC PSYCHIATRIST AS CLINICAL TEAM MEMBER

ASHLEY TRUST AND JAMES G. BAKER

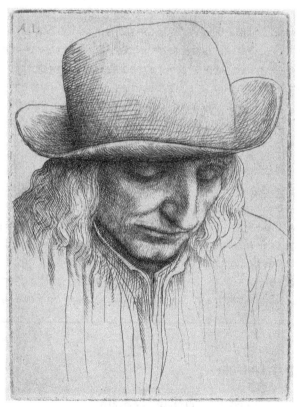

FIGURE 3.1 Alphonse Legros, *Peasant in a Round Hat*, etching.

Alphonse Legros (1837–1911) was a French painter, sculptor, and etcher who spent most of his career in London, where he created a niche for himself as a French traditionalist in a Victorian art scene and also taught art at University College in London. He had little formal education in early life, and his first job was painting houses to help his family make ends meet. He studied art in Paris, and from the beginning of his career, his work focused on the circumstances of his upbringing. He used a formula of traditional, rural French people placed within a seemingly authentic setting to appeal to his English clientele (Figure 3.1) (1).

CASE STUDY: INITIAL PRESENTATION

You are starting your first job serving as the community psychiatrist for an assertive community treatment (ACT) team that cares for mostly homeless, chronically mentally ill patients in an underserved urban area. You have limited experience on multidisciplinary teams but assume you will provide clinical leadership to the team once you begin. You are surprised to learn that a social worker serves as the team leader. Your role seems to be assessing the need for and prescribing medications, providing education on medications to patients and other team members, and participating in treatment planning meetings with other team members. You believe that your medical and residency training means that you should provide leadership for clinical decision-making on the team, while the social worker provides administrative supervision to the non-physician team members.

QUESTIONS
1. How might you approach resolution of the tension between your opinion of your clinical role and the treatment team's perceived needs of a team psychiatrist?
2. An alternative model would have you serving as a contracted psychiatrist, independent of the treatment team. What are the advantages and disadvantages of that model versus being a part of the multidisciplinary team?
3. What types of services, other than medication, might the patients treated by this ACT team require? What disciplinary roles and decision-making do those services require?

PSYCHIATRY AND LITERATURE

I Felt a Funeral, in My Brain
by Emily Dickinson

I felt a Funeral, in my Brain,
And Mourners to and fro
Kept treading—treading—till it seemed
That Sense was breaking through—

And when they all were seated,
A Service, like a Drum—
Kept beating—beating—till I thought
My mind was going numb—

And then I heard them lift a Box
And creak across my Soul
With those same Boots of Lead, again,
Then Space—began to toll,

As all the Heavens were a Bell,
And Being, but an Ear,
And I, and Silence, some strange Race,
Wrecked, solitary, here—

And then a Plank in Reason, broke,
And I dropped down, and down—
And hit a World, at every plunge,
And Finished knowing—then—

One of the greatest American poets, Emily Dickinson (born in 1830) was arguably one of the most original poets of all time. She lived a secluded life in her later years, and it has been thought that she perhaps suffered from a mood disorder or a severe anxiety disorder such as agoraphobia, but it may have been that she was simply absorbed in her responsibilities caring for her ailing mother (2).

PUBLIC PSYCHIATRISTS ON MULTIDISCIPLINARY TEAMS

Too much of a physician's training still implies that the physician always serves as the captain of the ship and, as such, needs to know how to do the job of every one of his shipmates. And so many public psychiatrists take that historic baggage into the community center setting with them. Historically, community mental health centers wanted psychiatrists to function in a variety of roles beyond prescribing medications, especially providing clinical guidance and training to other staff as well as help in policy development (3). But a number of factors, particularly the rising cost of psychiatrist time relative to reimbursement in the public sector, have tended to relegate many public psychiatrists into the role of "prescriber."

The problem is exacerbated by historic medical training of physicians that does not leave the physician well prepared for work on a multidisciplinary treatment team. Doctors may join the clinic with an assumption of authority that may not be shared by other professionals, creating conflict and inhibiting team building (4). This tension between self-perception of clinical role and the community center's perceived needs of the physician may be one reason why studies show that "line" psychiatrists are less satisfied with their jobs than are psychiatrists in leadership positions (5).

These tensions can play out in a multidisciplinary treatment team as well, in which historically the psychiatrist was, indeed, captain of the ship, often with final—or only—say on treatment plans. But that role has evolved, and so it behooves the public psychiatrist to get past her residual training and view the treatment team as a model for shared decision-making that can mirror the process of contemporary treatment planning for patients (6). After all, most of the disorders treated in public psychiatry are complicated by psychological and social challengers that demand intervention from a number of specialists on an interdisciplinary treatment team and that require differentiated disciplinary roles and decision-making in the context of the shared core task or improving the lives of the patients served.

THE CONTEMPORARY ROLE OF PSYCHIATRIST ON MULTIDISCIPLINARY TEAMS

One of the advantages of working in public psychiatry is the support in patient care provided through teamwork. It allows the psychiatrist to take a comprehensive view that puts each patient's psychiatric disorder in the context of his social network and challenges. It offers the patient a variety of skills beyond what the psychiatrist is trained to do, it allows for continuity of care between physician appointments, and it fosters mutual support and education. Indeed, there is little doubt that the psychiatrist working as part of a treatment team can offer much more to her patients than can a psychiatrist working in, for example, a single-discipline clinic (7). The depth and breadth of knowledge of treatment team members can be enriching for the psychiatrist as well.

The professional disciplines of a multidisciplinary team in a community center or a public mental health hospital vary from site to site but often include psychiatry, psychiatric nursing, social work, psychology, case management, and peer support.

Although they often have the least formal education and are the poorest paid members of the treatment team, case managers typically provide the most comprehensive service to patients, doing so in the community and in the patients' homes. They are often the most persistent advocates for the patient in the community, frequently making something happen for a patient when all other providers have failed to do so (8). Some community centers use case managers in a very hands-on way, solving patient problems for them. Others prefer a broker model, which emphasizes education and monitoring of patients in solving their own problems rather than actual delivery of care.

Social workers have a long history of adherence to the principles of the contemporary recovery movement in public psychiatry (9). By training, they offer a variety of potential interventions to patients, from collaborative problem-solving to evidence-based psychotherapy. The social work profession was a mainstay of the treatment team in the decades before deinstitutionalization, and from the beginnings of that movement, social workers played a critical role in the community mental health system. Indeed, treatment strategies in the deinstitutionalization era stemmed from earlier efforts by the social work profession to serve as the aftercare provider following hospital stays, focusing on the social needs of discharged patients and their families (10). Today, however, community centers rely on social workers (and other licensed professionals) to provide psychotherapies that require a license and to provide supervision to unlicensed case managers working in the community.

The clinical psychologist also provides clinical education and supervision to other members of the treatment team in the contemporary community center. At the beginning of the deinstitutionalization movement, psychologists were a major part of community centers. Today, they are underrepresented but are highly valuable in the public mental health setting. Their distinct skill set allows them to serve as managers and administrators, as well as to provide clinical supervision and training in evidence-based psychotherapies (11). Specific training in core competencies central to public mental health has been suggested as one strategy to increase the representation of psychology in community centers (12).

Mental health nurses' duties include internal coordination of care, monitoring clients' psychopathology, and patient outreach. They work with health care providers within and outside of the treatment team to find resolutions to patients' medical, psychiatric, and psychosocial problems. Psychiatric nurses screen for metabolic syndromes and other medical disorders, while also negotiating access to medical health care services, especially in non-integrated community centers (13). Nurses may also be responsible for medication education and management. In residential or inpatient settings, dispensation of medication is the responsibility of nursing staff as well (14).

Peer support specialists are people with lived experience of mental health challenges who are employed by community centers to use those experiences to support patients (15). Peer support specialists serve in a variety of roles depending on the center. Roles include offering individual support to patients in the clinic or community, facilitating or co-facilitating groups on psychoeducation or treatment, and being a patient advocate within the treatment team and organization (16). Peer support specialists can also be role models for patients by demonstrating the possibility for future recovery (17).

Engaging with the Treatment Team

Serving on a community mental health center treatment team offers a wealth of clinical expertise and support. Successful practice in public psychiatry depends on successful engagement with one's treatment team. A study of community mental health teams in the United Kingdom showed that the staff with highest job satisfaction and lowest burnout were those who had identification both with their assigned treatment team and with their profession and who were clear about their own role and the role of other team members (18). Herrman et al. (7) delineate five primary barriers to effective teamwork and collaboration: ambiguity or conflict over roles, conflict and confusion over leadership, differing understandings of responsibility and accountability, interprofessional misperceptions, and differing income and social status of various professions. They argue that psychiatrists along with clinicians from other disciplines need training in the principles of teamwork, including understanding the concepts of shared responsibility, accountability, and leadership. For this reason, psychiatrists considering a leadership role in public psychiatry might consider advanced training in administration, through a public psychiatry fellowship, pursuit of a degrees in health administration or business administration, or other psychiatric leadership training (19).

Leadership involves helping team members agree about what needs to be done and how to do it and then facilitating the team's effort, individually and collectively, to accomplish shared objectives (20). Rather than delegating leadership to the physician as might have occurred in the past, contemporary treatment teams use distributed leadership in which leadership is conceived as a collective process that emerges out of team member interaction. It reflects openness of leadership boundaries, recognizing that optimal care requires the expertise and treatment recommendations of all team members (21). However, leadership ambiguity must be managed when distributed. That is, whereas leadership boundaries may be diffuse, clinical role boundaries must be crystal clear, and team members must agree about which member assumes ultimate authority in various clinical areas and situations (22).

Inevitably, conflict arises in teams and must be managed in the best interest of the team's patients. Although we are quick to point to personality issues—in our teammates, not in ourselves—as the prime etiology of conflict, the literature suggests that it more likely that systemic problems, not personalities, drive team conflict. In addition to clinical role ambiguity, work environment, perceived lack of support from management, and poor communication are common reasons often enacted by treatment teams. Thus, although knowledge of conflict management techniques might be helpful when disagreements arise, a public psychiatrist who finds herself in a struggling treatment team might encourage the team to examine the context of its conflict, including workload, time pressures, and the emotional demands of the team's caseload (23).

A VIGNETTE: TEAM CONFLICT

The lead social worker on Dr. Collins' treatment team had long complained to the clinic medical director about the way Dr. Collins treated team members. He was often irritable, short, and demanding. When Dr. Collins left the clinic, the lead social worker was pleased that Dr. Masters was assigned the team because Dr. Masters was known to be respectful and engaging of team members. So the medical director was surprised when he began to receive complaints about Dr. Masters, too. Convinced that the issue must be systemic, the medical director began searching for possible issues and discovered that the problem team's caseload was decidedly higher in acuity and social needs than the other teams in the clinic. After adjusting the caseload by attrition and new-case assignment, the team complaints ceased.

Fostering High-Functioning Treatment Teams

Fostering cross-discipline collaboration requires understanding the systemic and interpersonal barriers (24). Mental health care teams that report strong interprofessional collaboration believe that it stems from mutual respect and shared goals among the different health professionals on the team. By contrast, team members who report unsatisfactory collaboration perceive that interprofessional input is not valued due to a professional hierarchy whereby the team psychiatrist makes most of the clinical decisions.

Collaboration is also hampered by poor understanding about professional roles, especially when team members are expected to function in clinical roles that do not fit well with their professional skills and training. Therefore, it is important for the public psychiatrist to understand the areas of expertise each team member brings to the team and can contribute to the treatment plan. Although the many roles of team members were described previously, it is still worthwhile to ask team members about their scopes of practice and to be clear about one's own (25).

In addition to exploring professional roles, it is important to explore clinical models with team members. It is safe to assume that different mental health disciplines, with their differing historical traditions and training, might hold equally differing models of mental illness and how to approach it. For example, Read et al. (26) found major differences, particularly in biological and social constructionist model endorsement, between psychiatrists and psychologists. Differing models of mental illness may lead to differing opinions about how best to serve patients and therefore could lead to conflict.

Finally, systemic pressures from outside the team can lead to conflict. Time pressures or even the documentation process of the team's electronic medical record might lead to poor communication. Or, organizational leadership may not be conducive to team cohesion. Lack of adequate resources to care for patients—poor staffing levels or poor service array—might lead to higher acuity and team stress that gets played out through team discord. Pressures for productivity and large caseloads leave little time to engage in team tasks, practice trust, and discuss differences in models and treatment approaches—all of which are important to foster mutual understanding of issues. It is important for the public psychiatrist to consider these systemic factors when addressing team conflict or fostering team member commitment.

CASE STUDY: CONTINUED

After a couple of weeks serving with your new team, you realize that a multidisciplinary approach is more effective for providing treatment of your patients and that the clinical talents brought to the team by its varied members warrant a shared decision-making approach to serving patients. However, your tolerance for shared decision-making is tested when a team case manager asks you to refill a medication for a patient who had not told the case manager that she had run out of medication several weeks ago. The case manager now understands why the patient seems to be functioning more poorly. Your schedule is full, and the notes in the medical record reflect some concerning side effects at the patient's last visit with the previous psychiatrist. The case worker states, "I am here to advocate for the patient and he needs the refill." You believe it is not best to dispense the medication without the patient being seen first.

QUESTIONS
1. How can you address your concern with the case manager in a manner that fosters shared decision-making?
2. Should the conflict be discussed at the next treatment team meeting? Why or why not?
3. What sort of systemic problems might provide context to the conflict between the case manager and you?
4. Are there, for example, service array additions that might help patients who are in this situation?

THE SERVICE ARRAY IN PUBLIC PSYCHIATRY

In addition to the advantages of working as part of a collegial, multidisciplinary treatment team, public psychiatry also offers the opportunity to work in a variety of evidence-based, treatment team models of care.

Assertive Community Treatment

Recovery-oriented ACT teams are the contemporary version of the extensively studied ACT model of care. ACT teams were initially developed to help keep patients with serious and persistent mental illness in the community and out of state psychiatric hospitals by providing them with outpatient services similar to those that they would have received if institutionalized (27). ACT focuses on low caseloads and service delivery in the community, not in the clinic. It uses strong multidisciplinary teams, including psychiatrists, nurses, social workers, supported employment and education specialists, and case managers. Psychiatrists working on ACT teams develop an intimate knowledge of the day-to-day challenges faced by their patients.

Although research long ago demonstrated the efficacy of ACT teams in keeping patients out of the hospital (28), recovery-oriented services have been used to augment the traditional ACT model because of its less-than-optimal impact on function in the community (29). Examples of these recovery-oriented services include cognitive–behavioral therapy, motivational interviewing, substance use services, and peer support services. However, successful development of a recovery-oriented care plan requires a shift from the psychiatrist-as-expert model to a model in which patient and family are treated as full partners (30).

ACT is also relatively expensive, and so there are also efforts to obtain the same outcomes with less expensive resources, such as the "flexible ACT team," which varies intensity of ACT team engagement with a patient based on relative acuity (31). Another variation, the forensic ACT team intended for patients with involvement in the criminal justice system, has shown evidence of efficacy in reducing jail time (32). In addition to working with the treatment team, the public psychiatrist serving on a forensic ACT team might work on behalf of patients directly with criminal court judges and attorneys, as well as with probation and parole officers.

Crisis Services

Public psychiatrists who work in crisis settings are the mental health equivalent of emergency room physicians. This work requires collaboration with other medical and mental health specialists. Given the mix of professionals, families, and patients involved in a psychiatric emergency room visit, the role of emergency psychiatrists has been described as that of a systems therapist (33). Public sector emergency psychiatrists also play a critical role in resource management of typically underfunded public mental health systems. They must be knowledgeable about community alternatives to inpatients hospitalization and develop a comfort level in using those alternatives as they triage patients into the appropriate level of care.

Outside of large urban areas, there are rarely freestanding mental health crisis units available for patients to access 24 hours a day. Consequently, medical emergency departments typically provide initial care to those in psychiatric crisis. However, there can often be barriers to assessment and care of psychiatric patients in a medical emergency department due to resource limitations, access blocks, and clinician knowledge deficits (29). Public psychiatrists should advocate for psychiatric emergency services colocated within medical/surgical emergency rooms so mental health specialists and medical clinicians can assess both psychiatric and medical comorbidities (34). A common cohort of patients who need evaluation from medical and psychiatric specialties are those with substance use disorders. Substance use assessments must be available in the emergency department, using the evidence-based screening, brief intervention, and referral to treatment model (35).

Crisis residential services are intended as a lower cost, patient-centered alternative to inpatient hospitalization for the resolution of mental health crises (36). A variety of services fall under the crisis residential categories, including short-term crisis units with 24-hour professional staff, crisis foster homes, peer-directed services, and informal nonclinical settings (37). Access to medical care, including psychiatric care, is generally reduced in crisis residential settings, but a public psychiatrist is often part of the treatment team and consults on medication regimens and treatment plan development. Studies of residential alternatives to acute care typically demonstrate clinical effectiveness equal to inpatient hospital stays and at a considerably lower cost. Patient satisfaction scores are typically higher as well (38).

A significant portion of community contacts with police officers, especially in urban areas, involve someone with a severe mental illness. Therefore, police are often the first responders in a mental health crisis. Although great strides have been made in educating law enforcement personnel on mental health issues that they face (39), it is still common for symptoms of a mental illness to be criminalized if for no other reason than to expedite a police officer's disposition of a call: Taking a misdemeanant to jail is much less time-consuming than taking a mentally ill patient to the psychiatric emergency room.

Mobile crisis services have been deployed as an alternative to emergency services transport of patients with psychiatric emergencies to emergency departments or mental health crisis units. These services typically are a partnership between law enforcement and the local community mental health center. Their purpose is to perform on-site assessment and crisis intervention, especially to determine the level of care needed to alleviate a mental health crisis. Members of a mobile crisis team are typically licensed mental health specialists, but frequently a mental health nurse and even a psychiatrist or advanced nurse practitioner will participate in a call, especially when medication questions are involved. In addition, clinic-based staff are responsible for receiving calls from law enforcement, determining appropriateness of mobile intervention, and then dispatching the mobile crisis team (40). Police officers, in particular, appreciate on-the-scene access to mental health care because it reduces the time spent on each mental health-related call (41).

Mobile crisis services have also been used to successfully engage patients who present to the emergency room with suicidal ideation by maintaining contact with patients after they leave the emergency room but before they are seen in an outpatient clinic (42). Mobile crisis assessment and intervention for children and adolescents can be provided at home or at school (43).

Co-occurring Substance Use Disorders

Substance use disorders occur in at least 40–50% of patients with emerging serious mental illness. Because co-occurring substance use and psychiatric disorders are associated with more functional impairment than either disorder alone, it is important to early and aggressively address the substance use. Treatment is difficult, and outcomes are not optimal (44).

Supported housing, especially the housing-first model, is likely the most successful intervention in co-occurring disorders, especially for patients who have endured long periods of homelessness and disengagement from traditional services (45). Housing-first programs provide permanent supported housing in scattered sites as the first step in treatment, providing access to ACT team-like services that provide recovery-oriented care (46). Housing-first programs do not require abstinence from drugs or even adherence to treatment for access to housing. Fidelity to the housing-first model has been shown to significantly improve success in keeping chronically homeless patients off the streets. Respect for patient wishes in choosing housing was especially important for success, as was the use of scattered site housing, rather than grouping patients together in a single housing project (47). In these programs, public psychiatrists serve as part of the intensive treatment team providing supported housing services.

A VIGNETTE: BEST-VALUE HOUSING

A local philanthropist wishes to help start a housing initiative for the homeless with mental illness in your community. As medical director of the community mental health center, you are asked to serve on an advisory committee to help design a program. Some on the committee members want to purchase a piece of property and build 50 apartments. Citing best practices, you advocate instead for simply leasing in various apartment complexes throughout the town. You also mention that the dollars would serve many more people through leasing than through building.

Jail-Based Care

The Bureau of Justice Statistics' 2011–2012 National Inmate Survey showed that one in four people in local jails had serious psychological distress, with major depression being the most common disorder (48). The cost of incarceration of people with serious mental illness, and especially their repeated incarceration, has led many urban, and even rural, jails to provide more aggressive treatment of mentally ill offenders while they are incarcerated.

Of course, the ideal goal both clinically and fiscally for treatment teams caring for mentally ill offenders is avoiding incarceration for people with mental illness who commit crimes related to their illness. Once detained, the team's goal should be to minimize time spent in jail. One strategy to attain these goals uses the sequential intercept model, which, in the sequence of a patient in the judicial system, identifies points of interception and diversion out of jail and into the health care system. Ideally, diversion will occur by, for example, mobile crisis teams before booking. However, diversion can also occur at hearings after incarcerated or as part of re-entry programming (49).

Even when a system of care fails in efforts to keep patients out of jail, the judicial system affords multiple opportunities to identify and serve patients. It is not uncommon for jail to serve as the place of initial presentation of severe mental illness (50). Identification and early engagement of patients into evidence-based treatment provide an opportunity to reduce future morbidity and incarcerations. Likewise, many jail stays are related to substance use disorders. Jails can offer motivational interviewing to engage patients into treatment, as well as offer initiation of medication-assisted treatment such as suboxone, when indicated. Treatment of these patients in a jail setting has the potential to stop rearrests.

Public psychiatrists are frequently engaged in the design of programs to identify and initiate treatment in jails, especially triage strategies for caring for inmates in underresourced, and therefore understaffed, jail settings. Public psychiatrists also provide psychiatric assessment, medication management, and even competency evaluations.

Hospital Transition Teams

Another strategy being used as a way of fostering engagement into outpatient services and to reduce readmission rates is the navigator or facilitated discharge team. Team members typically are called upon by the hospital treatment team to engage with the patient prior to discharge and then follow the patient transitionally until the patient is engaged with the outpatient treatment team. Facilitated discharge has been shown to reduce length of stay in the hospital but not reduce the rate of readmission (51).

CONTEMPORARY TREATMENT PLANNING

Regardless of the type of treatment team on which the public psychiatrist serves, the team bases its interventions on the elements of a service plan developed together by the team and the patient, identifying a comprehensive list of biopsychosocial factors responsible for patient difficulties and influencing his or her ability to achieve life goals and using this information to plan treatment.

Person-directed treatment planning emerged out of the developmental disability field at the time of the shift from institutional to community-based services, which was the first time that people with developmental disabilities had the opportunity for much choice in how they lived their lives as well as choice in the services they received in order to achieve their life goals (52). The expansion of person-centered treatment planning in mental health stemmed from the President's New Freedom Commission on Mental Health in 2003, which emphasized the development of individualized treatment plans to guide care and seek out supports oriented toward recovery and resilience (53).

The philosophy of person-directed care is that decisions about care are shared between the treatment team and the patient. The treatment team recognizes the capacity of patients to assess their own needs and actively participate in determining how the needs are met, and by what sort of practitioner. That is, the treatment planning process acknowledges and respects each patient's autonomy, capabilities, and rights.

In its most robust form, patient-directed care offers flexible benefits and individualized funding of service plans that may include nontraditional care, such as gym memberships or personal assistance. Patients may be allocated a certain percentage of their benefits in the form of flexible funds that they can use to implement their individualized service plans.

Person-centered treatment planning is intended to be focused on recovery and resiliency. Despite that contemporary preference, there is often confusion about what recovery means. Recovery is characterized as a process leading to clinical outcomes such as symptom remission, normative psychosocial functioning, and quality of life. Recovery focuses not on symptom management but, rather, on a program of rehabilitation based on the patient's assets and strengths (54).

Contemporary treatment planning must demonstrate cultural humility as well. It is well documented that racial and ethnic minorities in the United States have more difficulty accessing psychiatric services compared with White Americans (55). The manner in which patients present with psychiatric disorders—or whether they present at all—may relate to racial and ethnic differences in how culture characterizes symptoms and in how that culture experiences help-seeking for those symptoms (56). Public psychiatrists can lead efforts to improve access and quality of care by helping treatment teams focus on treatment planning and care that are culturally competent and that consider cultural factors that can impede access to services (57).

One approach to reducing disparities in access and care is to insist that treatment plans be culturally tailored (58). Simply ensuring professional translation services is a start, but changes in how service is delivered to specifically address important cultural issues may also be indicated. Even in the initial encounter with the patient, it is important to consider culturally derived differences in transactional style. For example, repeated directive questioning may be a routine part of the psychiatric examination but also may be considered disrespectful in some cultures. In treatment planning, it is important to identify strengths and supports that may be specific to a patient's culture, such as cultural pride or strong culturally identified interpersonal support systems. Likewise, it is important to ensure that treatment plans are sensitive to, rather than confronting of, core cultural beliefs (59).

A VIGNETTE

Donald is a 26-year-old African American male who has been seeing Dr. Smith, a Caucasian male, for the past year. Dr. Smith is frustrated that Donald continues be non-adherent with the medications prescribed, as well as inconsistent in attending appointments. Donald's depression continues to worsen, and Dr. Smith consistently tells him he has to be compliant with treatment in order to feel better.

Dr. Smith decides to schedule Donald into a psychiatric evaluation appointment slot in order to give time for a new treatment plan inclusive of a cultural formulation. Using open-ended questions and asking about Donald's beliefs and culture, Dr. Smith learns that Donald is both working full-time and attending college in the evenings, making it difficult for him to attend appointments. He also learns that Donald has been hesitant to take his medications because he was hopeful that prayer alone would be enough. Now cognizant of the importance of Donald's faith, Donald and Dr. Smith develop a person-centered plan of care that adjusted appointment frequency to account for his busy schedule, included his faith community, and helped him feel better about using both medication and prayer.

In working as part of the treatment team developing, along with the patient, a person-directed treatment plan focused on recovery and based on the patient's goals for herself and growing out of her assets and strengths, what should the public psychiatrist expect that treatment plan to look like (60)?

The plan should represent the basic mental health recovery principle that achieving wellness is possible, regardless of the severity of the illness. It should be written in a manner that reflects the inclusion of the individual in its development, with goals that are empowering and respectful of the individual and of her self-determination, not only with respect to the plan's content but also in her community.

The plan should have treatment goals that are beyond symptom management, with life goals written in the individual's own words and reflective of the individual vision for herself, regardless of the severity of the person's mental illnesses. It should reflect the person's interests, personally and socially, and draw on the individual's talents and expressed strengths, rather than delineating deficits.

Symptoms and impairments caused by mental illness should be reframed as barriers to attaining goals. Interventions such as medication, psychosocial rehabilitation, case management, and peer support should be framed as tools to help the individual overcome the barriers. In the plan, even medications prescribed by the public psychiatrist should target barriers to life goals such as syndrome symptoms rather than being listed as for "depression" or "schizophrenia."

Recovery planning must help the individual overcome not only the barriers inherent in her illness but also the social barriers related to living with a mental illness in communities that still stigmatize the disorders because of errant beliefs about them. Sometimes, the treatment team members must also work together to overcome their own implicit beliefs—that some people with mental illness make poor choices, that they lack motivation, or that they are too sick to be a true partner in recovery planning.

CASE STUDY: CONCLUSION

As the new member of the ACT team in this case, it is important to keep in mind the various individual and systemic dynamics that come to bear as the team cares for its patients. Then, when tackling the inevitable misunderstandings and conflicts that arise on a team, solutions should be discussed together in that context. For example, although your medical and residency training does prepare you to provide clinical leadership on the team, the reality is that the training and experience of other team members may have prepared them equally well. It is important to know the training and experience of your team members, as well as the biases that they (like you) bring to patient encounters and team meetings. Likewise, it is important to know the skills that each team member has to offer the team's patients because this will also help clarify who should have decision-making authority in various clinical situations.

Exploring the training, experience, and skills of the case manager will help resolve the conflict about when to write a refill for a patient who you believe needs to be seen. It is also important to review the current treatment plan for the patient to determine if there are already strategies in place to understand and address barriers to medication adherence. In this case, you might say, for example, "I agree with you, we need to do something differently for this patient. Can you help think of something else we can do until I am able to see him in order to address his symptoms?" Perhaps this would open a dialogue for information sharing that also allows you to share your concerns about prescribing the medication and allows for shared decision-making between you and the patient and you.

It would be helpful to discuss the conflict with the rest of the team, if done so in the context of the systemic pressures within which the team must function. For example, are there barriers that led to the patient going so long with medications and without being seen? Is there a need to advocate for non-emergent, walk-in clinics to ease access to refills when team-based physicians are swamped? The case might serve as a way to explore how the team might collectively develop plans of care that meet the goals of the patient in a way that everyone involved believes is both safe and effective and in which each team member's responsibility is clear. As this case reflects, although the public psychiatrist may not be directing all the moving parts associated with a patient's care, she can advocate for a team that works collectively to help the patient's progress toward his recovery goals. This is most likely to occur when a cohesive treatment team works alongside the patient and family to develop goals and strategies. It is also most likely to occur when the public psychiatrist recognizes that her role is not set in stone and can morph based on the needs of the team and patient population being treated.

REFERENCES

1. Berry M. Alphonse Legros and masculine identity construction in Victorian London. Vis Cult Br. 2015 Jul;16(2):186–199.
2. McDermott JF. Emily Dickinson revisited: A study of periodicity in her work. Am J Psychiatry. 2001 May 1;158(5):686–690.
3. Diamond RJ, Goldfinger SM, Pollack D, Silver M. The role of psychiatrists in community mental health centers: A survey of job descriptions. Community Ment Health J. 1995 Dec 1;31(6):571–577.
4. Norman IJ. Working together in adult community mental health services: An inter-professional dialogue. J Ment Health. 1999 Jan;8(3):217–230.
5. Ranz J, Stueve A, McQuistion HL. The role of the psychiatrist: Job satisfaction of medical directors and staff psychiatrists. Community Ment Health J. 2001 Dec 1;37(6):525–539.
6. Iqbal N, Rees M, Backer C. Decision making, responsibility and accountability in community mental health teams: Nasur Iqbal and colleagues clarify how roles have changed under the new ways of working in the health service. Ment Health Pract. 2014 Apr 9;17(7):26–28.
7. Herrman H, Trauer T, Warnock J. The roles and relationships of psychiatrists and other service providers in mental health services. Aust N Z J Psychiatry. 2002 Feb 1;36(1):75–80.
8. Lerbæk B, Aagaard J, Andersen MB, Buus N. Assertive community treatment (ACT) case managers' professional identities: A focus group study. Int J Ment Health Nurs. 2016 Dec 1;25(6):579–587.

9. Carpenter J. Mental health recovery paradigm: Implications for social work. Health Soc Work. 2002 May 1;27(2):86–94.

10. Vourlekis BS, Edinburg G, Knee R. The rise of social work in public mental health through aftercare of people with serious mental illness. Soc Work. 1998;43(6):567–575.

11. Carr ER, Miller R. Expanding our reach: Increasing the role of psychologists in public and community mental health. Psychol Serv. 2017 Aug;14(3):352–360.

12. Chu JP, Emmons L, Wong J, Goldblum P, Reiser R, Barrera AZ, et al. Public psychology: A competency model for professional psychologists in community mental health. Prof Psychol Res Pract. 2012 Feb;43(1):39–49.

13. Heslop B, Wynaden D, Tohotoa J, Heslop K. Mental health nurses' contributions to community mental health care: An Australian study. Int J Ment Health Nurs. 2016 Oct 1;25(5):426–433.

14. Tin-Fu Ng D, Chan SWC, MacKenzie A. Case management in the community psychiatric nursing service in Hong Kong: Describing the process. Perspect Psychiatr Care. 2000 Apr 1;36(2):59–66.

15. Holley J, Gillard S, Gibson S. Peer worker roles and risk in mental health services: A qualitative comparative case study. Community Ment Health J. 2015 May 1;51(4):477–490.

16. Chinman MJ, Weingarten R, Stayner D, Davidson L. Chronicity reconsidered: Improving person–environment fit through a consumer-run service. Community Ment Health J. 2001 Jun 1;37(3):215–229.

17. Salyers MP, Hicks LJ, McGuire AB, Baumgardner H, Ring K, Kim H-W. A pilot to enhance the recovery orientation of assertive community treatment through peer-provided illness management and recovery. Am J Psychiatr Rehabil. 2009 Aug 31;12(3):191–204.

18. Rosen A, Callaly T. Interdisciplinary teamwork and leadership: Issues for psychiatrists. Australas Psychiatry. 2005 Sep 1;13(3):234–240.

19. Sowers W, Pollack D, Everett A, Thompson KS, Ranz J, Primm A. Progress in workforce development since 2000: Advanced training opportunities in public and community psychiatry. Psychiatr Serv. 2011 Jul 1;62(7):782–788.

20. Yukl GA. Leadership in organizations. 6th ed. Upper Saddle River, NJ: Pearson/Prentice Hall; 2006.

21. Bolden R. Distributed leadership in organizations: A review of theory and research. Int J Manag Rev. 2011 Sep 1;13(3):251–269.

22. Chreim S, MacNaughton K. Distributed leadership in health care teams: Constellation role distribution and leadership practices. Health Care Manage Rev. 2016;41(3):200–212.

23. Almost J, Wolff AC, Stewart-Pyne A, McCormick LG, Strachan D, D'Souza C. Managing and mitigating conflict in healthcare teams: An integrative review. J Adv Nurs. 2016 Jul;72(7):1490–1505.

24. Chong WW, Aslani P, Chen TF. Shared decision-making and interprofessional collaboration in mental healthcare: A qualitative study exploring perceptions of barriers and facilitators. J Interprof Care. 2013 Sep 1;27(5):373–379.

25. McLoughlin KA, Geller JL. Interdisciplinary treatment planning in inpatient settings: From myth to model. Psychiatr Q. 2010 Sep 1;81(3):263–277.

26. Read R, Moberly NJ, Salter D, Broome MR. Concepts of mental disorders in trainee clinical psychologists. Clin Psychol Psychother. 2017 Mar 1;24(2):441–450.

27. Drake RE. Brief history, current status, and future place of assertive community treatment. Am J Orthopsychiatry. 1998;68(2):172–175.

28. Burns T, Catty J, Dash M, Roberts C, Lockwood A, Marshall M. Use of intensive case management to reduce time in hospital in people with severe mental illness: Systematic review and meta-regression. BMJ. 2007;335(7615):336–340.

29. Kidd SA, George L, O'Connell M, Sylvestre J, Kirkpatrick H, Browne G, et al. Recovery-oriented service provision and clinical outcomes in assertive community treatment. Psychiatr Rehabil J. 2011;34(3):194–201.

30. President's New Freedom Commission on Mental Health. Achieving the promise: Transforming mental health care in America: Final report. Rockville, MD: President's New Freedom Commission on Mental Health; 2003. Retrieved from http://hdl.handle.net/2027/mdp.39015060777912

31. Nugter MA, Engelsbel F, Bähler M, Keet R, Veldhuizen R van. Outcomes of FLEXIBLE Assertive Community Treatment (FACT) implementation: A prospective real life study. Community Ment Health J. 2016 Nov 1;52(8):898–907.

32. Smith RJ, Jennings JL, Cimino A. Forensic continuum of care with assertive community treatment (ACT) for persons recovering from co-occurring disabilities: Long-term outcomes. Psychiatr Rehabil J. 2010;33(3):207–218.

33. Sadler JZ. The emergency room psychiatrist as multiple agent: A family systems analysis. Fam Syst Med. 1986;4(4):367–375.

34. Baillargeon J, Thomas CR, Williams B, Begley CE, Sharma S, Pollock BH, et al. Medical emergency department utilization patterns among uninsured patients with psychiatric disorders. Psychiatr Serv. 2008 Jul 1;59(7):808–811.

35. Barbosa C, Cowell A, Bray J, Aldridge A. The cost-effectiveness of alcohol screening, brief intervention, and referral to treatment (SBIRT) in emergency and outpatient medical settings. J Subst Abuse Treat. 2015 Jun 1;53(Suppl C):1–8.

36. Lloyd-Evans B, Slade M, Jagielska D, Johnson S. Residential alternatives to acute psychiatric hospital admission: Systematic review. Br J Psychiatry. 2009 Aug 1;195(2):109–117.

37. Morant N, Lloyd-Evans B, Gilburt H, Slade M, Osborn D, Johnson S. Implementing successful residential alternatives to acute in-patient psychiatric services: Lessons from a multi-centre study of alternatives in England. Epidemiol Psychiatr Sci. 2012 Jun;21(2):175–185.

38. Thomas KA, Rickwood D. Clinical and cost-effectiveness of acute and subacute residential mental health services: A systematic review. Psychiatr Serv. 2013 Nov 1;64(11):1140–1149.

39. Tully T, Smith M. Officer perceptions of crisis intervention team training effectiveness. Police J. 2015 Mar 1;88(1):51–64.

40. Guo S, Biegel DE, Johnsen JA, Dyches H. Assessing the impact of community-based mobile crisis services on preventing hospitalization. Psychiatr Serv. 2001 Feb 1;52(2):223–228.

41. Kisely S, Campbell LA, Peddle S, Hare S, Pyche M, Spicer D, et al. A controlled before-and-after evaluation of a mobile crisis partnership between mental health and police services in Nova Scotia. Can J Psychiatry. 2010 Oct 1;55(10):662–668.

42. Currier GW, Fisher SG, Caine ED. Mobile crisis team intervention to enhance linkage of discharged suicidal emergency department patients to outpatient psychiatric services: A randomized controlled trial. Acad Emerg Med. 2010 Jan;17(1):36–43.

43. Vanderploeg JJ, Lu JJ, Marshall TM, Stevens K. Mobile crisis services for children and families: Advancing a community-based model in Connecticut. Child Youth Serv Rev. 2016 Dec 1;71(Suppl C):103–109.

44. Sheidow AJ, McCart M, Zajac K, Davis M. Prevalence and impact of substance use among emerging adults with serious mental health conditions. Psychiatr Rehabil J. 2012;35(3):235–243.

45. Tsemberis S, Gulcur L, Nakae M. Housing first, consumer choice, and harm reduction for homeless individuals with a dual diagnosis. Am J Public Health Wash. 2004 Apr;94(4):651–656.

46. Tsemberis S. From streets to homes: An innovative approach to supported housing for homeless adults with psychiatric disabilities. J Community Psychol. 1999;27(2):225–241. Retrieved November 20, 2017, from http://www.readcube.com/articles/10.1002/(SICI)1520-6629(199903)27:2<225:: AID-JCOP9>3.0.CO;2-Y

47. Gilmer TP, Stefancic A, Katz ML, Sklar M, Tsemberis S, Palinkas LA. Fidelity to the housing first model and effectiveness of permanent supported housing programs in California. Psychiatr Serv. 2014 Oct 31;65(11):1311–1317.

48. Bronson J, Berzofsky M. Indicators of mental health problems reported by prisoners and jail inmates, 2011–2012. Retrieved November 20, 2017, from https://www.bjs.gov/index.cfm?ty=pbdetail&iid=5946

49. Munetz MR, Griffin PA. Use of the sequential intercept model as an approach to decriminalization of people with serious mental illness. Psychiatr Serv. 2006 Apr 1;57(4):544–549.

50. Trestman RL, Ford J, Zhang W, Wiesbrock V. Current and lifetime psychiatric illness among inmates not identified as acutely mentally ill at intake in Connecticut's jails. J Am Acad Psychiatry Law Online. 2007 Dec 1;35(4):490–500.

51. Tulloch AD, Khondoker MR, Thornicroft G, David AS. Home treatment teams and facilitated discharge from psychiatric hospital. Epidemiol Psychiatr Sci Verona. 2015 Oct;24(5):402–414.

52. Powers LE, Sowers J-A, Singer GHS. A cross-disability analysis of person-directed, long-term services. J Disabil Policy Stud. 2006 Sep 1;17(2):66–76.

53. President's New Freedom Commission on Mental Health. Achieving the promise: Transforming mental health care in America: Final report. Rockville, MD: President's New Freedom Commission on Mental Health; 2003. Retrieved from http://hdl.handle.net/2027/mdp.39015060777912

54. Liberman RP, Kopelowicz A. Recovery from schizophrenia: A challenge for the 21st century. Int Rev Psychiatry. 2002 Jan;14(4):245–255.

55. Cook BL, Zuvekas SH, Carson N, Wayne GF, Vesper A, McGuire TG. Assessing racial/ethnic disparities in treatment across episodes of mental health care. Health Serv Res. 2014 Feb 1;49(1):206–229.

56. Bhugra D. Severe mental illness across cultures. Acta Psychiatr Scand. 2006 Feb 1;113(Suppl 429):17–23.

57. Betancourt JR, Green AR, Carrillo JE, Ananeh-Firempong O 2nd. Defining cultural competence: A practical framework for addressing racial/ethnic disparities in health and health care. Public Health Rep 2003;118(4):293–302.

58. Kohn-Wood LP., Hooper LM. Cultural competency, culturally tailored care, and the primary care setting: Possible solutions to reduce racial/ethnic disparities in mental health care. J Ment Health Couns. 2014 Apr;36(2):173–188.

59. Hays PA. Integrating evidence-based practice, cognitive–behavior therapy, and multicultural therapy: Ten steps for culturally competent practice. Prof Psychol Res Pract. 2009 Aug;40(4):354–360.

60. Matthews EB, Stanhope V, Choy-Brown M, Doherty M. Do providers know what they do not know? A correlational study of knowledge acquisition and person-centered care. Community Ment Health J. 2018 Jan 8;54(5):514–520.

THE PUBLIC PSYCHIATRIST AND THE PATIENT WITH INTELLECTUAL DISABILITY

EMILY MORSE, KELLY VINQUIST, AND JODI TATE

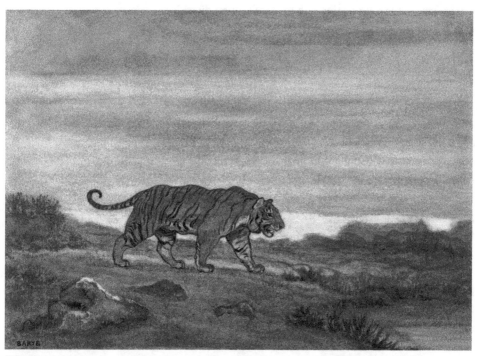

FIGURE 4.1 Antoine-Louis Barye, *Tiger Approaching Pool*, c. 1810–1875, watercolor.

Source: The Metropolitan Museum of Art, New York, https://www.metmuseum.org.

PSYCHIATRY AND LITERATURE

Antoine-Louis Barye (1795–1875) was a Parisian sculptor and painter whose primary subject was animals. He was known for his ability to depict anatomic detail and the struggles of living in the wild.

What a Tiger Can Do
by Vince Fiorilli

My oh my, what can a tiger do
If you believe in a tiger
they can make you brave and unstoppable
they can also make you smart and wise
you can even make a good guard
but the question is, do you want all that?
I'd say just do things your way, not the tiger way

Source: Reprinted with permission from *The Best of Cow Tipping Press: Volume 1*. Cow Tipping Press creates writing by people with developmental disabilities, giving audiences a new way to think about this rich form of human diversity.

CASE STUDY: INITIAL PRESENTATION

A 20-year-old male presents to the community mental health center for an initial visit, accompanied by staff from the group home where he lives. He is transitioning care from the child psychiatrist he had seen for many years. He is shy when you greet him in the waiting room, and as you walk him back to your office, he stops to examine each painting on the wall. A few moments after sitting in your office, he returns to the hallway to revisit one of the paintings. You offer to show him more artwork in your office, and he eventually agrees to return from the hall.

As he explores your office, his accompanying staff member begins to describe how things have been at home. He moved to this particular home 6 months ago from a setting in which there was a greater staff-to-resident ratio. Staff report that most days he does well. He enjoys visiting a nearby park and dancing to music. In the past few months, however, he has shown more aggressive and self-injurious behaviors, including hitting staff and himself. He has also run away from the house several times. You are provided with a long list of his current medications.

QUESTIONS

1. What strategies might assist you in building rapport with this patient and allowing him to feel comfortable in the clinic environment?
2. What etiologies for his recent challenging behaviors should be considered? How will you further assess each of them? How will these considerations influence your treatment plan?

INTELLECTUAL DISABILITY AND THE COMMUNITY PSYCHIATRIST

Individuals with intellectual disability (ID) comprise an estimated 1–3% of the population. Despite the many challenges those with ID face, their lives can be full and meaningful when provided with optimal support, empowerment, and social inclusion. Unfortunately, this population has been one of the most stigmatized and underserved groups in society.[1] Relative to individuals with other types of disability, those with ID face a heightened level of discrimination and isolation, including by the health care community. Lack of provider training in working with this population and a system that limits the provision of comprehensive assessment and care are just a few of the many barriers at both the individual level and the system level that limit access to health care services for individuals with ID.[2] Other determinants of health, including genetic, social, environmental, and behavioral factors, also contribute to excess morbidity and mortality among this population.[3]

Many individuals with ID will present for psychiatric care at some point in their lifetime. With the shift toward deinstitutionalization in recent decades, most of these individuals now reside in community-based settings and will receive their medical and psychiatric care in the communities in which they live. Rooted in its values of person-centeredness, team-based care, and advocacy, the field of community psychiatry has its foundation in the principles that are most needed in the care for individuals with ID.[4] However, a majority of psychiatrists believe their training in diagnosis and management of patients with ID is inadquate.[5] This chapter provides an overview of special considerations and potential challenges the community psychiatrist may encounter when working with this exceptional population.

Definitions

Intellectual disability is considered a subset of developmental disability (DD), which is defined as a severe, chronic disability with onset during childhood and resulting in substantial limitations in multiple functional domains. An individual may have DD without ID, and although they hold distinct meaning, the terms are sometimes used interchangeably. The scope of this chapter will focus primarily on care for individuals with ID.

The diagnosis of ID is characterized by deficits in intellectual and adaptive functioning, with onset during the developmental period and persisting throughout a person's lifetime.[6] Legislation passed in 2010 (Public Law 111-256; "Rosa's law") changed the previous vocabulary of "mental retardation" to "intellectual disability" in federal legislation and disability literature.[7] Prior to the most recent *Diagnostic and Statistical Manual of Mental Disorders* (DSM-5), IQ score was the primary basis on which the diagnosis and severity of ID were determined. The current diagnostic model takes a more comprehensive approach, taking into account the relative abilities and difficulties across multiple domains in characterizing the level of severity.[8] Assessment incorporates history from multiple informants regarding day-to-day function across each domain. Severity classification per DSM-5 guidelines is outlined in Table 4.1. Although IQ is generally considered nonprogressive over an individual's lifetime, adaptive functioning can be strengthened over time.

Epidemiology and Etiology

The prevalence of ID is estimated to be 1–3% of the general population, with higher rates found in lower socioeconomically resourced areas.[9] ID in the mild range accounts for approximately 85% of ID diagnoses, with prevalence decreasing as severity increases.[10] Life expectancy has been found to decrease with increasing severity of ID.[11,12]

There are many recognized etiologies for ID, yet for a substantial portion of individuals, no specific cause is ever identified. Estimates of the proportion of ID attributable to a genetic cause have ranged from 17% to 50%. Trisomy 21 is the most common known cause of ID, whereas fragile X syndrome is the most common inherited cause.[13] Other identified neurodevelopmental syndromes known to cause ID are listed in Table 4.2. Neonatal complications, including birth injury, hypoglycemia, hypoxia, and neonatal infection, as well as prenatal toxin exposures, are also risk factors.[14] Maternal factors such as advanced maternal age and low socioeconomic status have also been associated with ID, along with childhood risk factors including abuse and neglect.

TABLE 4.1 Severity Levels for Intellectual Disability

Severity Level	Conceptual Domain	Social Domain	Practical Domain
Mild	Early childhood: May be no discernable differences School-aged children: Difficulties with academic skills (reading, writing, arithmetic, time, money, etc.), with need for support in one or more areas Adults: Deficits in abstract thinking, executive function, short-term memory, and use of academic skills	May be immature in comparison with same-age peers Communication and language more concrete and immature Difficulties regulating emotion and behavior in age-appropriate manner Limited understanding of risk in social situations, posing risk for being manipulated	May function age-appropriately in personal care Need some support with complex daily living tasks (e.g., grocery shopping, transportation, and money management) Judgment related to well-being and organization may require support Employment often seen in jobs that do not emphasize conceptual skills Generally need support in health care and legal decisions Typically need support in raising a family
Moderate	Academic skills delayed at all ages Preschoolers: Language and pre-academic skills delayed School-age: Delayed in reading, writing, math, and understanding time and money Adults: Academic skills typically similar to elementary level; support needed for daily conceptual tasks	Marked differences in social and communicative behaviors across development Simple spoken language Misperceive social cues Limitations in social judgment and decision-making Relationships somewhat limited Social and communicative support needed in work settings	Able to care for personal needs with eating, dressing, elimination, and hygiene as an adult, although requires more time to become independent and may require reminders Household tasks may be achieved by adulthood but often need ongoing support Support needed for employment in jobs that require limited conceptual and communication skills
Severe	Limited attainment of conceptual skills Little understanding of written language or concepts involving numbers, time, and money Extensive support needed for problem-solving throughout life	Spoken language limited; may be single words or phrases Speech and communication focused on here and now Understand simple speech and gestures Relationships with family and familiar others	Requires support for all activities of daily living (meals, dressing, bathing, and elimination) Requires supervision at all times Assistance needed in all decision-making regarding well-being
Profound	Conceptual skills involve the physical world rather than symbolic processes Certain visuospatial skills, such as matching and sorting based on physical traits, may be learned	Very limited understanding of symbolic communication in speech or gesture Largely uses nonverbal, non-symbolic communication Enjoys relationships with well-known family and caretakers	Dependent for all aspects of daily physical care and safety, although may be able to participate in some activities Physical and sensory barriers often limiting

Source: Adapted from the American Psychiatric Association.[8]

CASE STUDY: CONTINUED

Through the initial portion of the interview, you notice that your patient speaks in three- to four-word sentences with simple vocabulary. He is easily distracted and makes very little eye contact. He appears nervous, scanning the room often and occasionally seeking reassurance from his support staff. You ask him about where he lives, and he describes living in a house with three roommates. When asked about things he does to care for himself, he states he brushes his teeth, takes a shower, and makes his bed each morning. You ask him about activities he enjoys, and he tells you he likes attending a day program during which he plays video games and going to the park. You observe that his physical appearance is notable for a long face, large ears, and prominent jaw.

QUESTIONS

1. Based on this initial history and observations of his communication and behavior, what early impressions do you have about his level of disability?
2. What, if any, genetic syndromes might be on your differential at this point? How might your differential(s) guide further assessment?

TABLE 4.2 Behavioral Phenotypes of 12 Intellectual Disability Syndromes

Syndrome/Etiology	Physical Phenotype	Behavioral Phenotype
Down syndrome	Short stature	Mild/severe ID
Trisomy 21	Cardiac defects	Relative strength in social function
	Hearing loss	Spared visuospatial abilities
	Broad neck	Self-talk
	Epicanthal folds	Mood and anxiety disorders
	Visual impairment	Alzheimer's dementia
	Dental problems	
	Thyroid dysfunction	
	Obesity	
Fetal alcohol spectrum disorder	Growth delay	Range in intellectual function
	Cardiac defects	Attention deficits
	Skeletal abnormalities	Executive dysfunction
	Renal problems	Social deficits
	Short palpebral fissures	Mood and anxiety disorders
	Smooth philtrum	Substance use disorders
	Thin upper lip	
	Maxillary hypoplasia	
	Ophthalmologic abnormalities	
	Hearing loss	

TABLE 4.2 (Continued)

Syndrome/Etiology	Physical Phenotype	Behavioral Phenotype

Williams syndrome
Microdeletion at 7q11.23
  chromosome
	Cardiac complications
	Hypertension
	Joint contractures
	Decreased muscle tone
	Short stature
	Vision impairment
	Stellate iris
	Hyperacusis
	Susceptibility to hernia/diverticuli
		Mild-moderate ID
		Strengths in verbal communication,
		  facial recognition, and
		  auditory memory
		Hypersociability/disinhibition
		Empathetic
		ADHD
		Anxiety and mood disorders

Fragile X syndrome
Trinucleotide expansion
  within the *FMR1* gene on
  the X chromosome
	Long face
	Large ears
	Macroorchidism
	Recurrent otitis/sinusitis
	Seizure disorder
	Aortic dilation
	Joint laxity
	Flat feet
		Shyness
		Executive dysfunction
		Stereotypic movements
		Sensitivity to noise
		ADHD
		Autism spectrum disorder
		Anxiety disorders

Angelman syndrome
Lack of maternally derived
  information on chromosome
  15q11–q13
	Microcephaly
	Seizure disorder
	GI/feeding problems
	Ataxic gait
	Glaucoma
		Moderate-profound ID
		Low linguistic ability
		Hyperactivity
		Happy demeanor with frequent
		  laughter unrelated to context
		Stereotyped behaviors
		Sleep disturbance

Prader–Willi syndrome
Lack of paternally derived
  information on chromosome
  15q11–q13
	Hypotonia early
	Short stature
	Hypogonadism
	High pain tolerance
	Hyperphagia leading to obesity
	Narrow nasal bridge
	Almond-shaped palpebral fissures
		Compulsive food-related behaviors
		Hyperphagia
		Perseverative speech
		Self-injury (skin-picking behavior)
		Impulsivity
		Tantrums

Rubinstein–Taybi syndrome Variable, often mapped to chromosome 16p13.3	Short stature Microcephaly Widely spaced eyes Beaked nose Cryptorchidism Broad thumbs and great toes Dental anomalies	Mild to severe ID Tic disorders Anxiety and mood disorders Obsessive–compulsive disorders Autism spectrum disorder Challenging behaviors Risk for NMS

TABLE 4.2 (Continued)

Syndrome/Etiology	Physical Phenotype	Behavioral Phenotype

Smith–Magenis syndrome
Gene deletion involving
    17p11.2
	Hypotonia/hypersomnolence
	    during infancy
	Brachycephaly
	Brachydactyly
	Heart defects
	Cleft palate
	Midface hypoplasia
	Urogenital abnormalities
	Peripheral neuropathy
		Mild-moderate ID
		Self-injury
		Onychotillomania (pulling out finger
		    and toe nails)
		Insertion of objects into body orifices
		Impulsivity
		Hyperactivity
		Stereotyped behaviors
		Sleep disturbance

Chromosome 15q11.2–13.1 duplication	Newborn hypotonia Seizure disorder Motor delays Epicanthal folds Flat nasal bridge Scoliosis	Cognitive delay or ID Autism spectrum disorder Hyperactivity Anxiety Emotional lability

Phenylketonuria
Mutation on chromosome
    12q22–24.1 that encodes
    for PAH enzyme
	Seizure disorder
	Gait abnormality
	Hypopigmentation
	Eczema
	"Mousy" odor
		Mild/severe ID
		Hyperactivity
		Stereotyped behavior
		Mood and anxiety disorders
		Autism spectrum disorder

Tuberous sclerosis complex
AD mutation in TSC1 on
    chromosome 9 or TSC2 on
    chromosome 16
	Facial angiofibromas
	Hypomelanotic macules
	    ("ash leaf spot"); shagreen patches
	Cortical tubers
	Seizures
	Retinal lesions
	Renal disease
		Average intellect to severe ID
		Challenging behavior
		Autism spectrum disorder
		ADHD
		Psychosis

22q11.2 deletion syndrome	Congenital cardiac malformations Cleft palate Narrow eyes Small ears Long pear-shaped nose Hypoparathyroidism Thymic hypoplasia Hearing loss Immune deficiency	Average intellect to moderate ID Emotional lability Social withdrawal Autism spectrum disorders Mood and anxiety disorders Psychotic disorders

AD, Alzheimer's disease; ADHD, attention-deficit/hyperactivity disorder; GI, gastrointestinal; ID, intellectual disability; NMS, neuroleptic malignant syndrome; PAH, phenylalanine hydroxylase.
Source: Adapted from Levitas et al.[15]

Clinical Assessment

The assessment of patients with ID should include all the usual elements of a comprehensive evaluation—a thorough history and mental status examination, review of prior treatment records, collateral history, and additional diagnostic testing as indicated. However, there are unique challenges that may be present in working with this population. Sovner described four specific challenges in assessment of individuals with ID (Table 4.3).[16]

Depending on the patient's cognitive function and expressive ability, he or she may be limited in providing a complete history. Nevertheless, the interviewer should work to engage and build rapport with the patient first, gathering as much information as possible through this interaction using both verbal and nonverbal approaches. This practice demonstrates respect for the patient, regardless of his or her communicative ability. Many patients have receptive abilities that exceed their expressive skills, and patience is essential. Using language that is understandable to the patient, allowing adequate time for response, asking one question at a time, and verifying that the question was understood are important practices. Interviewers must also be attentive to the tendency of patients with ID to respond in a way they think will please the provider and be wary of disproportionately affirmative responses.

Although collateral information is crucial in the assessment, providers must be mindful about managing potentially complex interactions between the patient, his or her family members, and other support staff who may be involved. Many individuals with ID express dissatisfaction with communication by providers and frequently feel excluded from discussion about their own care.[17] Interviewers should seek permission from the

TABLE 4.3 Challenges in Assessment

Baseline exaggeration	Frequency or intensity of pre-existing behaviors may escalate with onset or exacerbation of psychiatric or medical illness.
Cognitive disintegration	Susceptibility to decompensation in cognitive functioning in relation to stress or illness; may present as increasing disorganization and psychotic-like symptoms, although may be developmentally appropriate.
Intellectual distortion	Impairments in abstract thinking and communication affect comprehension of examiner questions and influence report of symptoms and emotional experience.
Psychosocial masking	Delays in development and limitations in intellectual function and life experience may influence presentation of psychiatric symptoms.

Source: Adapted from Sovner.[16]

patient before including accompanying individuals in the interview. It is common for caretakers to answer for the patient, and when time is limited, it can be easy to accept these responses and hurry the interview forward. Doing so may damage rapport and lead to missed information the patient may provide.

It is also worth keeping in mind that attending appointments can be a distressing experience and is disruptive to an individual's routine. Establishing expectations for how the visit will go and reassurance of safety may be helpful. Other strategies for managing distress may include bringing a familiar item to hold during the appointment, use of as needed medication for anxiety prior to the visit if appropriate, and maintaining a consistent routine with each subsequent visit.

DUAL DIAGNOSIS: COMORBID INTELLECTUAL DISABILITY AND MENTAL ILLNESS

Individuals with ID are affected by psychiatric disorders at higher rates than the general population. Dual diagnosis—the coexistence of ID and mental illness—occurs in approximately 40–60% of those with ID, with wide variation in the reported rate.[18,19] Historically, it was thought that individuals with ID could not have a mental illness. Although this attitude has shifted over time, diagnostic overshadowing—the misattribution of symptoms to the presence of intellectual disability—continues to compound the inherent challenges in properly diagnosing psychiatric illness in this population. In an effort to address some of these difficulties, the *Diagnostic Manual—Intellectual Disability (DM-ID): A Textbook of Diagnosis of Mental Disorders in Persons with Intellectual Disability* was published in 2007. Now in its second edition (DM-ID-2) to correspond with DSM-5, this text outlines adjusted diagnostic criteria that incorporate behavioral observations in place of self-reported symptoms, among other adaptations.[19]

Mood Disorders

Depressive disorders are often underrecognized among individuals with ID when subjective report of distress is considered a requisite symptom. Diagnostic consideration may instead revolve around caregiver observations of signs such as irritability, agitation, and change in behavior, all of which may represent a mood disorder. Stressful life events such as change in living arrangement, loss of or change in support staff, or death of a family member or peer are associated with heightened risk for development of depression. These events may be even more stressful in those with ID compared to the general population if coping resources and natural supports are limited. Clinicians should also be mindful that bereavement affects individuals with ID as well.

Adapted DSM-5 major depressive disorder diagnostic criteria for DM-ID-2 include requirement of *four* symptoms (rather than five), with at least one symptom being depressed mood or loss of interest or *irritable mood*.[20] Common presenting symptoms also include crying, anhedonia, withdrawal, and nighttime awakening.[21] There is little research on suicide among those with ID, yet assessment of suicidality and risk remains critical in this population, particularly among those with mild to moderate disability. Assessment of suicidality is nearly impossible in those with severe to profound disability, but risk assessment remains important.

Diagnosis of bipolar disorder in this population can also be challenging, particularly when mood lability and behavioral fluctuations have been long-standing. Common presenting symptoms that might suggest bipolar disorder include expansive or irritable mood; excessive laughing, singing, talking, or vocalizations; intrusiveness; exaggerated claims of skills or achievements (grandiosity); sleep disruption; increased motor activity; and excessive sexual behavior. Adaptation in diagnostic criteria for mania for DM-ID-2 includes need for only two of seven symptoms in addition to disturbance in mood and heightened energy, or three additional symptoms if mood is primarily irritable.[22] A similar reduction in symptom threshold is used for diagnosis of hypomania.

Psychotic Disorders

Psychotic disorders are estimated to occur at a rate of approximately 3–5% among those with ID.[19,23,24] Definitive diagnosis of psychotic disorders in this population is difficult, and an existing diagnosis in a patient should be explored and confirmed. Self-talk and stereotyped behaviors are common and may be difficult to differentiate from the presence of psychotic symptoms. Imaginary friends and fantasy play may also be developmentally appropriate behaviors and further confound assessment. Symptoms of autism spectrum disorder involving social impairment and repetitive behaviors can also be confused with psychosis.

It is important to establish understanding of an individual's baseline behavior and recognize emergence of new symptoms or behaviors or a change in the nature or content of baseline behaviors as more concerning for onset of psychiatric illness. However, mood disorders are more common than psychotic disorders and should be considered first as a cause for a behavioral change.[25]

Common presentation of symptoms of psychosis may include description of hallucinations that are inconsistent with baseline fantasy or self-talk; suspiciousness of support staff; persecutory, erotomanic, or somatic delusional content; disorganization of speech and behavior that is a change from baseline; and negative symptoms including decline in self-care or withdrawal from normal activities.

There is no adaptation of DSM-5 criteria for schizophrenia, schizoaffective disorder, or delusional disorder for individuals with ID. As with all patients, thorough evaluation to rule out physiological effects that may present with psychotic symptoms is imperative.

Anxiety/Obsessive–Compulsive Disorders

The reliance on subjective report of anxiety or worry again limits traditional diagnostic techniques in evaluating anxiety disorders in individuals with ID. Observations of behavior by care providers are one of the primary diagnostic tools, and the DSM-5 criteria for panic disorder, agoraphobia, and generalized anxiety disorder are adapted in DM-ID-2 such that observation of core symptoms may substitute for patient report.[26] There is no adaptation in criteria for obsessive–compulsive disorder, although it is not required that an obsession be interpreted as ego-dystonic given the challenge in assessing this.

Anxiety may present as avoidant behavior, fearfulness of previously tolerated situations, sleep disturbance, restlessness, increased irritability and challenging behaviors, vague somatic complaints, and regressive behaviors such as dependence and clinging to caregivers. Panic symptoms may include behavioral outbursts with aggression or self-injury and also physiologic signs such as flushing, sweating, hyperventilation, and muscle tension. Running away from anxiety-provoking situations or refusal to leave home may be signs of agoraphobia. Obsessions can be difficult to assess, particularly in more severe ID when communication of thoughts is significantly impaired. In milder ID, however, repetitive topics in speech may suggest obsessional thinking. Compulsive behaviors can be observed but must be differentiated from stereotypies. Compulsions more commonly consist of excessive washing/cleaning behaviors, counting rituals, hoarding objects, with challenging behaviors if ability to engage in compulsion is restricted.[27]

Autism Spectrum Disorder

Autism spectrum disorder (ASD) is a neurodevelopmental disorder involving impairments in communication and social interaction, along with restricted, repetitive patterns of behaviors. Onset of ASD occurs in early childhood, often prior to age 2 years. Deficits in communication include poor eye contact and inability to understand reciprocating social emotions. Rigid behavioral patterns, attachment to particular objects or ideas, preference for or aversion to certain textures, sensitivity to noise, and repetitive behaviors such as flapping or rocking may be additional features. Up to one-third of individuals with ASD exhibit challenging behaviors, including aggression and self-injury.

ASD affects approximately 1 in 59 children by most recent estimates and has been diagnosed at increasing rates.[28] Males are affected four times more often than females. Not all individuals with ASD have intellectual disability, although they are recognized as commonly co-occurring conditions. Approximately 30% of those with ASD have comorbid ID, with another 25% having borderline intellectual ability.[28] Teasing apart these diagnoses can be challenging because there can be substantial overlap between the impairments of each. DSM-5 requires that social communication deficits in individuals with ID exceed their predicted developmental level to meet a diagnosis of ASD.

Research suggests that ASD is highly heritable and that inheritance is multifactorial, involving a complex interaction among multiple genes and epigenetic and environmental factors.[29] Like ID, there are a number of identified genetic syndromes commonly associated with ASD, including fragile X syndrome (FXS), Rett syndrome, and tuberous sclerosis. Approximately 10% of individuals with ASD have an identified genetic association, with FXS being the most common single-gene cause of ASD. Among males with FXS, an estimated 50% carry a diagnosis of ASD.[30]

Treatment for ASD aims at improving the core features and management of medical and behavioral comorbidities. An interdisciplinary treatment plan should be devised to meet the individual's needs. Early intensive behavioral intervention (EIBI) is considered the behavioral treatment of choice.[31] Emphasizing training of functional skills, EIBI may incorporate speech, occupational, and behavioral therapies, along with training by parents and teachers. Other social skills training interventions may also be implemented in educational settings.

Pharmacologically, two second-generation antipsychotics, risperidone and aripiprazole, have US Food and Drug Administration approval for irritability in ASD, although these should generally only be considered when behavioral interventions have been ineffective.[32,33] Selective serotonin reuptake inhibitors may provide benefit for treating comorbid mood and anxiety disorders. Attention-deficit/hyperactivity disorder (ADHD) is also common in ASD. Treatment with stimulant medication may have utility, although close monitoring for side effects is merited.[33]

Treatment Considerations

There are limited published data regarding psychiatric treatments for individuals with ID because most treatment trials exclude this population. Expert consensus guidelines recommend use of the same treatment interventions as those used for individuals without ID, which may include medication, psychotherapy, and possibly electroconvulsive therapy (ECT). In prescribing medication, a conservative "start low, go slow" approach is recommended given the high propensity for side effects and paradoxical effects. The latter two treatments tend to be less commonly employed, particularly ECT, given the ethical challenges that may arise. When used for indications that would warrant its use for patients without ID, ECT has yielded positive response in the very limited literature that exists.[34] Psychotherapy should also not be overlooked as a treatment intervention and may be adapted to the individual's strengths and challenges. Behavioral therapy can be particularly helpful in building skills to manage illness.[35]

Polypharmacy is a common occurrence in this population and poses significant risks to individuals in whom risk for medical complications and side effects is already elevated.[36] Medications such as antipsychotics and mood stabilizers, which carry potential for major adverse effects, are prescribed at higher rates to patients with ID compared to patients without ID.[37] It is estimated that antipsychotics represent more than 50% of prescribed psychotropics for adults with ID.[23] It is therefore worth careful consideration when starting medication in this population. There must be a diligent effort to minimize polypharmacy and attentive monitoring for adverse effects.

CHALLENGING BEHAVIOR

Challenging behavior is the most common presenting concern among individuals with ID who present for psychiatric care.[37] Physical aggression, destruction of property, self-injury, verbal aggression, and elopement are examples of the challenging behaviors most often reported. These difficulties can cause significant stress to family and care providers and may jeopardize an individual's community living arrangement. Providers often feel compelled to act swiftly to mitigate this distress even though they have incomplete information. The primary goal should instead be to determine the underlying etiology for the behavior, which is often multifactorial. Frequently, providers mistakenly attribute the behavior to the intellectual disability itself rather than recognizing it as an indication of distress or way of expressing an unmet need or problem. Successful intervention is contingent on thorough assessment and accurate diagnosis of the underlying cause for the behaviors. Etiologies to consider include mental illness, medical illness, medication side effects, behavioral phenotypes of specific syndromes, behavioral/functional factors, and skill deficits, all of which are detailed in the following sections.

Mental Illness as Etiology

The extent to which behavioral disturbances represent symptom presentation of a primary psychiatric illness has been widely debated; however, a correlation between psychiatric morbidity and challenging behavior has been frequently reported.[19,38] Despite this correlation, it is generally accepted that challenging behavior is a means of expressing symptoms or distress related to a mental illness and is not a behavioral equivalent of illness itself.[39] Intervention for this etiology follows the standard treatment options for mental illness in the general population, with necessary modifications as described previously.

A VIGNETTE

A 30-year-old female with moderate ID presents to your office accompanied by staff from her group home. Staff report she has had more frequent aggression and self-harm, hitting staff and herself when prompted to do activities she previously enjoyed. She has been increasingly irritable and less communicative than is typical for her. She tells you her mood is "fine" but becomes tearful with no apparent trigger. Staff describe a change in her sleep pattern, with her sleeping late into the morning and napping in the afternoon, both of which are unusual for her. She has refused to leave the house to visit her favorite places. There has also been a decline in her appetite. You suspect a major depressive episode as the cause for the behavioral changes and initiate treatment with an antidepressant and weekly psychotherapy. Two months later, she has resumed her previous activities and restored a normal sleep pattern.

Medical Illness as Etiology

Individuals with ID receive less preventative health care than the general population.[3] Many conditions therefore go undetected until they are more advanced and potentially involve complications. Atypical presentations of symptoms also make timely diagnosis of medical illness a challenge. Due to limitations in communication skills, behavioral changes are often the first sign of a medical problem. For instance, biting of one's hand may be a sign of hand pain or dental, sinus, or ear problems.[40] The mental health clinician is frequently the first point of contact when there is a behavioral change and therefore plays a vital role in identifying and facilitating appropriate assessment and treatment of potential medical issues. Maintaining a consistent primary care provider who is familiar with a patient's health history and typical behavior can also be immensely helpful in uncovering new problems if they arise.

A number of medical conditions are found at relatively high rates among individuals with ID, including epilepsy, skin conditions, constipation, osteoporosis, poor oral health, sleep disturbance, and respiratory disorders.[3] High rates of obesity and related complications, such as heart disease and sleep apnea, are seen in this population due to a number of potential factors, including dietary habits, sedentary lifestyle, and the prevalent prescription of medications with metabolic side effects. Visual and hearing impairments are also common and frequently go undetected. Regular sensory screenings are therefore recommended to identify deficits at an early stage, and assessment for changes in vision or hearing should be considered when unexplained behavioral changes arise.[40]

A VIGNETTE

A 42-year-old male with severe ID presents to the clinic with significant worsening of aggression and self-harm behavior for the past week. He has limited verbal skills, and when asked, he denies having pain. Accompanying staff deny any recent changes in his daily routine or in his care providers. He seems to be sleeping normally at night. The staff does note that they have observed a few instances of rectal digging behavior in the past few days. Physical exam is limited but does not yield any notable findings. A visit to primary care is recommended for thorough medical assessment. Basic labs are ordered and are unremarkable. An abdominal X-ray is obtained and reveals significant distension of the colon and increased stool burden, consistent with constipation. An aggressive bowel regimen is implemented, and as his constipation improves, the challenging behaviors subside.

Medication Side Effect as Etiology

Polypharmacy is a widely recognized problem among individuals with ID. Vulnerability to adverse effects from medications and drug–drug interactions is heightened in this population, and challenging behaviors may arise as a manifestation of these effects. Sleep changes, fatigue, weight changes, and neurologic symptoms are among the most common adverse effects, and many patients experience more than one medication side effect.[41] Extrapyramidal side effects, including akathisia, parkinsonism, tardive dyskinesia, and acute dystonia, commonly develop in response to antipsychotics, although they may not be readily identified. Increased appetite may prompt challenging food-seeking and feeding behaviors. Cognitive slowing can impair an individual's ability to communicate. Given that this ability is already limited in individuals with an ID, any medication that causes further decline in cognitive skills can contribute to challenging behavior. Anticholinergic side effects not only cause cognitive slowing but also can cause or exacerbate constipation, both of which can lead to challenging behavior.

Careful review of a patient's current medications with particular attention to potential interactions and duplications of mechanisms, timing of medication initiation in relation to onset of behaviors, and adherence to medications is of utmost importance during evaluation of challenging behaviors. It is also vital to closely monitor blood levels for medications for which monitoring is available. When there is high suspicion for adverse effects contributing to behavioral challenges, a careful taper plan should be devised. Abrupt continuation can lead to worsening of symptoms (e.g., withdrawal dyskinesia) or discontinuation syndromes.

A VIGNETTE

A 32-year-old female with moderate ID, epilepsy, and a diagnosis of bipolar disorder presents with challenging behaviors consisting of increased motor activity and aggression if she is limited from pacing or moving. Staff also report spells of staring to the left side for up to 1 minute, during which time she is less responsive and after which she appears distressed. She has recently seen her neurologist and underwent electroencephalography monitoring, which showed there was no seizure activity during these spells. Her medication list is long and includes a moderately dosed first-generation antipsychotic. You suspect this may be inducing akathisia and dystonic reactions in the form of oculogyric crisis and recommend rapid taper of this medication with close monitoring of symptoms. She returns 2 weeks later and has been spell-free for 1 week and restlessness has improved.

Behavioral Phenotype Models

Behavioral phenotypes are characteristic cognitive and psychiatric patterns that typify a specific disorder. Behavioral and physical phenotypes have been defined for 12 syndromes associated with ID (see Table 4.2). Awareness of a known etiology for a patient's ID can guide the evaluation of behavior and raise suspicion for potential medical conditions that are common in a given syndrome.

A VIGNETTE

A 44-year-old male with mild intellectual disability presents to your clinic accompanied by care staff. He is short-statured and obese. His staff describes significant difficulties with food-related behaviors, including stealing food from the kitchen at the house where he lives, hoarding food in his room until it has spoiled, and eating excessively at meals—at times taking food from other roommates' plates. They have worked to keep the kitchen locked and restrict his access to food outside meals, but this has led to an increase in aggressive behaviors. You also observe him picking at his skin throughout the interview. You recognize this constellation of symptoms and behaviors as suggestive of Prader–Willi syndrome and ask if genetic testing has previously been completed.

Behavioral/Functional Models

Behavioral models recognize operant functions for challenging behaviors and aim to identify positive and/or negative reinforcement contingencies.[42] This approach to evaluating variables that maintain challenging behaviors is known as *functional behavior assessment*. Functions may include seeking of positive reinforcements such as attention, tangible items, or preferred activities. Avoidance of undesirable tasks or demands, escape from aversive stimuli, or social avoidance are examples of negative reinforcement contingencies. Automatic reinforcement is achieved through engaging in the behavior itself with no identified environmental influence. The function of a given behavior may vary across different settings. Intervention involves modification of the environmental contingencies that maintain the behaviors—for instance, by providing reinforcement for alternative behaviors, known as differential reinforcement.[42] For example, teaching a communication alternative such as asking for help rather than hitting and then providing the reinforcing response when verbal communication is used and offering no attention for hitting would be a strategy to modify this behavior. A behavioral analyst or psychologist with training in applied behavioral analysis, if available, can be particularly helpful in providing a comprehensive behavior assessment and designing a treatment plan.

A VIGNETTE

A 23-year-old female with moderate ID and history of depression presents to your clinic with recent challenging behaviors consisting of destruction to property. She has been eating and sleeping well and appears to be in a good mood outside of these episodes. She remains interested in activities she normally enjoys. Additional history reveals that a new roommate recently moved in who has a number of medical needs requiring a substantial amount of attention from staff. The timing of your patient's new behaviors corresponds to this change in her living arrangement, and you suspect her behaviors may be a means of accessing staff's attention. You discuss a plan with staff to withhold extra attention when she engages in property destruction and to provide extra attention when she demonstrates positive behaviors, thus providing differential reinforcement.

Lack of Skills

The deficits in adaptive and cognitive function that characterize an ID constitute additional sources of challenging behavior. From a developmental perspective, behavioral difficulties often represent lack of skills for managing internal states and responding to the environment.[43] Setting boundaries, recognizing social cues, and identifying potential environmental dangers are examples of possible skills deficits that may contribute to problematic behaviors.

A VIGNETTE

An 18-year-old male with moderate ID presents with increased self-injury behavior. Staff explain that since he was young, he has had a tendency to hug everyone he meets, including strangers, and attempts to touch their hair. As he has grown older, those around him have become less tolerable of this behavior. When his advances are not well received, he hits himself in the head repeatedly. Further assessment does not reveal additional symptoms to suggest a mental or medical illness, and you suspect the most likely cause for his recent behavior is lack of awareness of appropriate boundaries and social norms. You develop a plan with him and his staff involving education about healthy boundaries with the various people in his life.

Interventions

The intervention used for challenging behavior will naturally depend on the identified etiology. In many cases, the etiology is multifactorial, and a comprehensive treatment plan will incorporate multiple approaches. When possible, incorporating an interdisciplinary team including direct care staff, primary care physicians, psychologists, and/or speech pathologists can be instrumental in formulating the assessment and plan.

From a pharmacologic standpoint, there is limited evidence to support the use of psychotropic medications as a nonspecific treatment for challenging behaviors, particularly in the absence of thorough investigation to determine the underlying cause. However, expert consensus guidelines have been developed to guide medication use for this purpose. These guidelines outline a number of scenarios when medication may be indicated, including when nonpharmacologic interventions fail, behaviors pose significant danger to others, and provision of acute relief of symptoms so nonmedication strategies may be adequately tried.[44] Note that these indications are separate from the use of medication to target a suspected psychiatric illness. In those cases, regular prescribing practices should be utilized, as earlier described.

For nonspecific treatment of behaviors, consensus guidelines list atypical antipsychotics as first-line, followed by mood stabilizers and then selective serotonin reuptake inhibitors. The aim should be for use of these medications to be for a time-limited trial. Specific behavior targets should be tracked prior to initiation of treatment to establish a baseline and then remeasured at regular intervals during the course of treatment (this should also be done with other modes of intervention). Medications should be prescribed at the lowest possible dose and for the minimum duration, and gradual withdrawal of medication should be considered once behaviors stabilize or if there is no evidence of benefit. Routine monitoring of physical exams and laboratory monitoring should be carried out as recommended for each medication.[27] Long-term use of as-needed medications is not recommended because the potential for overutilization of these may mask other underlying problems. As previously emphasized, polypharmacy should be avoided, and diligent monitoring for adverse effects is essential.

CASE STUDY: CONTINUED

On further interview, you gather that your patient has been eating and sleeping normally. He seems to enjoy preferred activities such as playing video games and taking walks. You learn that he lived in his previous residence for 4 years, and he often asks about staff and roommates from there. At times when he is upset, he mentions wanting to return there. When you ask more about the circumstances in which challenging behaviors occur, staff report transitioning between activities or places tends to be a difficult time. Being in loud or crowded areas has also precipitated self-injury or running away. Staff note he sometimes has facial flushing, rapid breathing, and squeezes his eyes shut during these episodes. His medical history is significant for seizure disorder, constipation, and recurrent ear infections. His current medications include valproic acid, lamotrigine, risperidone, methylphenidate, fluoxetine, lorazepam, benztropine, allergy medication, and a stool softener.

QUESTIONS

1. You suspect the etiology of the described behaviors is multifactorial. What considerations would you include for each of the described etiologies (mental illness, medical illness, medication side effects, behavioral/functional, behavioral phenotype, and lack of skills)?
2. What concerns will you address first as part of a comprehensive treatment plan? What other professionals or natural supports might be helpful in evaluating and implementing treatment?

SPECIAL ISSUES

Deinstitutionalization in recent decades has required expansion of community-based services for individuals with ID. Notable legislation on this matter is the *Olmstead* decision, a Supreme Court ruling in 1999 that required states to support individuals with mental disabilities in their communities by providing public services "in the most integrated setting appropriate to the patient's needs."[45] Home and Community Based Services waivers are a funding source through Medicaid for a variety of in-home support services that allow individuals to remain in their own homes as opposed to institutions. Many individuals with ID receive supportive services within the community; these include case management, home health care, hourly staff support, day programming, vocational rehabilitation, and sheltered work. Living arrangements vary based on specific needs, but common settings include group homes, independent housing, family homes, and intermediate care facilities for individuals with ID. These options range in the frequency and intensity of supervision, and it is important to clarify the level of support an individual is receiving in a particular setting.

Although the shift from custodial models to a more person-based approach has been a positive advance, integrating complicated systems of care involving multiple service providers has proven to be a significant challenge. It is worth becoming familiar and establishing relationships with the available resources and agencies in your local area of practice to help patients and families navigate this complex system of care delivery.

Legal Issues

The disabilities right movement brought about a shift toward empowerment for individuals with ID. Decisions about guardianship, criminal responsibility, and ability to stand trial are not made on the sole premise of having an ID diagnosis. Instead, individualized assessment of a person's functional abilities and the specific demands in question is required.[46]

Guardianship

Guardianship is a legal mechanism through which the court concludes that an individual is unable to make certain decisions him- or herself and grants decision-making authority to someone else—the appointed guardian. A guardian may have full decision-making responsibility, or the scope of decision-making may be limited based on the individual's specific needs. For instance, a guardian may be appointed to make health care decisions but the individual retains rights over other decisions, such as managing finances. A copy of the court order designating guardianship should detail the scope of the guardian's authority. When medical decision-making is included, the guardian's consent must be obtained for medical treatment, even if the provider believes the individual has capacity to consent independently.

Interactions with Law Enforcement

Individuals with ID are overrepresented in the criminal justice system as both victims and offenders. Police involvement most often occurs in instances in which an individual with ID is in need of assistance, but it is frequently initiated related to challenging behaviors.[47] Once law enforcement becomes involved, outcomes vary, including but not limited to arrest, transport to an emergency department or other medical service, or on-scene resolution. Physical aggression and prior legal interactions are risk factors for arrest instead of other alternatives.[48]

Local jurisdictions vary in their response to crisis involving those with ID, including the degree to which they look to the individual or agency who sought assistance for input on the outcome. For instance, staff working with an individual with ID may call emergency services for additional assistance in de-escalating a situation but have no intent to initiate legal action. Many law enforcement agencies conduct training sessions that cover strategies for responding to situations involving individuals with ID and ASD. Psychiatrists and other behavioral health providers can offer invaluable assistance and support of law enforcement, particularly for patients under their care who have frequent encounters. Agencies often welcome input from care providers regarding approach, communication, and management techniques that may be helpful in keeping these interactions as safe as possible and minimizing distress for the individual.

Transitions in Care

Transition from pediatric to adult-based services is particularly difficult for both providers and individuals with ID. There is a sharp decline in service utilization across many levels of care in youths with ID and ASD in the transition period from pediatric to adult services, which may reflect lack of availability and access to services.[49] It is important to consider planning for transitions both within the school system and with medical and psychiatric providers well in advance. When shifts occur without planning, there may be prolonged periods of time without an established provider who is familiar with the patient's needs. Patients and families are often unfamiliar with adult services such as group homes, day programming, vocational services, and other available supports. Having an established case manager who can assist with navigating through this process can be helpful. Knowing that this can be a challenging time, there may be benefit to planning more frequent visits during a transitional period to monitor for difficulties and provide adequate time to address concerns as they arise.

CASE STUDY: CONCLUSION

This case illustrates a number of topics that are described in this chapter. As you conclude your initial visit, you summarize your formulation with your patient and his staff. Your patient presents with a number of phenotypic features of FXS. Genetic testing could confirm or rule out this diagnosis and may be worth pursuing if it has not been done previously. With this on your differential, you might consider the common behavioral features seen in FXS, such as ASD, ADHD, and anxiety disorders.

You recognize that a number of challenges seem to have arisen around the time of transition from his previous residence to his current one. Establishing care with you as his new provider is one additional transition that may be difficult for your patient, and building rapport with him may take a number of visits. Developing a routine for the appointments involving things he finds comforting can help ease this transition. Knowing that he recently transitioned from youth to adult services, it will be important to ensure he and his caregivers are aware of the available adult resources such as day programming and vocational support. Establishing a structured schedule can be helpful when individuals are moving out of the educational system and the structure it provides.

The etiology for the challenging behaviors described is likely multifactorial. A differential might include each of the following:

1. Mental illness: Considerations might include panic disorder, ASD, and ADHD. Grief related to loss of contact with his past staff and roommates may be an additional consideration.
2. Medical illness: He has a seizure disorder, and it is important to clarify the type of seizures he experiences and to ensure these are well controlled because some seizure variants may appear with behavioral symptoms. Frequency of ear infections and constipation should both be considered as well.
3. Medication side effects: His current regimen poses risk for a number of side effects and drug–drug interactions.
4. Behavioral phenotype: If FXS is confirmed, consider the phenotypic features, including shyness, sensitivity to noise, stereotyped behavior, ADHD, ASD, and anxiety disorders.
5. Behavioral/functional: An escape function may be considered with the description of running away and self-injury in relation to crowded areas. Elopement from his home may also be an attempt to return to his previous residence. Knowing his new home has a greater client-to-staff ratio, access to staff attention might be an additional function to explore.
6. Lack of skills: Communication deficits and identifying dangers related to running away are skills to target. Others may be identified as well.

Identifying the target behaviors of physical aggression, self-harm, and elopement, a treatment plan can be devised to address each of the previous concerns. Carrying out such a plan will be a process done over time and multiple visits; however, discussing these possible etiologies with the patient and staff and identifying mutual priorities at the initial visit will build a strong foundation from which to work moving forward. Often, choosing one or two areas to focus on for the period between visits is sufficient. If accessible, incorporating an interdisciplinary team including a primary care provider, psychologist, and/or speech therapist will enhance the support of the patient and his care providers and ultimately help improve his quality of life.

Providing optimal psychiatric care to individuals with ID is undoubtedly a complex and at times challenging undertaking. When confined by managed-care reimbursement systems to the narrow role of a psychopharmacologist, working with this population can feel frustrating and unsatisfying as repeated trials of escalating doses of medication fail to alleviate the presenting concerns. The community psychiatrist who is instead able to embrace a broader view of his or her role, drawing on his or her full range of expertise to collaborate with patients, their support systems, and other professionals involved in their care to implement meaningful, comprehensive treatment plans will find much greater fulfillment in this work. The clinician will inevitably face great clinical uncertainty when working with this population and may feel pressured to allay the anxiety that comes with uncertainty with premature prescription of medication. Often, this tension may be better managed by acknowledging the presence of uncertainty and joining with the patient, family, and care team to develop a wise course of action, which may sometimes involve therapeutic inaction, or a careful "watchful waiting" strategy.[50] As is true in all psychiatric work, the value of therapeutic alliance cannot be overemphasized, and in difficult times, having this foundation in which uncertainty may be shared and validated can alleviate a substantial degree of fear and frustration for all involved.

REFERENCES

1. Ditchman, N., Werner, S., Kosyluk, K., et al. (2013). Stigma and intellectual disability: Potential application of mental illness research. *Rehabil Psychol*, 58(2), 206–216. doi:10.1037/a0032466

2. Williamson, H. J., Contreras, G. M., Rodriguez, E. S., et al. (2017). Health care access for adults with intellectual and developmental disabilities: A scoping review. *OTJR*, 37(4), 227–236. doi:10.1177/1539449217714148

3. Krahn, G. L., Hammond, L., & Turner, A. (2006). A cascade of disparities: Health and health care access for people with intellectual disabilities. *Ment Retard Dev Disabil Res Rev*, 12(1), 70–82. doi:10.1002/mrdd.20098

4. McQuistion, H. L., Sowers, W. E., Ranz, J. M., et al. (2012). The present and future of community psychiatry: An introduction. In H. McQuistion, W. Sowers, J. Ranz, & J. M. Feldman (Eds.), *Handbook of community psychiatry* (pp. 3–10). New York, NY: Springer.

5. Werner, S., Stawski, M., Polakiewicz, Y., et al. (2013). Psychiatrists' knowledge, training and attitudes regarding the care of individuals with intellectual disability. *J Intellect Disabil Res*, 57(8), 774–782. doi:10.1111/j.1365-2788.2012.01604.x

6. American Association on Intellectual and Developmental Disabilities. (2018). Definition of intellectual disability. Retrieved July 6, 2018, from https://aaidd.org/intellectual-disability/definition#.Wz-i3C2ZPOQ

7. 111th Congress. (2010). Public Law 111–256.

8. American Psychiatric Association. (2013). *Diagnostic and statistical manual of mental disorders* (5th ed.). Arlington, VA: American Psychiatric Publishing.

9. Maulik, P. K., Mascarenhas, M. N., Mathers, C. D., et al. (2011). Prevalence of intellectual disability: A meta-analysis of population-based studies. *Res Dev Disabil*, 32(2), 419–436. doi:10.1016/j.ridd.2010.12.018

10. King, B. H., Toth, K. E., Hodapp, R. M., & Dykens, E. M. (2009). Intellectual disability. In B. J. Sadock, V. A. Sadock, & P. Ruiz (Eds.), *Comprehensive textbook of psychiatry* (9th ed., pp. 3444–3474). Philadelphia, PA: Lippincott Williams & Wilkins.

11. Patja, K., Iivanainen, M., Vesala, H., et al. (2000). Life expectancy of people with intellectual disability: A 35-year follow-up study. *J Intellect Disabil Res*, 44(Pt 5), 591–599.

12. Bittles, A. H., Petterson, B. A., Sullivan, S. G., et al. (2002). The influence of intellectual disability on life expectancy. *J Gerontol A Biol Sci Med Sci*, 57(7), M470–M472.

13. Rauch, A., Hoyer, J., Guth, S., et al. (2006). Diagnostic yield of various genetic approaches in patients with unexplained developmental delay or mental retardation. *Am J Med Genet A*, 140(19), 2063–2074. doi:10.1002/ajmg.a.31416

14. Karam, S. M., Barros, A. J., Matijasevich, A., et al. (2016). Intellectual disability in a birth cohort: Prevalence, etiology, and determinants at the age of 4 years. *Public Health Genomics*, 19(5), 290–297. doi:10.1159/000448912

15. Levitas, A., Finucane, B., Simon, E. W., et al. (2013). Behavioral phenotypes of neurodevelopmental disorders. In R. J.Fletcher, J. Barnhill, & S. A. Cooper (Eds.), *Diagnostic manual—Intellectual disability (DM-ID-2)* (2nd ed., pp. 35–74). New York, NY: National Association for the Dually Diagnosed.

16. Sovner, R. (1986). Limiting factors in the use of DSM-III criteria with mentally ill/mentally retarded persons. *Psychopharmacol Bull, 22*(4), 1055–1059.

17. Wullink, M., Veldhuijzen, W., Lantman-de Valk, H. M., et al. (2009). Doctor–patient communication with people with intellectual disability—A qualitative study. *BMC Fam Pract, 10*, 82. doi:10.1186/1471-2296-10-82

18. Cooper, S. A., Smiley, E., Morrison, J., et al. (2007). Mental ill-health in adults with intellectual disabilities: Prevalence and associated factors. *Br J Psychiatry, 190*, 27–35. doi:10.1192/bjp.bp.106.022483

19. Fletcher, R. J., Barnhill, J., & Cooper, S. A. (2017). *Diagnostic manual—Intellectual disability 2 (DM-ID): A textbook of diagnosis of mental disorders in persons with intellectual disability* (2nd ed.). New York, NY: National Association for the Dually Diagnosed.

20. Charlot, L. R., Benson, B. A., Fox, S., et al. (2013). Depressive disorders. In R. J. Fletcher, J. Barnhill, & S. A. Cooper (Eds.), *Diagnostic manual–Intellectual disability (DM-ID-2)* (2nd ed., pp. 265–302). New York, NY: National Association for the Dually Diagnosed.

21. Hurley, A. D. (2008). Depression in adults with intellectual disability: Symptoms and challenging behaviour. *J Intellect Disabil Res, 52*(11), 905–916. doi:10.1111/j.1365-2788.2008.01113.x

22. Pary, R. J., Charlot, L. R., Fox, S., et al. (2013). Bipolar and related disorders. In R. J. Fletcher, J. Barnhill, & S. A. Cooper (Eds.), *Diagnostic manual—Intellectual disability (DM-ID-2)* (2nd ed., pp. 245–264). New York, NY: National Association of the Dually Diagnosed.

23. Tsiouris, J. A. (2010). Pharmacotherapy for aggressive behaviours in persons with intellectual disabilities: Treatment or mistreatment? *J Intellect Disabil Res, 54*(1), 1–16. doi:10.1111/j.1365-2788.2009.01232.x

24. Hassiotis, A, Fodor-Wynne, L, Fleisher, MH, et al. (2016). Schizophrenia and Other Psychotic Disorders. In R. J. Fletcher, J. Barnhill, & S. A. Cooper (Eds.), *Diagnostic manual—Intellectual disability (DM-ID-2)* (2nd ed., pp. 231–244). New York, NY: National Association for the Dually Diagnosed.

25. Cowan, A. E. (2012). Psychotic disorders. In J. Gentile & P. M. Gillig (Eds.), *Psychiatry of intellectual disability: A practical manual* (pp. 161–190). Hoboken, NJ: Wiley.

26. Cooray, S., Andrews, T., Bailey, N. M., et al. (2016). Anxiety disorders. In R. J. Fletcher, J. Barnhill, & S. A. Cooper (Eds.), *Diagnostic manual—Intellectual disability (DM-ID-2)* (2nd ed., pp. 303–328). New York, NY: National Association for the Dually Diagnosed.

27. Blankenship, K. M. (2012). Anxiety disorders. In J. Gentile & P. M. Gillig (Eds.), *Psychiatry of intellectual disability: A practical manual* (pp. 146–160). Hoboken, NJ: Wiley.

28. Baio, J., Wiggens, L., Christensen, D. L., et al. (2018). Prevalence of autism spectrum disorder among children aged 8 years—Autism and Developmental Disabilities Monitoring Network, 11 Sites, United States, 2014. *MMWR Surveill Summ, 67*(No. SS-6), 1–23. Retrieved August 9, 2018, from http://dx.doi.org/10.15585/mmwr.ss6706a1.

29. Ivanov, H. Y., Stoyanova, V. K., Popov, N. T., et al. (2015). Autism spectrum disorder—A complex genetic disorder. *Folia Med (Plovdiv), 57*(1), 19–28. doi:10.1515/folmed-2015-0015

30. Abbeduto, L., McDuffie, A., & Thurman, A. J. (2014). The fragile X syndrome–autism comorbidity: What do we really know? *Front Genet, 5*, 355. doi:10.3389/fgene.2014.00355

31. Reichow, B. (2012). Overview of meta-analyses on early intensive behavioral intervention for young children with autism spectrum disorders. *J Autism Dev Disord, 42*(4), 512–520. doi:10.1007/s10803-011-1218-9

32. Fung, L. K., Mahajan, R., Nozzolillo, A., et al. (2016). Pharmacologic treatment of severe irritability and problem behaviors in autism: A systematic review and meta-analysis. *Pediatrics, 137*(Suppl 2), S124–S135. doi:10.1542/peds.2015-2851K

33. Baribeau, D. A., & Anagnostou, E. (2014). An update on medication management of behavioral disorders in autism. *Curr Psychiatry Rep, 16*(3), 437. doi:10.1007/s11920-014-0437-0

34. Little, J. D., McFarlane, J., & Ducharme, H. M. (2002). ECT use delayed in the presence of comorbid mental retardation: A review of clinical and ethical issues. *J ECT, 18*(4), 218–222.

35. Morrison, A. K., & Weston, C. (2012). Mood disorders. In J. P. Gentile & P. M. Gillig (Eds.), *Psychiatry of intellectual disability: A practical manual* (pp. 125–145). Hoboken, NJ: Wiley.

36. Lunsky, Y., & Modi, M. (2018). Predictors of psychotropic polypharmacy among outpatients with psychiatric disorders and intellectual disability. *Psychiatr Serv, 69*(2), 242–246. doi:10.1176/appi.ps.201700032

37. Hurley, A. D., Folstein, M., & Lam, N. (2003). Patients with and without intellectual disability seeking outpatient psychiatric services: Diagnoses and prescribing pattern. *J Intellect Disabil Res, 47*(Pt 1), 39–50.

38. Felce, D., Kerr, M., & Hastings, R. P. (2009). A general practice-based study of the relationship between indicators of mental illness and challenging behaviour among adults with intellectual disabilities. *J Intellect Disabil Res, 53*(3), 243–254. doi:10.1111/j.1365-2788.2008.01131.x

39. Allen, D., & Davies, D. (2007). Challenging behaviour and psychiatric disorder in intellectual disability. *Curr Opin Psychiatry, 20*(5), 450–455. doi:10.1097/YCO.0b013e32826fb332

40. Gentile, J. P., & Monroe, M. A. (2012). Medical assessment. In J. Gentile & P. Gillig (Eds.), *Psychiatry of intellectual disability: A practical manual* (pp. 26–50). Hoboken, NJ: Wiley.

41. Scheifes, A., Walraven, S., Stolker, J. J., et al. (2016). Adverse events and the relation with quality of life in adults with intellectual disability and challenging behaviour using psychotropic drugs. *Res Dev Disabil, 49–50*, 13–21. doi:10.1016/j.ridd.2015.11.017

42. Lloyd, B. P., & Kennedy, C. H. (2014). Assessment and treatment of challenging behaviour for individuals with intellectual disability: A research review. *J Appl Res Intellect Disabil, 27*(3), 187–199. doi:10.1111/jar.12089

43. Dosen, A. (2005). Applying the developmental perspective in the psychiatric assessment and diagnosis of persons with intellectual disability: Part II—Diagnosis. *J Intellect Disabil Res, 49*(Pt 1), 9–15. doi:10.1111/j.1365-2788.2005.00657.x

44. Manetta, C. T., & Gentile, J. P. (2012). Psychotropic medications. In J. P. Gentile & P. M. Gillig (Eds.), *Psychiatry of intellectual disability: A practical manual* (pp. 250–277). Hoboken, NJ: Wiley.

45. Opinion of the Court. (1999). Olmstead, Commissioner, Georgia Department of Human Resources, et al. v. L.C. States. Supreme Court of the United, 98–536.

46. Cox, J. (2012). Legal issues for treatment providers and evaluators. In J. P. Gentile & P. M. Gillig (Eds.), *Psychiatry of intellectual disability: A practical manual* (pp. 325–337). Hoboken, NJ: Wiley.

47. Henshaw, M., & Thomas, S. (2012). Police encounters with people with intellectual disability: Prevalence, characteristics and challenges. *J Intellect Disabil Res, 56*(6), 620–631. doi:10.1111/j.1365-2788.2011.01502.x

48. Raina, P., Arenovich, T., Jones, J., et al. (2013). Pathways into the criminal justice system for individuals with intellectual disability. *J Appl Res Intellect Disabil, 26*(5), 404–409. doi:10.1111/jar.12039

49. Nathenson, R. A., & Zablotsky, B. (2017). The transition to the adult health care system among youths with autism spectrum disorder. *Psychiatr Serv, 68*(7), 735–738. doi:10.1176/appi.ps.201600239

50. Hauser M. J. (1997). The role of the psychiatrist in mental retardation. *Psychiatric Annals, 27*(3), 170–174.

///5/// THE PUBLIC PSYCHIATRIST AND INTEGRATED HEALTH

HELENA WINSTON AND
ELIZABETH LOWDERMILK

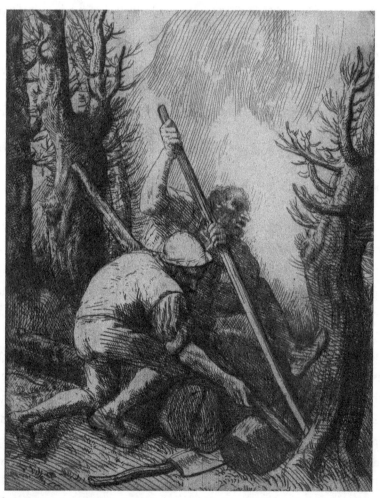

FIGURE 5.1 Alphonse Legros, *Woodcutters*, third plate (*Les bucherons*), date unknown.

Alphonse Legros learned the art of etching by watching a colleague in Paris (1) and refined the skill through practice. Figure 5.1 depicts two men working together to harvest a tree. Although not necessarily intended, it can also be seen as a portrayal of collaboration in the pursuit of rooting out something decaying in order to transform it into something else.

CASE STUDY: INITIAL PRESENTATION

Jim is a 38-year-old Caucasian male who has been feeling down. He has lost interest in his favorite pastime (playing classical music), feels guilty all the time about not being a good enough husband, cannot concentrate at work, has no energy, and does not sleep well. He is not having suicidal thoughts but does feel hopeless, and sometimes he hears a voice telling him he is worthless. He would like to see a psychiatrist, so he calls the local community mental health center, but it has a 2-month wait list. Jim is worried that his work is suffering and does not want to be fired. He calls private psychiatrists, but they all want him to pay cash and he cannot afford their rates.

QUESTIONS
1. What are some of the challenges that patients today face in accessing mental health services?
2. What are some strategies for addressing the impact that psychiatrist shortages have on access to care?
3. What are some models that primary care physicians and psychiatrists could use to collaborate?
4. What are the strengths of the various models of integrated care?

Integrated care takes as its motivation the reality that many people desperately in need of psychiatric care are never seen in the current mental health system and that even with expansion and some structural change, it is unlikely that the mental health system will soon be able to accommodate or treat all of them (2). Integrated care seeks to maximize, or leverage, the role of the psychiatric treatment to improve overall medical and mental health, as the two are so intertwined as to be inseparable.

The term *integrated care* is used in a variety of settings and so can have different meanings. Most commonly, it refers to a primary care setting in which there is a behavioral health team that is fully integrated into the clinic. It usually takes a population health perspective with the goal of improving care or targeting metrics for an identified population—for example, people with depression seen in a primary care setting. It may refer not just to care of mental illnesses but also to behavioral interventions designed to improve other aspects of health, such as quitting smoking, exercising, and medication adherence to improve treatment of heart disease, hypertension, obesity, and diabetes. Integrated care may also be performed with a small behavioral health team (or individual) in place at a clinic and a psychiatrist located remotely and seeing patients via video (telepsychiatry) or with the psychiatrist visiting the clinic a limited number of times per week (or month). Finally, integrated care may refer to specialized psychiatrists functioning much as those in primary care integrated clinics function but located at specialized clinics, such as dermatology, HIV, or peripartum clinics. These psychiatrists are performing mental health care for a defined target community subpopulation. In these specialized clinics, the consulting psychiatrists may be trained in consult-liaison psychiatry, highlighting how the boundaries between medical specialties and psychiatry—and between psychiatric subspecialties—are further blurring in today's dynamic health care system that seeks to care for the individual patient and for communities.

Integrated care is also defined in opposition to co-located care, in which a psychiatrist or small mental health team is located at, but functions largely independently of, the primary care clinic. In co-located care, patients have the convenience of seeing a psychiatrist at their primary care location, and the primary care provider (PCP) and psychiatrist are in close proximity, enabling rapid and easy communication. In co-located care, the psychiatrist performs care as usual, and as a result, wait lists may be long and treatment times lengthy.

There are multiple reasons why not all people with mental health problems are seen in the current mental health system. Many are not seen at all in any mental health setting (2), perhaps because they do not want help, they are afraid of the stigma of seeking help, their families are not supportive of pursuing help, they do not know how to access care, they do not have coverage for appropriate care, they may not realize care is available, or they may not realize they need care at all. However, many of these same people *are* seen in primary care (2). Therefore, if psychiatrists are connected to a primary care clinic, they may be able to access this population. In addition, many people who are seen in primary care and referred to see mental health providers do not follow through with the referral. This may be due to fear or stigma of seeking mental health care, the additional cost of doing so, the location of the psychiatric clinic, or the unavailability of psychiatric care providers. It may also be that the kind of care provided by available psychiatrists is not the type of care that the patient is seeking (2). For example, some patients may want long-term therapy but can only find medication management services. All of this suggests that if mental health care is embedded into primary care, access and use will likely be improved.

PSYCHIATRY AND LITERATURE

If I Can Stop One Heart from Breaking
by Emily Dickinson

If I can stop one heart from breaking,
I shall not live in vain;
If I can ease one life the aching,
Or cool one pain,
Or help one fainting robin
Unto his nest again,
I shall not live in vain.

INTEGRATED CARE: THE GOAL

Integrated care is an attempt to shore up the inadequacies of the current mental health system and make the greatest use of limited resources. For example, a study of access to psychiatric care in 2009 and 2010 showed that almost half of psychiatrists did not accept commercial insurance, and more than half did not accept Medicare or Medicaid (3). A 2017 report on the shortage of psychiatrists showed a 10% reduction in psychiatrists working with public sector and insured populations during the 10 years ending in 2013 (4). This report stated that "aging of the current workforce, low rates of reimbursement, burnout, burdensome documentation requirements and restrictive regulations around sharing clinical information necessary to coordinate care are some of the reasons" for the reduced access (p. 5). For example, more than 50% of currently practicing psychiatrists are older than age 55 years, compared to less than 40% of all physicians (5). Collaborative care has been noted as a possible solution to this crisis in access to psychiatric care (4).

A VIGNETTE

Min is a 75-year-old Chinese American woman with a history of major depressive disorder. Her depression is treated in a federally qualified health center clinic that utilizes a collaborative care model. The clinic uses objective measures of depression in its treatment protocol and can demonstrate not only improving depression scores for their patients but a likely containment in their overall health care costs. Min's depression, like that of many other people served by the clinic, demonstrably improves.

Integrated care, and especially the collaborative care model of integrated care, has been studied in more than 80 trials, and results are positive (2). Not only do patients show measurable improvements in their mental health but also studies show that their costs may be reduced. For example, a study of the 4-year effect of collaborative care for late-life depression found that those who participated in the IMPACT (Improving Mood—Promoting Access to Collaborative Treatment) program (discussed later) had lower mean total health care costs compared with usual care patients during this time period ($29,422 vs. $32,785, respectively) (6).

INTEGRATED CARE MODELS FOR PRIMARY CARE

There are two major models for integrating mental health care in primary care: the collaborative care model (CCM) and the primary care behavioral health (PCBH) model. They share a focus on behavior as a major facet of mental and physical health. Behavior is directly influenced by mental state and affects all aspects of health. Thus, the integrated care provider is interested not just in the psychological well-being of the patient but also in how this affects a patient's behavior and how that behavior impacts his or her physical and mental health. Interventions are designed to improve all of these aspects.

The Collaborative Care Model

The CCM is described in detail by Raney et al. in *Integrated Care: A Guide for Effective Implementation,* a book that focuses, as noted in the title, on guiding implementation of such a model in a primary care clinic (2). CCM has been studied more than any other integrated care model and thus has the most evidence to support it. It has been largely proven to improve defined outcomes and contain costs. CCM consists of four key components: team-driven care, population-focused care, measurement-guided care, and evidence-based care (7).

A VIGNETTE

Janie is a 67-year-old African American woman who has moderate major depressive disorder. Janie decides to see her PCP at the local public hospital's outpatient clinic. She calls and gets an appointment for the next day. Her clinic administers a Patient Health Questionnaire-9 (PHQ-9), and the results are consistent with moderate depression. Janie and her primary care physician decide to start low-dose fluoxetine. The PCP calls in the clinic's psychiatric social worker to see Janie. The PCP steps out to see her next patient, and the social worker talks to Janie about the causes of depression and reviews some brief cognitive–behavioral therapy techniques. They make a plan for Janie to return in 2 weeks, at which time the social worker will perform another PHQ-9. After the visit, the social worker enters the case in a registry of the clinic's depression patients used to track their depression scores. Later in the week, the social worker reviews Janie's case with a consulting psychiatrist.

CCM is based on the IMPACT study that was performed at the University of Washington. IMPACT was a 2-year randomized controlled trial that investigated a collaborative integrated care model for the treatment of depression in the elderly in primary care settings versus care as usual. It found that CCM led to a twofold increase in the efficacy of depression treatment (8, 9) Care as usual included interventions such as medications only or referral to a specialty mental health clinic.

The CCM used in the IMPACT studies is stepped care that uses a behavioral health provider or consultant in the primary clinic and a consulting psychiatrist working indirectly to oversee the mental health care. In a typical scenario, a patient is seen by the PCP, who identifies a problem such as depression. The patient is then introduced to the clinic's behavioral health consultant, who sees the patient either then or as soon as possible, preferably the former, and added to a clinic depression registry. The behavioral health consultant may perform brief psychotherapeutic interventions such as psychoeducation, or supportive or behavioral therapies, and sees the patient at regularly scheduled future visits to track progress using standardized assessment tools such as the PHQ-9 and the General Anxiety Disorder 7-item scale (GAD-7).

Key to the IMPACT model is the use of a registry that lists all the clinic's patients who are being treated for depression and tracks their progress and outcomes. The registry is essential to the CCM in general; without it, progress and outcomes cannot be followed and interventions targeting patients lagging behind others cannot be introduced. Registries are regularly reviewed by the behavioral health consultant in conjunction with a consulting psychiatrist. Patients who are not showing improvement in the time frames expected are reviewed by the consulting psychiatrist, who makes recommendations to the behavioral health consultant and the PCP. Only occasionally, the psychiatrist may see the patient to help with diagnostic clarification. Rarely, a case may be severe enough to warrant the psychiatrist's referral to a specialty mental health clinic. Prescribing control is maintained by the PCP. Algorithm-driven treatment iterations continue until target depression outcome is achieved.

The results of the IMPACT study were very impressive. Regardless of primary care setting (including traditional fee-for-service clinics, one inner-city public health clinic, two Veterans Administration clinics, and health maintenance organizations), depression outcomes improved. After 1 year of treatment with IMPACT CCM, approximately 50% of patients had a 50% reduction in depressive symptoms versus 19% receiving care-as-usual. Patients receiving IMPACT CCM treatment had 100 additional depression-free days over 2 years compared to those receiving care-as-usual, and an intent-to-treat analysis found ongoing benefits from IMPACT CCM. The IMPACT model has been expanded to treat those with cancer and diabetes and has had positive results (8, 9).

Problems with the Collaborative Care Model

The CCM has several drawbacks. The first problem is that it was designed to treat mild to moderate depression in the elderly, although its application has been expanded to other populations over time. It is not intended as a treatment for serious mental illnesses such as depression with psychotic features, bipolar disorder, refractory obsessive–compulsive disorder, or any of the psychotic spectrum disorders. People with serious mental illness often have difficulty attending regular appointments and with treatment adherence, especially when in decompensated states, and thus may have inherent difficulty attending appointments crucial to the success of CCM.

Second, not all primary clinics have ready access to the kind of data warehouse needed to create registries. Registries may need to be created outside of the electronic medical record, which has potential legal and privacy implications, and non-integrated databases may be unwieldy and impractical, thus slowing implementation of integrated care.

The third drawback of the model is that the ideal behavioral health consultant, one with a broad and impressive skill set, can be difficult to find, and because of the intensity of interventions, a typical behavioral health consultant may carry a large caseload of patients at any one time. Therefore, a busy primary care practice will need to recruit several behavioral health consultants or else serve only a very small number of patients in need. Finally, CCM requires a major culture shift within many primary care clinics, and culture takes years to change (10).

Variations on the Collaborative Care Model

There are examples of variations on the original IMPACT study models of CCM that address the previously mentioned problems and that seem to work well. Although not studied in random controlled trials, they have the advantage of having been implemented and studied in real-world settings. Two examples are DIAMOND (Depression Initiative Across Minnesota, Offering a New Direction) and RESPECT-Mil (Re-Engineering Systems of Primary Care Treatment of PTSD and Depression in the Military) (22).

DIAMOND is exceptional because it was designed with the help of insurance companies in Minnesota to appropriately plan for reimbursement. Eighty clinics were transitioned to the DIAMOND model over 6 months each. Each clinic had a registry and tracked patient response via the PHQ-9. Each clinic's registry was kept online as part of a central database so that the different clinics' results could be compared. The registries were not necessarily within each clinic's electronic medical record. The behavioral health consultants in this model were mostly registered nurses, each with a caseload of 50–100 depression patients. The consulting psychiatrist reviewed the entire caseload and made recommendations when required, and any patient found to be lacking in improvement was reviewed in detail by the psychiatrist for potential interventions. Although "DIAMOND sites consistently outperformed other primary care sites on 6- and 12-month response and remission rates as measured by the PHQ-9" (7), cost savings were not immediately or universally apparent.

The RESPECT-Mil program used the CCM to treat both post-traumatic stress disorder and depression, not just depression. Results were tracked using the PTSD Checklist and PHQ-9. It was a very large study, inclusive of more than 3.5 million visits to nearly 100 primary care Veterans Administration clinics, and led to major changes within the Veterans Administration health care model, which now requires implementation of both CCM and co-located care in each of its medical centers and community-based outpatient clinics that have more than 5,000 patients (7).

The Primary Care Mental Health Model

The PCBH model is described in detail by Robinson and Reiter in their book titled *Behavioral Consultation and Primary Care: A Guide to Integrating Services* (11). Like Raney's book on collaborative care, this book focuses on guiding implementation. PCBH is not as evidenced based as CCM, but it may be easier to implement because it does not require a registry, and it is easier to adapt because it makes use of systems that are already in place in a site clinic (11).

A VIGNETTE

Janie, the previously discussed 67-year-old woman who has moderate major depressive disorder, has multiple medical comorbidities. Janie decides to see her PCP. She calls and gets an appointment for the next day. The PCP prescribes an antidepressant and has a social worker see her to provide psychoeducation on depression and diabetes. The social worker agrees to see her for a few cognitive–behavioral therapy appointments. Janie's case is not entered into a registry, and after she completes her sessions with the social worker, depression care returns to her PCP. Janie's care is kept within the primary care clinic for as long as possible to reserve referral to specialty mental health for extreme cases.

Despite being considered more adaptable, PCBH does have a fairly defined model. PCBH takes as its inspiration the common-sense view that a patient-centered medical home should directly address behavior and mental health and that a behavioral health provider therefore should be included in the multidisciplinary team for all patients (11). PCBH does not define a role for a psychiatrist. Instead, it advocates for a behavioral health specialist who is highly trained in providing a variety of mental health interventions. Hypothetically, this provider could be a psychiatrist but is more likely to be a social worker, psychologist, or other provider who is not as costly as a psychiatrist. However, adaptations of the model are far from fixed, and psychiatrists may find themselves functioning in models that are drawn from PCBH but that include positions and roles for them. For example, the Cherokee Health Systems implementation employs multiple psychiatrists in its integrated care system, in addition to its psychologists (12).

The behavioral health consultant in the PCBH model is a consultant only and has limited contact with the patient. The PCP refers patients to the behavioral health consultant, who would be available on demand but also have some scheduled appointments on any given day. The behavioral health consultant is physically located in the same clinic as the PCP and his or her team—that is, readily visible and available for questions or for in-person patient consultations. The behavioral health consultant is viewed as benefitting from the "aura" of the PCP's lengthier and more intimate relationship with the patient, so an individual patient–consultant therapeutic relationship is actually discouraged. The behavioral health consultant deals with whatever arises in clinic that requires behavioral or mental health intervention, and then he or she refers to specialty mental health when necessary. PCBH does not set as its goal the attainment of specific targets for defined population groups as is done in collaborative care but instead works with the entire population of the primary care clinic (11).

The benefits of the PCBH model include its adaptability to a busy primary clinic that sees patients with multiple mental health challenges, because it is flexible to work with a variety of problems and patients. The electronic medical record also does not have to be able to track a specific subpopulation ("registry") of patients, which may make this model more appropriate for rural or smaller practices. In addition, the model does not necessarily require the added cost of an expensive psychiatric consultant, although most PCBH models do employ psychiatrists.

Although there are some random controlled trials on the PCBH model, there are none on which the model is directly based (11). Research studies have investigated the efficacy of its varied forms. For example, Blue Cross/Blue Shield examined "outcomes in the *behaviorally enhanced* PCMH of Cherokee Health Systems, in Tennessee, [and] found that . . .Cherokee patients used emergency rooms, medical specialists, and hospital care significantly less; and the overall cost of Cherokee's patients was significantly and substantially lower" than other comparable primary care systems (11, p. 26).

Choosing and Adapting Integrated Care Models

The public psychiatrist asked to work for, or consult to, an integrated care setting should carefully examine the model in place and be sure to ask as many questions as possible regarding expectations and roles. The psychiatrist may be expected to grow the mental health integrated care program from the ground up or may be stepping into an already fully formed program. Regardless, the psychiatrist will be in a position to help the primary care practice find a model of care best suited to the clinic and its patients. Many factors influence the chosen specific model or adaptation of a model.

A VIGNETTE

Kim is a 45-year-old woman with a long history of severe bipolar depression with rapid-cycling manic episodes. She has had a positive effect from fluoxetine in the past but stopped her medications several weeks ago, and she is currently in a depressive episode that is getting worse. Because she is not sleeping, her husband calls the local community mental health center to make an appointment to see her former psychiatrist, but there is a 2-month wait list. Kim agrees to see her PCP at the local federally qualified community health center, and so she gets an appointment for the next day.

A primary clinic with abundant local resources for substance use disorders—methadone clinics, buprenorphine prescribers, dual diagnosis treatment programs, and residential treatment—in addition to a robust community mental health center may choose a model that focuses on a specific subset of patients who are most likely to improve with integrated care. In this model, the psychiatrist may function in a purely consulting role, reviewing caseloads and ensuring that all patients are progressing. Patients with more severe mental illnesses or a severe substance use disorder who are not part of the target population could easily be referred out to one of the local resources.

Not all clinics have this luxury, however, whether due to a lack of state funding for mental health services or location (e.g., a rural setting). In these cases, a clinic may choose an adapted PCBH model with a psychiatrist who comes to the clinic infrequently to consult on complex cases and may follow a subset of severely ill patients. Similarly, in areas in which patients are of a lower socioeconomic status, a model that combines as many services as possible at the primary care clinic might be preferred. Such a clinic might incorporate case managers to help patients find housing and employment, or it might have clinic-based substance abuse counselors but only an infrequent consulting psychiatrist.

Primary care practices should be encouraged to expand and modify integrated health care models to fit their setting and the needs of their patients with mental health issues. For example, in the previous vignette, a rigorous CCM may not be best for addressing the patient's bipolar depression, especially if the CCM practice does not have a registry for bipolar disorder. CCM may also be less suited to treat this case because there are fewer standardized tools for assessing progress in the treatment of bipolar disorder. Instead, a variant of CCM might be used that, for example, provides psychoeducation about bipolar disorder and teaches some coping skills to the patient and her husband. The clinic's behavioral health consultant might staff the case with a consulting psychiatrist who could make a recommendation to introduce a mood stabilizer, for example. Or in a modified version of PCBH, there may be a consulting psychiatrist on the team who could see this complex patient and make recommendations to the team about ongoing care.

Regardless of the integrated model used, the consulting psychiatrist should encourage primary care clinicians to measure the impact of their interventions. Measurement tools such as the PHQ-9 and GAD-7 are available and validated, and there are many other brief, structured symptom rating scales in the public domain that primary clinicians may use in their day-to-day practices (13). Primary clinicians also can be encouraged to use implementation science to track and study the effects of their adaptations of integrated care models. No model fits every situation perfectly, and real-world situations and insights drive innovation and progress as much as fidelity to the original model (14). Implementation and evidence-based care have a bidirectional relationship. Other possible metrics that can be tracked to measure impact are PCP satisfaction and willingness to ask about mental health conditions. Focusing on measurable symptoms and treating to target (a core tenet of CCM) not only improves outcomes but also empowers physicians by allowing them to see the results of their interventions and providing fodder for quality improvement innovations (13).

Reverse Integrated Care

In the public sector, reverse integration is the incorporation of a medical provider into a community mental health center. Such physicians help treat the medical comorbidities of individuals with severe psychiatric illnesses who often do not make it to a primary care clinic. The goal in embedding a PCP in a mental health clinic is to help patients whose medical health negatively impacts their psychiatric health with the hope of improving health in both realms. The ideal model would incorporate the primary care clinician into the multidisciplinary treatment team, with the team using a single electronic medical record. Unfortunately, co-located primary care is much more common that integrated care (15). Although reverse integrated care may improve the outcomes of patients within a mental health clinic, it does not address the problems of those who are not seen in psychiatric care centers at all.

TEAM MEMBER ROLES

In addition to gaining a full understanding of the particular integrated care model that a primary care clinic has in place (or is considering), the psychiatrist should understand the proposed place for the psychiatrist within the treatment team, as well as the role of other team members. Integrated care models use a team to care for each patient. The main team members are the primary care physician and his or her clinical staff, the behavioral health consultant, and, depending on the version/adaptation of model, the consulting psychiatrist.

The primary care physician identifies psychiatric illnesses or problems with a behavioral component using a screening instrument such as the PHQ-2, possibly administered by a medical assistant. The primary care physician then makes referrals to either a behavioral health consultant or a team-based psychiatrist, typically through a warm handoff in which the PCP introduces the mental health clinician to the patient. Given the way that appointments are scheduled in primary care, the primary care physician does not have enough time to do a full mental health assessment and treat all behavioral or mental health problems, so they are tasked to other team members.

Behavioral health consultants may be licensed or unlicensed mental health providers. Many practices use master's or doctoral-level licensed professionals in social work or psychology, or a licensed professional counselor. Some integrated care practices use a nurse or nurse practitioner with behavioral health training, and some use bachelor's level care or case managers with training in mental health interventions (2).

Regardless of their training, behavioral health consultants are familiar with psychiatric assessment, and advanced licensed clinicians may work up a full psychiatric diagnosis. Behavioral health consultants also perform crisis evaluations to decide, for example, whether a patient might need a crisis stabilization unit or inpatient mental health treatment. They also link patients to external services and, depending on the integrated model, might provide a brief therapy course with a targeted goal or counsel patients on health behavior modification, such as performing motivational interviewing for weight loss, smoking cessation, or medication/treatment adherence. Behavioral health consultants may also recommend and identify appropriate group treatments for a particular patient.

In the research-validated CCM, the behavioral health consultant has a very defined role. The consultant is focused on behavior change and as such works to educate patients, provide brief interventions, and support the primary care physician. Raney et al. (2) describe five "core functions": patient engagement (forming a quick relationship with a patient, drawing on the established relationship between the patient and the PCP); assessment and triage, including differential diagnosis in 5- to 10-minute assessments; treatment intervention, such as motivational interviewing, behavioral activation, solution-focused brief therapy, problem-solving treatment, mindfulness-based stress reduction, or acceptance and commitment therapy; follow-up and referral coordination; and data management in preparation for review with the consulting psychiatrist.

Additional team members may include a patient navigator or case manager who can help the patient with social factors that interfere with the patient's progress. These individuals may help the patient file for Medicaid, obtain transportation vouchers, or search for affordable housing options. They may also help the patient make appointments at other facilities. A substance abuse counselor can focus on substance abuse treatment resources and provide motivational interviewing for cessation/decreasing use or psychoeducation about the effects of prolonged drug abuse. A clinical pharmacist may review the patient's medication list and identify ways to streamline medications or save the patient money when resources are scarce.

PSYCHIATRIST ROLES

Regardless of the integrated care, much of the assessment and management of identified mental health issues are delegated to behavioral health consultants or other team members. This may leave the psychiatrist interested in integrated care wondering what his or her responsibilities include. Again, this is dependent on the model of care. In CCM, the psychiatrist has a defined role. According to Raney et al. (2), the consulting psychiatrist serves as a *leader*, helping organize the course of integrated care in the clinic and serving as an inspirational role model for the culture change that necessitates medical and mental providers working hand-in-hand. The psychiatrist is also a *consultant*, providing guidance on caseloads and individual cases both indirectly through curbside consults and supervision of the behavioral health consultants and (rarely) by directly seeing patients but resisting any pressure to take over care of the patients. Finally, the psychiatrist is also an *educator*, making use of his or her expertise to maximize care of a large number of individuals.

In PCBH and its adaptations, the psychiatrist may serve as a supervisor, consultant, and teacher. The psychiatrist may find him- or herself advising the behavioral health consultant on treatment, coordinating care among multiple providers, or evaluating patients directly and making recommendations. When consulting on an individual case, the psychiatrist may be asked to provide further diagnostic clarification, initiate more complex medication recommendations and coordinate titration schedules, or investigate the complex interplay of psychiatric and medical problems.

When in the clinic, integrated psychiatrists may also find themselves answering curbside questions or being called into the primary care examination room to see a patient with whom a primary care physician is having problems. Although the behavioral health consultant does not necessarily have to screen every patient whom a psychiatrist is to directly see, doing so will increase the efficient use of the more costly psychiatrist's time. The integrated psychiatrist may also answer questions that arrive via the electronic medical record system. If a registry is kept, the psychiatrist may manage this as well, reviewing the registered patients on a regular basis to ensure treatment goals are being attained. The psychiatrist may review individual cases to make specific recommendations, including frequency of visits with the behavioral health consultant or whether the patient should, indeed, see a psychiatrist.

In integrated care models, one of the main roles the psychiatrist plays is teacher, a role crucial to fostering a multiplier effect of the psychiatrist's knowledge within the practice. The goal is to increase the knowledge and comfort of the behavioral health consultant and the primary care physician so that they require increasingly less psychiatric consultation on routine cases. Just-in-time learning is the best way to do this, providing direct educational information about a patient who the behavioral health consultant or primary care physician is seeing. Psychiatrists may also teach other team members, including medical students, residents in both medicine and psychiatry, and pharmacy students and providers. By expanding these individuals' knowledge base about psychiatry, care becomes streamlined and the psychiatrist will ultimately find him- or herself consulting on only the most difficult cases.

Next, several vignettes are presented that illustrate the various roles of the psychiatrist in public sector integrated care settings.

A VIGNETTE

Dr. Nguyen is a psychiatrist whose employer, the local community mental health center, has asked him to serve as integrated care consulting psychiatrist at the local federally qualified health center. As the consulting psychiatrist, Dr. Nguyen talks once a week by video conference to the social workers who serve as behavioral health consultants to review caseloads. He also visits the health center every other week. During his clinical time there, Dr. Nguyen sees a few complex patients and connects with the primary care staff. The staff know the basics of psychiatric care but seem to get anxious when serving patients who do not have straightforward mental health issues.

One possible approach to the primary care staff's issue is for the consulting psychiatrist to offer brown bag lunches during which he reviews topics such as complex depression, anxiety, schizophrenia, and personality disorders. He might also cover common and severe psychiatric medication side effects, how to monitor psychiatric medications, and capacity and safety evaluations. The psychiatrist could also use the sessions to reassure the staff of his availability by phone or through the electronic medical record for confusing and emergency situations. In-person lunches would also help build rapport between the psychiatrist and the behavioral health consultants so that they might view him as a knowledgeable and trusted supervisor.

A VIGNETTE

Dr. Smith is a PCP in an integrated clinic using the CCM. She has told the clinic's consulting psychiatrist that she feels confident about diagnosing uncomplicated major depression, but she is unsure how to use adjunctive medications when first-line medications are not achieving treatment goals. The behavioral health consultant has suggested to Dr. Smith to consider adjunctive medications in these situations and relays Dr. Smith's reluctance with the consulting psychiatrist during their weekly caseload/registry review.

In this case, the consulting psychiatrist may want to consider providing the primary care physician with a handout outlining the basic adjuncts for major depression. She may also give the primary care physician a summary of the STAR*D trial, including the medication algorithm and outcomes information. The psychiatrist would still review all depression cases and make individual recommendations if necessary, especially if a specific patient did not improve. The psychiatrist can also reaffirm her availability to the primary care physician by phone or electronic health record message for discussion of individual recommendations.

A VIGNETTE

Dr. Pritchard, who serves as a PCP in an integrated outpatient clinic inside a public hospital, is seeing a 25-year-old patient with insomnia who has tried diphenhydramine, melatonin, and trazodone without effect. He is hesitant to start zolpidem due to the patient's history of sleepwalking and is worried about weight gain with mirtazapine. He remembers that the clinic's consulting psychiatrist has offered to be available by phone for such situations, so he sends the consultant a text message asking her to call when she has time.

In this case, the request for consultation can be used to educate the primary care physician about other alternatives for the treatment of insomnia (e.g., low dose of doxepin), including an explanation as to why it is recommended for this particular patient. The consulting psychiatrist could also educate the primary care physician about other treatment modalities, such as group cognitive–behavioral therapy for insomnia, perhaps offered at the local community mental health center. In addition, she could offer to send information on the evidence-based treatment of insomnia. The consultation need not be telephonic. The consulting psychiatrist could review the patient's medical record remotely and send a message to the primary care physician through the electronic medical record, attaching an article about evidence-based care.

A VIGNETTE

Dr. Jones serves as a primary care physician in a federally qualified health center. She has been following a patient who was diagnosed with schizoaffective disorder, bipolar type, during a hospitalization many months ago. Worried about the patient's ongoing stability, Dr. Jones asks the clinic's consulting psychiatrist, Dr. Yang, to see the patient. Dr. Yang is integrated into the clinic 1 day each week. On Dr. Yang's clinic day, Dr. Jones performs a warm handoff to Dr. Yang in the examination room and then departs. Dr. Yang evaluates the patient and believes that she is continuing to do quite well.

In this case, the consulting psychiatrist might ask the clinic's behavioral health consultant into the room and explain why she thinks it is still appropriate for the patient to be cared for in the primary care clinic. Unless the primary care physician is available to discuss the case, the consulting psychiatrist might also write a concise and clear note in the electronic medical record that describes her reasoning in making the recommendation that the patient continue to be seen in the primary care clinic. When time allows, the psychiatrist might try to understand what led to the primary care physician's concerns about the patient and provide education regarding the reasons for their different experiences of the patient's stability.

LEGAL LIABILITY

When first exposed to integrated care models, it is very common for consulting psychiatrists to raise questions about their risk from a medicolegal perspective. The degree of delegation to other behavioral health providers may be uncomfortable for psychiatrists who are used to performing psychiatric evaluations and risk assessments themselves. They also may not be used to the informal nature of curbside consults in the CCM. This different mode of practice may leave psychiatrists feeling vulnerable to, and liable for, the mistakes that other might make.

However, the consensus in general case law is that the risk for lawsuits stemming from curbside consultations is minimal. Because generally only the primary care physician prescribes medications in the CCM, authority, and therefore liability, primarily falls to him or her. Team care actually decreases overall risk because many clinicians have been consulted and have had a chance to weigh in on the care decisions. Team discussions should also be documented, including the caseload reviews that the consulting psychiatrist does with the behavioral health consultants. For these reviews, the note should include a statement that the patient was not seen. When a psychiatrist serving in an integrated setting does a face-to-face evaluation of a patient, the risk of a lawsuit does increase, and so the encounter should be documented in the medical record. A good rule of thumb is to document all discussions and interactions and to include qualifying statements in all written documents, including email (7).

INTEGRATED MODELS IN SPECIAL SITUATIONS

Specialty Care

Integrated mental health care is spreading beyond primary care, so it is likely that public psychiatrists may be approached about providing care or consultations in a specialty care clinic, including post- or peripartum psychiatric care clinics, pediatric care clinics, on-cologic care clinics, infectious disease/HIV clinics, or clinics that specialize in the medical care to the homeless. Even a dermatology clinic can use a consulting psychiatrist if, for example, a patient with delusional parasitosis consumes an inordinate amount of dermatologic care while declining to go to a mental health clinic. Psychiatrists serving in integrated specialty clinics are often trained in consultation liaison psychiatry and have specialized knowledge about the specialty in which they serve, but especially in a public sector setting, a psychiatrist may find him- or herself filling such a niche without specialized training.

Consulting psychiatrists who serve in specialty clinics typically provide direct care to more patients because they initially present as complex referrals. However, integrated models in specialty clinics will still have behavioral health consultants working with patients as well, including in groups. Specialty clinics pose unique challenges to traditional integrated care models. For example, it may not be as easy to provide longitudinal care to patients because the frequency of clinic visits is often less than in primary care. In addition, the psychiatrist may experience more pushback from specialist physicians regarding prescribing outside their area of expertise. This may lead to two prescribing physicians: the specialist doctor and the consulting psychiatrist. Alternatively, the specialty may employ advanced nurse practitioners as the prescribers. These challenges increase the potential for confusion and error, and so communications must be strong in these settings and include regular meetings between specialist providers and consulting psychiatrists.

Telepsychiatry in Integrated Care

Telepsychiatry is becoming an important component of integrated care models. Especially in rural areas, it may be difficult for a consulting psychiatrist to get to the primary care clinic. In this model variation, all of the functions of the consulting psychiatrist remain intact, but they are performed remotely. For example, rapport with the clinic team and its behavioral health consultants is developed primarily through video and phone conferencing along with infrequent in-person meetings. The consulting psychiatrist can also see patients via videoconferencing.

Public psychiatrists committed to increasing access to patients to primary care in rural settings may initially be uncomfortable with the use of telepsychiatry to do so. However, this medium can afford certain benefits. It increases the efficiency of a busy public sector physician by allowing the consulting psychiatrist to be visible to patients and staff at the remote clinic without the travel time. Telepsychiatry also allows for easier cross-referencing of medical records during team meetings, and it is easier to type team meeting notes during discussions with the behavioral health consultants or patient visits notes during the appointment, both of which save the psychiatrist valuable time. The legalities of telepsychiatry must be considered as well, especially because laws on its use vary by institution and state. Conferencing system security must be explored, and insurance coverage for telepsychiatry may vary by plan as well. All of these elements must be addressed prior to engaging in integrated telepsychiatry.

Project ECHO (Extension for Community Healthcare Outcomes), which was developed at the University of New Mexico, provides an example of a model for integrated care through telepsychiatry. Originally developed to extend the reach of specialists in the treatment of hepatitis to rural areas of New Mexico, ECHO connects PCPs with online and telemedicine providers who are at a remote hub located at the university. The specialists serve not only as consultants but also as educators of PCPs to maximize specialist knowledge dissemination. Project ECHO has an entire telemedicine clinic devoted to integrated addiction and psychiatric care in New Mexico. This model has been expanded to other states and to other subspecialties in psychiatry, including pediatric psychiatry (16).

Serious Mental Illness in Integrated Care

The major models for integrated care were developed to treat conditions such as anxiety and depression that are commonly seen in primary care settings. As such, they would not seem to be well suited to treat serious mental illness in integrated primary care settings. Indeed, there are no randomized controlled trials that have investigated the use of primary care integration to serve people with schizophrenia or schizophreniform disorders (17).

However, because psychotic disorders in particular are profoundly undertreated (18), working with PCPs to allow stabilized schizophrenia to be managed in primary care settings is one strategy to increase the reach of limited public sector psychiatrist time. For example, Lowdermilk et al. (19) have described a model for treating psychotic spectrum disorders in integrated clinics instead of immediately referring patients to specialty mental health clinics. They note that although primary care physicians may initially feel uncomfortable treating psychosis, this may be ameliorated through an integrated care model that includes ongoing educational sessions for primary care staff and that uses behavioral health consultants and a consulting psychiatrist.

Patients with a history of psychotic disorders may find this sort of model of care in primary care settings less threatening if, for example, they associate mental health clinics with past involuntary inpatient treatment. The stigma of a psychotic spectrum diagnosis also may discourage patients from seeking treatment in a mental health facility.

A team-based model incorporating behavioral health consultants and a consulting psychiatrist offers an alternative, primary care setting to treat such individuals. Early identification and engagement of patients with psychosis may also be enhanced by engaging primary care settings.

CONSIDERATIONS FOR CHOOSING A CAREER IN INTEGRATED CARE

The Emily Dickinson poem at the beginning of this chapter reflects, among other things, some of the reasons that a student might choose to go into medicine, generally, or into psychiatry, in particular. In that context, the public psychiatrist considering work in an integrated care setting, especially one in which service is primarily as a consultant and not direct interaction with patients, may view the consultant role as counterintuitive—that is, as contrary to the reason for going into psychiatry in the first place: connecting and treating patients directly (2). However, psychiatrists working in this capacity are generally satisfied with the choice; find the role intellectually stimulating; and get a sense of professional fulfillment through educating others, interacting with multiple colleagues, and knowing that they are helping expand access to care for the community. For example, Norfleet et al. (20) surveyed a convenience sample of 52 psychiatrists who worked in integrated care and found most to be happy working as supervisory consultants overseeing behavioral health consultants. They found the work to offer opportunities for innovation and personal growth, and they enjoyed working in a patient-centered care model, working with a team, and serving as an educator. It is also important to note that most psychiatrists do not serve solely as integrated care consultants. Typically, psychiatrists add a few hours of integrated care work to a direct care practice.

A VIGNETTE

Dr. Ngalie is a fourth-year psychiatry resident who is considering practicing in an integrated care setting after completing his residency. He enjoys multitasking and being engaged in multiple projects. For example, he prefers inpatient work because of the variety of tasks performed during the day: talking to other providers, families, and patients. He does not mind it when nurses interrupt him with patient care issues, and he can easily go back to his work. He also enjoys teaching the medical students and watching their appreciation for psychiatry grow. In addition, nothing is more professionally satisfying to him than stabilizing acutely ill patients so that they are well enough to leave the hospital.

Dr. Ngalie's co-resident, Dr. Samuelson, also thinks she might be interested in practicing in an integrated care setting after residency. She is attracted to the idea of spreading her reach by helping a community access mental health care through a public primary care clinic. Her favorite part of her training has been her outpatient practice, and especially her psychotherapy practice, in which she can learn about patients in-depth. The part of outpatient practice she does not like is the time required for collateral calls and prior authorizations that she could be using to sit with patients instead. Nothing is more professionally satisfying to her than the relationships she has made with her patients and the progress she has seen them make throughout the years.

Certain personal characteristics and professional preferences appear to be correlated with success and happiness for the psychiatrist working in an integrated care setting (2, 11). It is important to have the ability to focus on details of patient care but without being a micromanager. Integrated care psychiatrists keep track of details as well as the big picture, but they allow the behavioral health consultants to perform their roles and do not take over care of patients from the primary care physician. They should be energetic, flexible, and interruptible—able to handle unexpected events and change course easily. They are friendly, outgoing, and possibly extroverted. They are capable of working independently, remaining motivated and engaged even without seeing patients on a regular basis. They need to be comfortable with consulting on patients without the in-depth information one might have in a usual psychiatrist–patient relationship, including the information that one might desire from a medicolegal perspective.

Understanding and having knowledge about the mental health system in the clinic, city, and state of practice are important. Integrated care psychiatrists must be adaptable to serving patients outside a narrow area of expertise, with a willingness to learn about novel treatment topics without obtaining formal training in them. Individuals interested in integrated psychiatry should enjoy teaching people on a variety of mental health topics and performing in a variety of roles. If working in a specialty clinic, it can be helpful to appreciate making connections with, and have some knowledge about, the specialty of interest.

Consulting psychiatrists serve as clinical supervisors to behavioral health consultants, and so they must be comfortable in a leadership role, including helping staff think about "the big picture." Teamwork is critical in integrated care, so the psychiatrist must find teams exciting and energizing. Integrated care psychiatrists should be able to recognize team members' strengths and weaknesses in order to appropriately delegate responsibility.

These attributes, characteristics, interests, and abilities are noted by most experts in integrated care. Parinda Khatri, PhD, Director of Integrated Care at Cherokee Health Systems, also describes characteristics needed of a behavioral health consultant. Such a person needs to be a team player; a good communicator; and someone who enjoys high-energy, fast-paced, and flexible environments. Amanda Lentz, a nurse practitioner with

Cherokee Health Systems, also stresses the importance of being able to function outside of one's routine to succeed in this type of setting (21).

A VIGNETTE—CONTINUED

Dr. Ngalie completes an integrated care rotation and finds that it fits his personality perfectly and professional needs in many ways. He finds a position that allows him to combine an inpatient practice with a few hours at a local federally qualified health center as a psychiatric consultant. He looks forward to working with physicians from other disciplines and to supervising several behavioral health consultants.

Dr. Samuelson completes an integrated care rotation and realizes that she still prefers direct patient care to the consultant role. She finds a place to open her own private practice. She plans to accept Medicaid in order to meet her desire to treat underserved patients in the community who are desperately in need of care, while also allowing her to do what she enjoys and believes she does best.

CASE STUDY: CONCLUSION

After unsuccessfully searching for a psychiatrist, Jim made an appointment at the clinic affiliated with the local public hospital. He was started on escitalopram by a primary care physician in the clinic, and he was introduced to a behavioral health consultant, who provided brief supportive therapy during the next several months. When Jim was feeling confident and trusted the behavioral health consultant, he confessed to hearing disparaging voices. With the consultation of the integrated care psychiatrist, the primary care physician agreed to add and manage aripiprazole for the psychotic features. Jim was added to a new registry of patients with psychosis that tracked important labs pertinent to those on antipsychotics. Through a modification of integrated care models, Jim's depression and psychotic symptoms remitted without him ever seeing a psychiatrist.

Patients dependent on the safety net system for health care face many barriers, both internal and external, to accessing mental health care. Even if their housing and income are stable, patients may be afraid of the stigma associated with mental illness—stigma that can come from the community or their families. They may not know that their symptoms represent a mental illness or, if they do, they may not know how to access mental health care. When they do realize they need care and know how to access it, costs may be excessive or distances to a psychiatric provider prohibitive. Even when insured to help with the costs, patients may have difficulty getting in to see a psychiatrist promptly, as happened to the patient in this case.

Given all of these barriers, and in the context of the shortages of psychiatrists described previously, integrated care represents a powerful way to improve access to care while also allowing the interested public psychiatrist to operate at the top of his or her skill set through consultation and supervision of a larger cohort of patients than he or she could serve alone. Other models of care—for example, co-location and reverse co-location—might address some limitations in access to mental health care, but these do not leverage available psychiatrist time toward improving population health as powerfully as integrated care.

In this case, the patient was offered care in an adaptation of the two major models for integrated care described in this chapter. Both of these models—the CCM and the PCBH model—allow a consulting psychiatrist to help provide care to a large caseload of patients in a primary care, or even specialty care, practice. The CCM has the strength of being strongly researched as a systematic evidence-based way to implement treatment of common mental health disorders in primary care. The PCBH model's strength is its flexibility to the needs of individual clinics and their patients in implementing best practices, especially when there are significant barriers to data-intensive approaches such as the CCM's registries.

This case demonstrates an adaptation of these model to offer services to a severely ill patient who otherwise may have waited weeks for care or perhaps would have deteriorated to the point of requiring hospitalization before accessing care. For a community psychiatrist, typically with a strong interest in strategies to improve population mental health, the case represents the potential power of integrated models of care. Indeed, the rapid progress in implementing integrated mental health in a multitude of settings—primary and specialty, urban and rural—offers community psychiatrists the opportunity to be at the forefront in this revolution in medical (including mental) health care, not only in their local communities but also regionally or nationally through the use of emerging technologies such as telepsychiatry.

REFERENCES

1. Access Community Health Centers. Primary care behavioral health: MH care redesign. October 30, 2008. Retrieved from https://www.youtube.com/watch?v=t0MsDjlTQfo
2. Raney LE, Lasky GB, Scott C. Integrated care: A guide for effective implementation. Arlington, VA: American Psychiatric Association Publishing; 2017.
3. Bishop TF, Press MJ, Keyhani S, Pincus HA. Acceptance of insurance by psychiatrists and the implication for access to mental health care. JAMA Psychiatry. 2014;71(2):176–181.
4. National Council Medical Director Institute. The psychiatric shortage: Causes and solutions. March 29, 2017. Retrieved from https://www.thenationalcouncil.org/wp-content/uploads/2018/04/Revised-Final-Access-Paper.pdf
5. Insel T. Psychiatry: Where are we going? National Institute of Mental Health. June 3, 2011. Retrieved from http://www.nimh.nih.gov/about/director/2011/psychiatry-where-are-we-going.shtml
6. Unützer J, Katon WJ, Fan M-Y, et al. Long-term cost effects of collaborative care for late-life depression. American Journal of Managed Care. 2008;14(2):95–100.
7. Annex Galleries. Alphonse Legros. Retrieved February 2019 from https://www.annexgalleries.com/artists/biography/1371/Legros/Alphonse
8. AIMS Center. IMPACT: Improving Mood—Promoting Access to Collaborative Treatment. Retrieved from https://aims.uw.edu/impact-improving-mood-promoting-access-collaborative-treatment
9. Unützer J, Katon W, Callahan CM, et al. Collaborative care management of late-life depression in a primary care setting: A randomized controlled trial. JAMA. 2002;288(22):2836–2845.

10. Katzenbach JR, Steffen I, Kronley C. Cultural change that sticks. Harvard Business Review. July–August 2012. Retrieved from https://hbr.org/2012/07/cultural-change-that-sticks ƒref

11. Robinson PJ, Reiter JT. Behavioral consultation and primary care: A guide to integrating services (2nd ed.). New York, NY: Springer; 2016.

12. Cherokee Health Systems. Retrieved from https://www.cherokeehealth.com

13. Fortney JC, Unützer J, Wreen G, et al. A tipping point for measurement-based care. Psychiatric Services. 2017;68(2):179–188.

14. Oslin D, Dixon L, Adler DA, et al. Adaptation in delivery integrated care: The tension between care and evidence based practice. Psychiatric Services. 2018;69(9):appips201800028.

15. Manderscheid R, Kathol R. Fostering sustainable, integrated medical and behavioral health services in medical settings. Annals of Internal Medicine. 2014;160:61–65.

16. University of New Mexico School of Medicine. Project ECHO: A revolution in medical education and care delivery. Retrieved from http://echo.unm.edu

17. Reilly S, Planner C, Gask L, et al. Collaborative care approaches for people with severe mental illness. Cochrane Database of Systematic Reviews. 2013;10(11):1–58.

18. Kohn R, Saxena S, Itzhak L, Saraceno B. The treatment gap in mental health care. Bulletin of the World Health Organization. 2004;82(11):858–866

19. Lowdermilk E, Joseph N, Feinstein RE. The treatment of schizophrenia spectrum and other psychotic disorders in integrated primary care. In RE Feinstein, J Connell, M Feinstein (Eds.), *Integrating behavioral health and primary care* (pp. 199–222). New York, NY: Oxford University Press; 2017.

20. Norfleet KR, Ratzliff AD, Chan YF, et al. The role of the integrated care psychiatrist in community settings: A survey of psychiatrists' perspectives. Psychiatric Services. 2016;67(3):346–349.

21. Health Care Best Practice: Cherokee Health Systems. Disparities: Mental health—Electronic medical record. Published by Richard Gooden, National Center for Primary Care, July 25, 2008. Retrieved from https://www.youtube.com/watch?v=OtqMPhDH5TU&feature=channel_video_title

22. American Psychiatric Association and Academy of Psychosomatic Medicine. Dissemination of integrated care within adult primary care settings: The collaborative care model. 2016. Retrieved from https://www.integration.samhsa.gov/integrated-care-models/APA-APM-Dissemination-Integrated-Care-Report.pdf

23. Bardach NS, Coker TR, Zima BT, et al. Common and costly hospitalizations for pediatric mental health disorders. Pediatrics. 2014;133:602–609.

24. Crowley RA, Kirschner N. The integration of care for mental health, substance abuse, and other behavioral health conditions into primary care: Executive summary of an American College of Physicians position paper. Annals of Internal Medicine. 2015;163(4):298–299, appendix.

25. SAMHSA-HRSA Center for Integrated Health Solutions. Behavioral health in primary care. Retrieved from https://www.integration.samhsa.gov/integrated-care-models/behavioral-health-in-primary-care

26. University of Colorado Hospital, Outpatient Clinic. Retrieved from http://www.ucdenver.edu/academics/colleges/medicalschool/departments/psychiatry/PatientCare/outpatient/Pages/Services.aspx.

27. The Working Party Group on Integrated Behavioral Healthcare. Joint principles: Integrating behavioral health care into the patient-centered medical home. Annals of Family Medicine. 2014; 12(2):183–185.

///6/// THE PUBLIC PSYCHIATRIST AS A LEADER

MICHAEL D. ROSS AND
OCTAVIO N. MARTINEZ, JR.

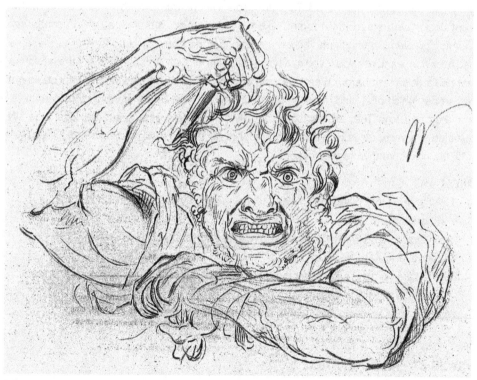

FIGURE 6.1 Charles Bell, *Anatomical Expression of Rage.*

Source: From Essays on the Anatomy of Expression in Painting. London: Longman; 1806.

Trained as a surgeon, the artist Sir Charles Bell (for whom Bell's palsy is named) taught anatomy and helped write a four-volume work titled *The Anatomy of the Human Body*. Regarding *Essays on the Anatomy of Expression in Painting* (1), Bell said that it was his interest in the art of expression that led to his discoveries in neurology (Figure 6.1) (2).

CASE STUDY: INITIAL PRESENTATION

You serve as medical director for your local community mental health center, where you supervise three other physicians and provide clinical leadership to the center, as well as lead the center's quality management team. You are also a child and adolescent psychiatrist and spend approximately 50% of your time in direct clinical care. Today, you will see John, a 12-year-old boy with a history of attention-deficit/hyperactivity disorder (ADHD) who was doing well on a stimulant until he moved to your Southern community from his family's home in New England. You are hopeful that this will be a straightforward case of ADHD, until John's parents start by saying they have several issues that they would like to address with you.

First, they mention to you their difficulty getting John to see you. They were on a waiting list for several weeks, and John has been without his medication, and so his behavior and grades at school have worsened. They are especially frustrated by the way the staff at the front desk have treated them today, "like we are lucky to get seen, at all." Second, they mention problems getting John accommodations at his current school similar to those he had back home and ask you if you can help make this happen. Third, they state that at John's last pediatrician visit before the move, one of John's thyroid values was off (they could not remember which one), and he was started on thyroid medication of which they cannot remember the name. They are having an equally difficult time getting into the local federally qualified health center, and so John is also out of his thyroid medication. They ask if you will refill the unknown thyroid medication.

QUESTIONS
1. What are some systemic challenges facing the physician leader in a community mental health clinic?
2. What are some ways that a physician leader can approach the challenges faced by John's family at the clinic?
3. What are some ways that a physician leader can approach the challenges faced by John's family in the community?

PSYCHIATRY AND LITERATURE

The Burial of the Dead
by T. S. Eliot (3)

April is the cruelest month, breeding
Lilacs out of the dead land, mixing
Memory and desire, stirring
Dull roots with spring rain.
Winter kept us warm, covering
Earth in forgotten snow, feeding
A little life with dried tubers . . .

The actions of leaders have consequences, both good and bad. Good leadership in a public mental health organization can be felt even among staff who rarely interact with the executive team. People understand the vision, and they feel engaged in achieving the goals of the organization and are committed to the organization. Poor leadership impacts morale and leads to high turnover and poor quality of care. Taken metaphorically, Eliot's opening to *The Waste Land* may well be referencing the devastation caused by the poor leadership that led to World War I. But Eliot was also known to suffer from mental illness, most likely depression, and so these lines could just as well reflect his own mindset. Indeed, they were written after Eliot spent 3 weeks convalescing for his depression and subsequently sought treatment at Lausanne with the psychoanalyst Roger Vittoz (4).

LEADING IN PUBLIC PSYCHIATRY

Many community psychiatrists enjoy, and obtain great job satisfaction from, spending their full days caring for patients in the office. However, some community psychiatrists wish to make an impact on public mental health for patients whom they do not directly serve through leadership in their clinic and their community. There are various roles in which a community psychiatrist can provide that important service of leadership, and there is evidence that taking on these roles leads to higher job satisfaction and less burnout (5).

Leading as a Unit Medical Director

Because of the shortage of psychiatrists, especially in the public sector, even new graduates can expect to be asked to take a leadership role on a unit in a hospital or in a partial hospital program. The medical director title may seem daunting at first, but there are tasks in running an inpatient unit for which staff will look to a psychiatrist for leadership (6).

One of those tasks is consulting on the milieu of the unit. Even though lengths of stay have become markedly shorted, sometimes the milieu treatments on inpatient units still reflect the standards of care when stays were much longer (7). For example, much time and energy have been expended to reduce seclusions and restraints, but until recently, less have been spent on understanding and changing historic practices on inpatient units that may contribute to behavior leading to seclusion or restraint. Unit medical directors can help ensure that care is evidence-based, especially with regard to the management of agitated behavior. For example, unit medical directors can advocate for staff education—starting at new-employee orientation—on evidence-based management of agitated behavior to reduce episodes of seclusion and restraint (8). Medical directors can encourage conversion of inpatient unit management to the principles of evidence-based, trauma-informed care models—a systemic approach that can be used to drive the integration of various unit interventions, unit psychotherapies, medication management, and even discharge planning (9).

Some physicians may believe they should function as captain of the ship and may come away from residency believing they will have ultimate authority over all clinical decisions on their unit. Contemporary clinical management uses a shared decision-making philosophy, engaging other clinical staff—and especially the patient—as a team in treatment planning. Nonetheless, the community psychiatrist can still play an important role in fostering collegial multidisciplinary team-building that improves patient outcomes and staff job satisfaction. Fostering cross-discipline collaboration requires understanding the systemic and interpersonal barriers, which is explored in-depth in Chapter 3.

Sometimes unexpected barriers arise to team cohesiveness.

A VIGNETTE

Upon completion of her residency, Dr. Jones joins the local community mental health center as medical director of its partial hospitalization program. On the unit, she will be sharing the patient load with and supervising Dr. Jefferson, who prefers patient care to administration and so did not want the medical director position when it came open. Yet almost immediately it becomes apparent to Dr. Jones that her senior colleague resents having a younger and less experienced physician supervisor. She worries about the impact that resentment will have on team cohesiveness and patient care.

Physicians in leadership positions are often called upon to provide both clinical and administrative supervision of fellow physicians. It is not unusual for fellow physicians to have been in practice for a longer period of time and/or worked at the facility longer, especially if they are doctors who prefer to spend their days in direct patient care or do not want the added responsibility of administrative medicine. It may take a different skill set to navigate these relationships in a way that balances respect for your colleagues with the role of the medical director. For example, it would be important for Dr. Jones to resist taking Dr. Jefferson's opinions personally. She would want to maintain open and respectful communication and specifically engage her clinical peer in decision-making in areas that fall under her authority, such as medical policy. Non-administrative medical staff members need to know that their experience and opinions are valued in clinical policymaking (10, 11).

Leading as a Hospital or Clinic Medical Director

Both public sector hospitals and community mental health outpatient centers typically have a psychiatrist serving as a medical director and, as such, providing senior medical leadership to the institution. Although responsibilities of a medical director may vary (12), they typically include recruiting and supervising medical staff, leading medical policymaking and often quality management, and serving as a key member of the leadership team.

Inquiries from physicians seeking employment are typically routed first to the medical director, who does the initial screening of applicants and reaches out to inquiring physicians and ultimately makes recommendations to the human resource department about hires. Once hired, physicians usually administratively report to the medical director or, in large organizations, to an associate medical director. The human resource responsibilities typically include annual performance evaluations and ongoing performance management. Medical directors match physician interests to clinical needs of their organizations. They set work and call schedules, and they ensure expectations regarding availability and workloads are met. In addition, they advocate for the individual and collective needs of the medical staff.

Medical directors offer guidance to organizational leadership on medical policy. These policy roles allow public psychiatrists the opportunity to influence the service array and quality of care that patients receive from their organizations. For example, standards of practice regarding the use of psychotropic medications are set with the medical director's guidance. One of the main responsibilities of a psychiatric medical director is to promote high-quality behavioral health care. This may seem like a major responsibility, but medical directors often work in conjunction with other department heads—the chief executive officer (CEO), chief financial officer, human resource director, and others—to create an efficiently run workplace. It is also not unusual for the medical director to provide executive leadership to the quality management initiatives of hospitals and mental health clinics, including leading quality management meetings.

As a member of the hospital's or clinic's executive team, the medical director helps set the strategic direction of the center or hospital and helps develop professional, clinical, and ethical standards for clinical staff. The medical director also represents the organization to other physicians in the community, including the local medical society and, in centers and hospitals with academic affiliations, the department of psychiatry. The medical director often serves as the liaison to the residency training and medical student clerkship directors and may also serve as one of the clinical supervisors of trainees, offering opportunities to teach medical students and residents about the various clinical, administrative, and advocacy roles of the administrative community psychiatrist.

Although the psychiatrist serving as state hospital or community mental health center medical director has many roles that are similar to the role of psychiatrist as clinician, many emerging physician leaders move into administrative psychiatry with little knowledge of, and limited experience in, administrative theory, especially regarding what has been described as "systems literacy" (13). That is, the contemporary public mental health medical director needs to understand the business aspects of administering a health care organization, including how Medicaid and other insurance products are structured and contracted, the organization's costs for providing care, principles in managing medical staff efficiency, and the organization's human resource policy.

The ability to read financial statements helps the medical director understand the fiscal health of her organization overall, the impact of physician services on that health, and the overall business practices of the organization. Most important is the income statement, which is typically presented to the governing body of the organization (typically its board of trustees or directors) on a monthly to quarterly basis. The income statement shows the profit and losses of the organization for the time period reported. It shows all of the sources of revenue and all of the expenses of the clinic or hospital. The chief financial officer can drill down the revenue and expenses to show the impact of physician services. The medical director can use these data to help the medical staff serve patients more efficiently and effectively (14).

It may be helpful to the medical director to participate in, and learn, the business office's strategies for negotiating provider contracts with insurance companies. Factors such as the number of mental health providers in the community and the size of the organization can affect negotiated rates for physician services, but the rates that the organization agrees upon can greatly impact its ability to hire adequate physician staff to provide high-quality care. If the rates are too low, then physician services do not pay for themselves, and physicians become a financial liability to the organization. The organization may therefore become hesitant to bring on adequate medical staffing, which in turn negatively effects caseloads and quality of care (15, 16).

Medical directors need to be familiar with human resource management. Hiring physicians who are good fits to the job, ensuring they have the training and support they need, and advocating for pay and rewards that foster organizational commitment and good patient care are all part of the medical director's role (17). Medical directors also need to be familiar with human resource law, including requirements on interviewing and discrimination in hiring, disability rights, sexual harassment and hostile workplace, and performance management (18). In managing fellow physicians, the medical director must also recognize the important differences between the therapeutic contract used with patients and the administrative contract used with supervisees. The latter focuses much more on building a team of employees to accomplish a similar goal and providing supervision and leadership as well as applying rewards and sanctions when necessary. Therefore, "interpersonal literacy"—the ability to effectively communicate organizational goals to medical staff and medical staff needs to leadership, to coach, and to provide feedback—is critical to success (13).

Contemporary hospitals and outpatient mental health clinics use adaptations of the techniques developed in the manufacturing industry to measure and modify their workflows. This work to standardize clinical processes is intended to improve system efficiency (and thereby improve patient access to care) and quality of care (19). These strategies can be applied to physician services under the direction of the medical director as well. For example, standardized workflows can optimize use of nursing and other licensed clinical staff so that physicians spend their time doing tasks that only physicians can do.

A VIGNETTE—CONTINUED

After 1 year of service as medical director of the partial hospitalization program, Dr. Jones applies for the position of, and is appointed, hospital medical director. Several weeks into the new job, she receives an email from the hospital CEO complaining about the medical staff's contribution to the poor financial performance of the hospital, which is losing money. Dr. Jones realizes that she does not know much about how the hospital is paid for patient care provided by her medical staff.

The medical director's job is sometimes described as working collegially with medical staff to find ways to provide cost-effective care without compromising the quality of the care delivered. In the vignette, the medical director might ask for a meeting with her CEO and/or the chief financial officer to review the hospital finances during the past several quarters and to obtain an understanding of the CEO's concerns. The knowledge obtained may help the medical director guide her staff toward optimizing reimbursement or improving their efficiency in caring for their patients.

Leading as a State-Level Medical Director

Most state governments, through their mental health authority role, hire public psychiatrists to serve in state-level policy roles (20). Typically, these psychiatrists are employed by the health and human services department of state government. There are many state mental health authority roles for psychiatrists—for example, chief medical officer for a state psychiatric hospital system, medical policy leader for the state community mental health system, and policy advisor for the state's Medicaid mental health program. In all these roles, the psychiatrist advises both political and bureaucratic leaders on medical aspects of current and proposed policy and/or law.

A VIGNETTE—CONTINUED

After several years of service as hospital medical director, Dr. Jones moves to her state's capital city and begins service as state medical director for behavioral health. A bill is filed in the house of representatives that would require every state prison to offer buprenorphine, along with substance use counseling, to prisoners diagnosed with opioid use disorder. The local community mental health centers in the state would be required to continue the medication once prisoners were released to the community. The governor asks Dr. Jones' boss, the commissioner of health, whether he should support the bill. The commissioner, in turn, asks Dr. Jones for her opinion.

State-level positions may offer an important opportunity to influence state policy that impacts patient care; to lead statewide clinical innovation; and to advocate for new laws and health policies that support best practices, optimal care for patients, and improved mental health for people throughout the state. In the vignette, Dr. Jones might conduct a current literature review on the efficacy of medication-assisted treatment of opioid use disorder, particularly in forensic populations. One of the concerns that the legislature may have is the cost of the proposed treatment, so Dr. Jones might look for research to determine if the proposed intervention might lead to reductions in costs to state government, perhaps in the form of reduced jail recidivism or reduced overall health care costs, that would offset the cost of the proposal. She might consider summarizing this information on a 1-page, bullet-point paper that is easy for a busy policymaker to understand.

Leading Quality Management

Regardless of the leadership role played by the public psychiatrist, he or she will likely have an important role in quality management. In some ways, psychiatry's quality management processes have been slower to evolve in comparison to those of other medical specialties, perhaps due to a historic lack of clear measures for what is considered quality care, lack of outcome measures with high validity and reliability, and the profession's historic "expert knows best" mentality. Nonetheless, having effective ways to analyze and improve treatment outcomes is an important issue that still needs to be solved. In addition, advances in information technology make it easier to track and analyze quality measurements (21).

A World Health Organization (WHO) report on quality improvement for mental health advocates for a quality management approach focused on several areas, including preserving the dignity of individuals with mental diagnoses, offering recommendations that aim to reduce the impact of disease while simultaneously improving quality of life for individuals suffering from mental disorders, fostering cost-effective mental health care to preserve scarce mental health resources, helping individuals with mental diagnoses cope with their disabilities, and improving quality of care in all areas (22). In order to attain these goals, the report advocates for designing a set of service standards that are measurable and policies to ensure that quality improvement is integrated into the current delivery of services.

The literature offers guidance to the public mental health medical director leading a quality management program who wants to achieve the WHO goals. For example, Lauriks et al. (23) have collated many quality indicators for psychiatry from the literature. They note that in the United States, the Healthcare Effectiveness Data and Information Set (HEDIS) is the most widely recognized quality indicator system. It includes mental health care performance measures that are commonly used in non-psychiatric settings. Metrics applicable to psychiatric care include adherence to antipsychotic medications in schizophrenia, metabolic screening of patients on antipsychotics, and follow-up for children prescribed psychostimulants. The latest measures can be found on the website of the National Committee for Quality Assurance.

Quality measures should strive to focus on actual outcomes (e.g., remission of symptoms and ability to develop meaningful relationships) as opposed to measuring processes (e.g., engagement in outpatient treatment after acute stay and substance use screening rates). Possible outcome measures include symptom improvement, patient functioning, quality of life, and patient satisfaction. The quality management process should also incorporate regular feedback of information to clinicians, in part to help the system of care improve but also to keep staff engaged by showing them the results of their efforts (21). Finally, although it is important that the primary focus of the quality management plan and measures be improving quality of care and treatment effectiveness, ethical contemporary practice in public psychiatry demands optimal use of limited funding and so cost-effectiveness of care must also be a focus.

A VIGNETTE

Dr. Rogers serves as medical director for a state psychiatric hospital with 300 patients. Increasing acuity of admissions has led to more episodes of agitation and, consequently, to an unwanted increase in seclusion and restraints. Recognizing the danger to patients in this pattern, he asks the quality management council of the hospital to focus on a reduction of seclusion and restraints. He is able to obtain data on census numbers and seclusion/restraints numbers during the past several years at the hospital, and so he is able to calculate seclusion/restraint rates. However, there are few data on the nature of the seclusions and restraints to guide new quality management initiatives.

In this vignette, the medical director could ask the quality management council to develop data elements for the hospital to collect on seclusion/restraints; these data elements would extend beyond rote events to include measures such as time of day, staffing patterns when restraints/seclusions occur, and diagnoses of patients involved. In terms of interventions, even before the data are available, the council might develop education programs for staff on alternatives to seclusion/restraint and perhaps training on trauma-informed care (9).

Team approaches to quality management that use outcome assessments and apply the WHO principles of quality management daily will likely result in more efficient, effective, and affordable health care with overall improved patient satisfaction.

Leading Integrated Mental Health

The integrated care model has gained traction during the past several years. It has been suggested that evolving systems of care into integrated care models can improve patient outcomes and also make sense financially through the prevention of unnecessary use of emergency and acute health care services. Indeed, the effectiveness of integrated care models is well established (24, 25). Psychiatrists in leadership positions therefore may be called upon to facilitate the implementation of one or many of the various integrated care models in public systems—for example, in federally qualified health centers. Many of the leadership skills required of psychiatrist administrators generally can be applied to leadership of integrated care initiatives.

Practice facilitation, the use of a consultant to help a practice through a major change, has emerged as an evidence-based method for facilitating change in primary care practices, and so its principles are also good guidelines for the public psychiatrist helping integrate a primary care setting. Facilitators serve as external change agents to foster incorporation of innovations into operations with the goal of ensuring the changes are sustained once the facilitator withdraws. Studies suggest that using practice facilitation as a change management strategy nearly triples the likelihood of implementation of evidence-based guidelines (26). Research in practice facilitation identifies the critical leadership skills that a public psychiatrist might bring to an integration initiative. The public psychiatrist must be viewed by clinical and administrative leaders as credible—that is, knowledgeable about integrated care and about the evidence in favor of the model of care. She also must be a good communicator because she will be called upon to communicate with, and educate, providers across other specialties. Finally, the public psychiatrist must be flexible and responsive to the needs of the clinical and administrative leadership (27).

Research in practice facilitation also suggests the roles of the psychiatrist leader in integrated care implementation. These include engagement of the clinic's clinical and administrative leaders in the change process, providing education on the principles of the chosen model of integrated care, fostering measurement-based care, encouraging auditing and feedback on fidelity to the chosen model, and providing ongoing problem-solving and support. Again, all of these are intended to help the team in the primary care setting modify its work processes to incorporate, and sustain, an evidence-based integrated mental health model (26).

Finally, beyond the change management processes, there are very concrete issues that need to be addressed in a mental health integration that the psychiatrist leader needs to facilitate. Most important is the establishment of high-quality, functional interdisciplinary treatment teams. This means finding social workers, psychologists, and other behavioral health clinicians with expertise in evidence-based, brief, and solution-focused interventions that will be required in a primary care setting. It also means determining how those clinicians and the primary care staff will work together to meet patient needs. Morning huddles or other structured meetings are a typical way to ensure communication, but it is also important to consider how space is allocated, how patients flow through the clinic, and how information is gathered and stored in the medical record. Working through these issues will help ensure that mental health issues are identified; that care flows readily between primary care and behavioral health clinicians; and that, when needed, appropriate referrals can be made for patients who need longer term or more intensive care (28).

One of the barriers to integrated care that must be addressed in any implementation is how to pay for it. One possible solution is funding alternative payment models. One example of an alternative payment model is the recent inclusion of payment for the evidence-based collaborative care model of integrated behavioral health by Medicare (29). Medicare's alternative payment model pays a monthly rate for integrated care services provided by behavioral health workers as well as for indirect psychiatric consultation time (30). This payment model allows the workers to provide case management services that may not always be billable services with face-to-face service codes.

The integration of mental health services into primary care settings offers the opportunity for the leader in public psychiatry to extend the reach of a limited mental health workforce and thereby improve access to psychiatric care for patients who might otherwise go without it. It is an opportunity for the public psychiatrist to provide leadership that impacts population health in his or her community.

Leading Physician Well-Being

The challenges to physician well-being are many, including career dissatisfaction, high rates of depression, and even suicide. Because of concern for physicians and their patients, guiding principles have been offered to assist physicians and physician leaders in addressing physician well-being (31). In particular, physician burnout—a recognized syndrome characterized by fatigue, lack of engagement, and cynicism—is known to negatively impact the quality of care provided by physicians, as well as lead to increased turnover. Just as in the rest of medicine, the impact of burnout is a significant issue for psychiatrists in leadership positions in public mental health. Research shows that the risk of burnout is greater for psychiatrists, including early career psychiatrists, than for other physicians (32). In addition, burnout is an issue among other mental health clinicians who might be working in the clinic or hospital (33). Because of these negative effects, public psychiatrists in leadership positions must take ownership of the problem rather than viewing burnout as an issue for individual physicians to address themselves (34).

A meta-analysis of studies on physician burnout showed that it doubles the likelihood of unsafe care, unprofessional behaviors, and/or low patient satisfaction (35). In addition to the impact on patients, the psychiatrists and other clinicians with burnout suffer personally, through reduced physical and emotional well-being. They also self-report more depression, anxiety, sleep disturbance, and memory impairment (36). Finally, burnout has been identified as a key factor driving turnover in public sector mental health clinics and hospitals (37). For the medical director of a community mental health center, for example, turnover means time spent funding, recruiting, hiring, and training a new physician for the clinic's team—a time-consuming and expensive process.

In order to develop strategies to address the problem of burnout, it is important to understand its possible roots. Factors associated with burnout in mental health settings include self-reports of high workloads, long hours, aggressive management, and lack of support from administration (38). Clinicians also note the barriers to quality care as factors, including inadequate facilities, poor funding, and the challenges of working with difficult patients (39). One pilot study also noted an association of burnout with the amount of time spent charting in electronic medical records (40). By contrast, physicians with a high sense of calling are less likely to report burnout (41). Other protective factors against burnout in psychiatrists include supportive relationships, extracurricular activities, and a variety in workplace tasks (42).

However, data concerning interventions for physician burnout are insufficient to recommend particular interventions (43). Two types of interventions are usually employed. Organization-directed interventions aim to remove the causes of job stress. Examples include across-the-board work-hour reductions, task restructuring, work evaluation, supervision aimed at identifying ways to restructure job duties or workflow to reduce stress and frustration, increasing job autonomy, and increasing the level of participation in decision-making. The other approach is person-directed interventions. Examples include enhancement of job competencies; building coping skills; and working to improve resilience through, for example, cognitive approaches to frustration and negative emotions (44).

Resources available to leaders working to develop interventions include the American Psychiatric Association's Workgroup on Psychiatrist Well-being and Burnout. It offers a website with an extensive list of individual interventions for burnout and links to the Stanford Medicine WellMD Center (45). The first step in ensuring patients served by public mental health hospitals and clinics receive excellent care is to ensure the well-being of the physicians who care for them. Leaders in public psychiatry can help increase well-being and reduce physician burnout by fostering collaborative efforts between the physician staff and the hospital or clinic to help physicians succeed in their personal commitments to patients and to the organization's mission (31).

Training for Psychiatrist Leaders

Community psychiatrists often find themselves serving in leadership positions based on their strong clinical performance in the clinic rather than on any demonstrable administrative training or experience. Thrown into the new role with few skills in how to be an effective administrator and leader, it would seem easy for psychiatrists to feel overwhelmed and inadequate to the task.

It has been suggested that this problem might be addressed by incorporating leadership training into residency training. Indeed, the curriculum of many psychiatry residency programs includes some seminar material on the administrative aspects of psychiatric practice. However, topics such as finance, workflow management, business law, human resource policy, and information technology are seldom taught in any detail. In addition, the lack of consensus on what constitutes leadership, or essential training therein, can lead to challenges in training physicians for leadership roles (46, 47).

However, psychiatrists who find themselves in public sector leadership positions can pursue other educational strategies, including a public psychiatry fellowship, or pursue a degree in health administration or business administration (48). Pursuit of a second degree in business or health administration is a particularly popular goal. Studies suggest that physicians with a degree in health or business administration are in a better position to face their leadership challenges. One study of physicians who earned a master's degree in business administration showed that more than 80% found the added degree to be very useful in career advancement (49, 50).

EXEMPLARY LEADERS IN PUBLIC PSYCHIATRY

Current and past community psychiatrists who have taken on leadership roles can serve as inspiration to young psychiatrists seeking to make a difference in their communities. Reaching out to find mentorship may help identify and develop skills that allow public psychiatrists to be viewed as leaders in their organizations and communities (48). Similarly, reviewing the stories of historical leaders may help public psychiatrists develop a personal vision as well as consider various career pathways that might foster the attainment of their leadership goals. Some exemplary histories are presented here.

Benjamin Rush

Due to his role in the Congress of 1776 and his signature on the Declaration of Independence, Benjamin Rush is probably the most famous American physician of the 1700s. But for many years, Rush led Pennsylvania Hospital, affiliated with the College of Philadelphia, where he was on faculty. Distraught at the dismal conditions in the hospital for the mentally ill, he advocated for the construction of a separate ward intended to provide amenities for longer term living—an asylum for the stigmatized. At a time when stigma toward the mentally ill meant that they were often treated worse than criminals (restraint using chains was not uncommon), Rush advocated for less violent ways of providing care. He was strongly invested in ensuring that patients' psychosocial needs— housing, clothing, and food—were met as well. At a time long before substance use disorders were known to be chronic diseases, he advocated for "sober houses" as treatment facilities (51). He was an abolitionist, against capital punishment, and an advocate of penal reform (52).

Rush was a graduate of the College of New Jersey. For his medical training, he apprenticed with physicians affiliated with the College of Philadelphia and then received a medical degree from the University of Edinburgh. After training, he returned to Philadelphia and joined the faculty at the College of Philadelphia, where he spent most of his medical career (53).

The "father of American psychiatry," Rush was a leader in every sense of the word. Within his organization, he helped improve the quality of care received by people with mental illness. Within his community, he urged that social determinants of health be addressed. And, of course, he was a political leader during the formation of the United States.

Adolf Meyer

Adolf Meyer was arguably the most well-known psychiatrist in the United States in the first half of the 20th century. He served as the CEO of the Johns Hopkins Hospital psychiatric clinic in the days when the positions of medical director and CEO were combined. He is probably best known in psychiatry for leading the movement that transitioned preeminence in psychiatry from the state psychiatric hospitals into academia. He trained generations of psychiatrists and consulted to government and academia in ways that continue to influence public policy and training in psychiatry until this day.

As an exemplary leader for the contemporary public psychiatrist, Meyer is even more important for his extraordinary ability to leverage partnerships with other mental health care reformers toward improving the lives of people with mental illness. Meyer is viewed, for example, as one of the founders of occupational therapy. When Meyer started the Johns Hopkins Hospital psychiatry clinic, he immediately hired Eleanor Clark Slagle, who was a major leader in the early days of occupational therapy. Meyer and Slagle shared an orientation toward occupational therapy as a discipline about socialization rather than making things and thus could be used as a tool in the treatment of some of the social sequelae of mental illness (54).

Most famously, Meyer linked up with Clifford Beers, who was a former patient of both private and public hospitals. Beers was a vocal advocate for state mental hospital reform, and Meyers helped channel Beers' focus from raising awareness of the poor conditions in hospitals to advocating for prevention through a focus on what they termed "mental hygiene." The organization known today as Mental Health America stemmed from their work together (55).

Based on his training and early career goals, Meyer seemed unlikely to become a national leader in public psychiatry. He emigrated to the United Stated from Switzerland soon after earning his doctoral degree. He was actually a neuropathologist, and his first job was as a pathologist for a state hospital in Illinois. He then served (after a sabbatical spent studying with Emil Kraepelin) at Worcester State Hospital in Massachusetts, after which he worked for the state of New York as the lead of pathology for the entire state psychiatric system. Frustrated by his inability to perform a good autopsy in the state psychiatric hospitals because of the quality of the medical care and recordkeeping, he gained a reputation for championing the application of scientific principles to the treatment of diseases seen in the New York hospital system. When the steel magnate Henry Phipps provided money to build a psychiatric clinic at Johns Hopkins, Meyer was chosen to lead it (56).

Meyer's work offers an example of the importance of collaborative work with other advocates and stakeholders when seeking to improve care for people with mental illness. Collective voices are often more powerful than a single one. Meyer's career demonstrates the unexpected pathways along which an emerging passion might lead.

Gloria Johnson-Powell

Gloria Johnson-Powell was a medical student at Meharry Medical College in Nashville, Tennessee, when she became distracted by her participation in nonviolent workshops with many emerging student civil rights leaders. She was pivotal in the formation of the Student Nonviolent Coordinating Committee, "accepting the challenge and throwing down the gauntlet that would ultimately prevail in bringing at least partial end to the long, dark night of America's racial rottenness" (57). She was among the leaders of the freedom rides, helping to lead sit-ins, kneel-ins, and voter registration drives of the 1960s. That work with several other student civil rights workers is chronicled in David Halberstam's 1999 book, *The Children*.

Like Meyer, Johnson-Powell did not immediately gravitate to psychiatry. She did her undergraduate training at Mount Holyoke College before medical school. Consumed by her civil rights work, she finished medical school only after being admonished by

Martin Luther King, Jr., to do so. She completed her residency in psychiatry and fellowship in child psychiatry at the Neuropsychiatric Institute at the University of California in Los Angeles and then taught there for many years before joining the faculty at Harvard Medical School and, later, the University of Wisconsin, where she was Dean for Cultural Diversity. She continued her advocacy throughout her psychiatric career. Indeed, it was her work that led to the creation of the National Center on Minority Health Disparities, a division of the National Institutes of Health (58).

Like Rush, Johnson-Powell served as an important leader on issues outside of mental health. Like Meyer, her career trajectory into psychiatry was not a straight one, but her experiences also allowed her to be a powerful voice on, for example, the impact of segregation and child abuse on children and their mental health.

LEADERSHIP ETHICS

Ethics are the cornerstone of leadership. The nature of the work in public psychiatry, especially its focus on service to people with chronic illnesses who also face difficult psychosocial challenges such as housing and income, brings special challenges in leadership ethics beyond the broader leadership issues of "doing the right thing," ensuring that others in the organization do so as well, and fostering the well-being of the organization as a whole for the sake of the patients it serves (59).

Because of these unique issues, the American Association of Psychiatric Administrators developed a more specific set of annotations to ethical principles applicable to physicians. Although those principles reassert the leader's primary commitment to patients (inclusive of broader issues such as maintaining boundaries and confidentiality), the principles also emphasize the responsibility of the psychiatrist leader to the clinicians and other workers who serve those patients, including insisting upon their primary commitment to patients but also to their own well-being. They also call upon the psychiatrist leader to insist upon legal and honest behavior, high character, and clinical competence in herself and in other staff. The principles take into consideration pressures that public sector psychiatrists experience due to poor funding and encourage the psychiatric leader to help ensure that the organization provides the best possible care given the resource limitations. Advocacy for quality improvement planning and outcome measures is also an important role of the psychiatrist in leadership. Finally, the principles emphasize the important role of psychiatrist leaders in fighting the stigma about mental illness and in helping their communities address the social determinants of mental health (59).

A VIGNETTE

Dr. Adams serves as medical director of a public psychiatric hospital. The director of nursing approaches her about Dr. Bell, one of the psychiatrists who provides weekend coverage only. The weekend nursing staff report that Dr. Bell frequently forgets to order medications for patients and orders inappropriate dosages that he readily changes when confronted. Dr. Bell has a long-standing and very positive reputation in the community, where he served on the medical school faculty prior to his retirement. Indeed, he was a supervisor to Dr. Adams during her medical school rotation in psychiatry. No issues with Dr. Bell have been raised through routine medical records reviews.

Physicians in leadership roles may have difficultly confronting concerns related to their ethical responsibilities to ensure staff competency, generally, but it is especially difficult when it is a senior colleague who has served as a mentor in the past. Nonetheless, physicians have an obligation—especially when in a leadership position—to address concerns about physician competency, whether the concerns are cognitive, substance related, medical problems, or psychosocial distractions. However, leaders also have an obligation to act ethically toward physicians identified as possibly impaired. Decisions that may affect the physician's ability to continue to practice medicine can have a significant impact on the physician's self-worth and autonomy, which in turn may affect overall health.

In the previous vignette, there are many possible reasons for the nursing staff's concerns. Therefore, the medical director might meet with the physician to give him feedback about the nursing staff's concerns and get his perspective. If a physician is not yet ready to acknowledge an identified problem, other steps may have to be taken, such as insisting on a medical or psychiatric evaluation as a stipulation for continuing to practice in the hospital or even a referral for formal peer review.

Public psychiatrists must wrestle with ethics related to societal issues as well. For example, a community mental health center may struggle with the balance between rationing access to services offered to the community and meeting the needs of current patients.

A VIGNETTE

Dr. Elder is the medical director of a clinic that is having problems with a high no-show rate. In leadership meetings, the question arises as to how much time and effort should be spent trying to find and engage patients struggling with making appointments, especially because the community mental health center has no funding allocated to case management that is not provided face-to-face. The chief financial officer, worried about the center's tight budget, advocates for using clinician time to care for patients who are coming to clinic and making progress on their treatment plans. She argues that they are most likely to benefit from the limited dollars available for services (60).

This vignette reflects the possible ethical dilemma of balancing the community's needs with finite resources that taxpayers, through their elected representatives, have chosen to allocate to the center. Although there is no right or wrong solution to this problem, it does reinforce the physician leader's responsibility to optimize stewardship of available resources so that the most good can be done for the most people. For example, some argue that leaders have an ethical responsibility to educate themselves about clinical operations and quality management that optimize access to care and quality in funding-constrained clinics (61). In the vignette, the medical director therefore might work to ensure that workflow in the clinic is efficient, allowing the same staff to see more patients or else make time for the outreach services. Similarly, some argue for the ethical imperative upon public health physicians to advocate for policy and law changes to impact those whom they serve, including adequate funding not only for mental health care but also for housing and employment for the challenged in our communities (60). In the vignette, the medical director might, for example, get involved in advocating for changes in the policies that disallow reimbursement for outreach services that are not face-to-face.

The vignette also demonstrates that the organizational and community activities in which the psychiatrist leader chooses to engage can be ethical and still highly personal choices, as the principles described previously acknowledge. However, the psychiatrist leader would, at the very least, seem to have an obligation to put his training and experience to work within his organization and community to help find acceptable answers to the ethical dilemmas faced by organizations and communities committed to serving people with mental illness (59).

CASE STUDY: CONCLUSION

As medical director of the clinic where John and his family present for care, your role in his care goes beyond the prescribing of medication for his ADHD. You will also play a leadership role in addressing systemic challenges that the community mental health center faces, including issues such as access to care (e.g., the wait list that John was on), balancing available funding for care with the community needs, community attitudes toward mental illness, and even the attitude of front desk staff in your clinic. You may also have the opportunity to address the balance between access to care and quality of care by encouraging center leadership to optimize clinic efficiencies through workflow changes and ensuring that all clinicians are working at the top of their respective licenses.

Externally, you might also serve as an advocate for adequate funding to ensure ready access to care, or you might help local public sector health centers, such as the federally qualified health center in this case, to develop integrated models of care that increase access in the community. On the other hand, in order to deal with John's difficulty accessing medical care, you might advocate for integrated care in your center, perhaps revamping clinical care to further take on an integrated medicine approach as a more cost-effective approach while also providing higher quality care for patients. Integrating medical and psychiatric care would make it much easier to manage the patient's thyroid abnormalities and determine the extent to which these may be contributing to his psychiatric presentation.

REFERENCES

1. Charles Bell, essays on the anatomy of. Wellcome Collection. Retrieved January 3, 2019, from https://wellcomecollection.org/works/p7pfamk7
2. A. Neher. Sir Charles Bell and the anatomy of expression. *RACAR: Revue d'art Canadienne/Canadian Art Review.* 2008:33(1–2);59–65.
3. Poetry Foundation. The Waste Land by T. S. Eliot. January 3, 2019. Retrieved January 4, 2019, from https://www.poetryfoundation.org/poems/47311/the-waste-land
4. A. J. Harris. T. S. Eliot's Mental Hygiene. *Journal of Modern Literature.* 2006;29(4):44–56.
5. J. Ranz, A. Stueve, & H. L. McQuistion. The role of the psychiatrist: Job satisfaction of medical directors and staff psychiatrists. *Community Mental Health Journal.* 2002;37(6):525–539.
6. J. Ranz & A. Stueve. The role of the psychiatrist as program medical director. *Psychiatric Services.* 1998;49(9):1203–1207.
7. S. Isobel. "Because that's the way it's always been done": Reviewing the nurse-initiated rules in a mental health unit as a step toward trauma-informed care. *Issues in Mental Health Nursing.* 2015;36(4):272–278.
8. L. Espinosa et al. Milieu improvement in psychiatry using evidence-based practices: The long and winding road of culture change. *Archives of Psychiatric Nursing.* 2015;29(4):202–207.
9. C. Muskett. Trauma-informed care in inpatient mental health settings: A review of the literature. *International Journal of Mental Health Nursing.* 2014;23(1):51–59.
10. R. Knight. When your boss is younger than you. *Harvard Business Review.* Oct. 2015.
11. T. Erickson. On young bosses and older direct reports. *Harvard Business Review.* Mar. 2008.
12. J. Ranz, H. L. McQuistion, & A. Stueve. The role of the community psychiatrist as medical director: A delineation of job types. *Psychiatric Services.* 2000;51(7):930–932.
13. L. Rosenstein, R. Sadun, & A. Jena. Why doctors need leadership training. *Harvard Business Review.* Oct. 2018.
14. D. P. Tarantino. Understanding financial statements. *Physician Executive.* 2001:27(5);72.
15. C. Spears. Negotiating insurance contracts—Is there any hope? *Urologic Clinics of North America.* 2005;32(3):271–273.
16. R. Town, R. Feldman, & J. Kralewski. Market power and contract form: Evidence from physician group practices. *International Journal of Health Care Finance and Economics.* 2011;11(2):115–132.
17. D. Ramadevi, A. Gunasekaran, B. K. Rai, S. A. Senthilkumar, & M. Roy. Human resource management in a healthcare environment: Framework and case study. *Industrial and Commercial Training.* 2016;48(8):387–393.
18. P. E. French. Employment laws and the public sector employer: Lessons to be learned from a review of lawsuits filed against local governments. *Public Administration Review.* 2009;69(1):92–103.

19. A. Chandrasekaran, C. Senot, & K. K. Boyer. Process management impact on clinical and experiential quality: Managing tensions between safe and patient-centered healthcare. *Manufacturing & Service Operations Management*. 2012;14(4):548–566.

20. National Association of State Mental Health Program Directors. The role of the medical director in a state mental health authority: A guide for policymakers. Dec. 2009. Retrieved from https://www.nasmhpd.org/sites/default/files/The%20Role%20of%20the%20Medical%20Director%20-%2012-09.pdf

21. B. M. McGrath & R. P. Tempier. Implementing quality management in psychiatry: From theory to practice—Shifting focus from process to outcome. *Canadian Journal of Psychiatry*. 2003;48(7):467–474.

22. World Health Organization. Quality improvement for mental health. 2003. Retrieved from https://www.who.int/mental_health/policy/services/essentialpackage1v8/en

23. S. Lauriks, M. C. Buster, M. A. de Wit, O. A. Arah, & N. S. Klazinga. Performance indicators for public mental healthcare: A systematic international inventory. *BMC Public Health*. 2012;12(1):214.

24. C. J. Miller, A. Grogan-Kaylor, B. E. Perron, A. M. Kilbourne, E. Woltmann, & M. S. Bauer. Collaborative chronic care models for mental health conditions: Cumulative meta-analysis and metaregression to guide future research and implementation. *Medical Care*. 2013;51(10):922–930.

25. J. R. Asarnow, M. Rozenman, J. Wiblin, & L. Zeltzer. Integrated medical–behavioral care compared with usual primary care for child and adolescent behavioral health: A meta-analysis. *JAMA Pediatrics*. 2015;169(10):929–937.

26. N. B. Baskerville, C. Liddy, & W. Hogg. Systematic review and meta-analysis of practice facilitation within primary care settings. *Annals of Family Medicine*. 2012;10(1):63–74.

27. C. B. Stetler et al. Role of "external facilitation" in implementation of research findings: A qualitative evaluation of facilitation experiences in the Veterans Health Administration. *Implementation Science*. 2006;1(1):23.

28. W. P. Dickinson. Strategies to support the integration of behavioral health and primary care: What have we learned thus far? *Journal of the American Board of Family Medicine*. 2015;28(Suppl 1):S102–S106.

29. J. Archer et al. Collaborative care for depression and anxiety problems. *Cochrane Database of Systematic Reviews*. 2012;28(10).

30. Center for Medicare and Medicaid Services. Behavioral health integration services. *Medicare Learning Network*. Jan 2018;ICN 909432.

31. L. R. Thomas, J. A. Ripp, & C. P. West. Charter on physician well-being. *JAMA*. 2018;319(15):1541–1542

32. I. J. Deary, R. M. Agius, & A. Sadler. Personality and stress in consultant psychiatrists. *International Journal of Social Psychiatry*. 1996;42(2):112–123.

33. G. Morse, M. Salyers, A. Rollins, M. Monroe-DeVita, & C. Pfahler. Burnout in mental health services: A review of the problem and its remediation. *Administration and Policy in Mental Health and Mental Health Services Research*. 2012;39(5):341–352.

34. T. D. Shanafelt & J. H. Noseworthy. Executive leadership and physician well-being: Nine organizational strategies to promote engagement and reduce burnout. *Mayo Clinic Proceedings*. 2017;92(1):129.

35. M. Panagioti et al. Association between physician burnout and patient safety, professionalism, and patient satisfaction: A systematic review and meta-analysis. *JAMA Internal Medicine*. 2018;178(10):1317–1330.

36. U. Peterson, E. Demerouti, G. Bergström, M. Samuelsson, M. Åsberg, & Å. Nygren. Burnout and physical and mental health among Swedish healthcare workers. *Journal of Advanced Nursing*. 2008;62(1):84–95.

37. M. A. Hoge et al. A national action plan for workforce development in behavioral health. *Psychiatric Services*. 2009;60(7):883–887.

38. S. Kumar, S. Hatcher, G. Dutu, J. Fischer, & E. Ma'u. Stresses experienced by psychiatrists and their role in burnout: A national follow-up study. *International Journal of Social Psychiatry*. 2011;57(2):166–179.

39. C. Bressi et al. Burnout among psychiatrists in Milan: A multicenter survey. *Psychiatric Services*. 2009;60(7):985–988.

40. N. M. Domaney, J. Torous, & W. E. Greenberg. Exploring the association between electronic health record use and burnout among psychiatry residents and faculty: A pilot survey study. *Academic Psychiatry*. 2018;42(5):648–652.

41. J. Yoon, B. Daley, & F. Curlin. The association between a sense of calling and physician well-being: A national study of primary care physicians and psychiatrists. *Academic Psychiatry*. 2017;41(2):167–173.

42. J. Fischer, S. Kumar, & S. Hatcher. What makes psychiatry such a stressful profession? A qualitative study. *Australas Psychiatry*. 2007;15(5):417–421.

43. S. Kalani, P. Azadfallah, H. Oreyzi, & P. Adibi. Interventions for physician burnout: A systematic review of systematic reviews. *International Journal of Preventive Medicine*. 2018;9(1):81.

44. W. L. Awa, M. Plaumann, & U. Walter. Burnout prevention: A review of intervention programs. *Patient Education and Counseling*. 2010;78(2):184–190.

45. Well-being and burnout. Retrieved January 11, 2019, from https://www.psychiatry.org/psychiatrists/practice/well-being-and-burnout

46. F. Mohyuddin, A. J. Mathai, P. Weinberg, & S. A. Saeed. Career paths and trends: How does one become a leader in psychiatric administration? Implications for residency training. *Psychiatric Quarterly*. 2015;86(3):325–335.

47. R. Yu-Chin. Teaching administration and management within psychiatric residency training. *Academic Psychiatry*. 2002;26(4):245–252.

48. W. Sowers, D. Pollack, A. Everett, K. S. Thompson, J. Ranz, & A. Primm. Progress in workforce development since 2000: Advanced training opportunities in public and community psychiatry. *Psychiatric Services*. 2011;62(7):782–788.

49. A. D. Turner, S. P. Stawicki, & W. A. Guo. Competitive advantage of MBA for physician executives: A systematic literature review. *World Journal of Surgery*. 2018;42(6):1655–1665.

50. S. G. Parekh & B. Singh. An MBA: The utility and effect on physicians' careers. *Journal of Bone & Joint Surgery*. 2007;89(2):442–447.

51. F. Wittels. The contribution of Benjamin Rush to psychiatry. *Bulletin of the History of Medicine*. 1946;20(2):157–166.

52. S. Altschuler & C. J. Bilodeau. Ecce homo! The figure of Benjamin Rush. *Early American Studies*. 2017;15(2):233–251.

53. D. Hosack. Biography: Art. XIII. A tribute to the memory of the late Dr. Benjamin Rush. *Philadelphia Journal of the Medical and Physical Sciences (1820–1827)*. 1823;7(13):162.

54. S. Lamb. Social skills: Adolf Meyer's revision of clinical skill for the new psychiatry of the twentieth century. *Medical History*. 2015;59(3):443–464.

55. E. E. Winters. Adolf Meyer and Clifford Beers, 1907–1910. *Bulletin of the History of Medicine*. 1969;43(5):414–443.

56. S. Lamb. "The most important professorship in the English-speaking domain": Adolf Meyer and the beginnings of clinical psychiatry in the United States. *Journal of Nervous and Mental Disease*. 2012;200(12):1061–1066.

57. W. Campbell. The children shall lead. *Sojourners*. 1998;27(3):42–46.

58. J. Stanley. Passing the movement's torch. *Philadelphia Tribune*. January 16, 2011;2C, 6C.

59. H. Steven Moffic, S. A. Saeed, S. Silver, & S. Koh. Ethical challenges in psychiatric administration and leadership. *Psychiatric Quarterly*. 2015;86(3):343–354.

60. A. Everett & C. Huffine. Ethics in contemporary community psychiatry. *Psychiatric Clinics of North America*. 2009;32(2):329–341.

61. J. P. Merlino, J. Petit, L. Weisser, & J. Bowen. Leading with lean: Getting the outcomes we need with the funding we have. *Psychiatric Quarterly*. 2015;86(3):301–310.

7

THE PUBLIC PSYCHIATRIST AS EDUCATOR

SARAH E. BAKER AND ADAM BRENNER

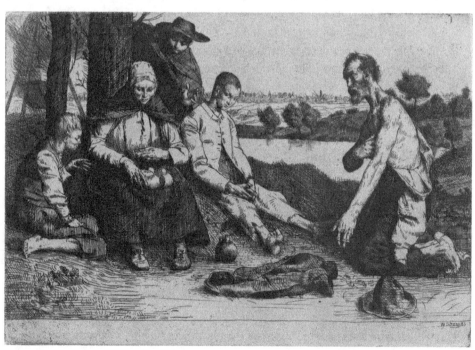

FIGURE 7.1 William Strang, *Meal Time*, 1883, etching.

William Strang was a Scottish printmaker of the late 19th and early 20th centuries. His teacher was Alphonse Legros, whose etchings are featured in other chapters of this book, and his sympathy for the poor has been compared to that of Legros (Figure 7.1) (1).

CASE STUDY: INITIAL PRESENTATION

You are recruited across country to become the medical director of a large urban community mental health center. You did your residency training in a program that had strong community psychiatry rotations and didactics, and these experiences led to your interest and career in public psychiatry. Upon accepting your current position, you were surprised to learn that you would not be working with any trainees. In fact, there are no trainees rotating through the center despite the two medical schools in the city. You have noted the reports of a shortage of community psychiatrists in the state and wonder whether the lack of training opportunities might be contributing. You decide to look into creating an opportunity for medical students and psychiatry residents to train in your center.

QUESTIONS
1. What are some reasons for the shortage in community psychiatrists?
2. What are the benefits of training programs for recruitment to community psychiatry? What other benefits do these training opportunities provide?
3. What might a training opportunity look like in a community setting?
4. What are the challenges that must be addressed in setting up clerkships and rotations in a public sector community mental health center?

PSYCHIATRY AND LITERATURE

On Teaching
by Kahlil Gibran (2)

Then said a teacher, Speak to us of Teaching.
And he said:
No man can reveal to you aught but that which already lies half asleep in the dawning of your knowledge.
The teacher who walks in the shadow of the temple, among his followers, gives not of his wisdom but rather of his faith and his lovingness.
If he is indeed wise he does not bid you enter the house of his wisdom, but rather leads you to the threshold of your own mind.
The astronomer may speak to you of his understanding of space, but he cannot give you his understanding.

The musician may sing to you of the rhythm which is in all space, but he cannot give you the ear which arrests the rhythm nor the voice that echoes it.

And he who is versed in the science of numbers can tell of the regions of weight and measure, but he cannot conduct you thither.

For the vision of one man lends not its wings to another man.

And even as each one of you stands alone in God's knowledge, so must each one of you be alone in his knowledge of God and in his understanding of the earth.

Kahlil Gibran was born in 1883 in Lebanon but emigrated at age 2 years to live in a Lebanese community in Boston. In 1923, he published what would become his most famous work, *The Prophet*. Although not critically acclaimed, it became popular in the 1960s as an alternative to established religion because it offered a less dogmatic form of spirituality (3).

INTRODUCTION

The public psychiatrist is a teacher in many contexts. She provides education to patients about their illnesses and about strategies for recovery. She answers questions from fellow clinical staff on topics such as medications. She adds her voice to leadership discussions about the quality of care from her unique perspective. And she is called upon by advocates and community leaders to educate the community on mental health and mental illness. These are all important roles that help reduce stigmatization, encourage understanding, and foster adherence to treatment plans. In addition to these important educator roles, the community psychiatrist may also be called upon to serve as a teacher for trainees in the medical profession, a role that is the subject of this chapter.

Academic–community partnership arose in the 1970s out of growing concern about the struggles of an underfunded public mental health system to meet the needs of the chronically mentally ill in state hospitals and in the community. Collaborations of academic medicine with community mental health centers and state hospitals were considered as a solution to the increasing need for psychiatrists in the public sector as well as a way to foster quality of care for the chronically mentally ill. The collaborations were also viewed as potentially offering additional opportunities for research and as a means to offer cutting-edge treatment to public sector populations (4). In addition to these historic reasons for partnering, there are other reasons to foster training in community settings, all of which can be used by public psychiatrists in making the case for educational partnership to psychiatry department chairs and community center chief executive officers. These are discussed later.

PUBLIC SECTOR WORKFORCE DEVELOPMENT

Educational experiences in community psychiatry have repeatedly been linked with a higher likelihood that trainees will practice in a public setting after graduation. For example, the Maryland Plan, a joint initiative between the Maryland Mental Hygiene Administration and the University of Maryland's Department of Psychiatry, was intended to "'destigmatize' state psychiatry by recruiting large numbers of graduates of university psychiatric training programs into state service" (5). Before the initiation of the project, 7 out of 57 residents (12%) entered practice in a public setting immediately after graduation. In the first 15 years of the program, 78 of 164 graduates (48%) entered public sector practice.

This result is not unique to Maryland. Oregon's investment in public sector training opportunities was also successful. After the development of a community psychiatry training program, 73% of residents involved with the program took positions in public sector psychiatry (6). In South Carolina, after the addition of public psychiatry electives, the time residency graduates spent in public sector during their first year out of training more than doubled (7). In New York, 92% of graduates of Columbia University's Public Psychiatry Fellowship work in public settings (8).

Early exposure to community psychiatry may be especially important to recruitment. A study from Columbia University asked psychiatry residents throughout the country (and from all 4 years of training) about their interest in community psychiatry. The study found that trainees in their first and second years of postgraduate training were more likely to express an interest in fellowship training in community psychiatry compared with third- and fourth-year residents. The authors indicated that this could be due to initial excitement about psychiatry found early on in training and suggested that residency training could capitalize on this enthusiasm by providing early clinical experiences in community psychiatry (9).

ACADEMIC ACCREDITATION REQUIREMENTS

Training in community psychiatry is a core requirement of the Accreditation Council for Graduate Medical Education (ACGME). Although the clinical requirements are not specific, residents are required to have exposure to public sector populations, including exposure to community-based case management and work within multidisciplinary systems of care (10).

Community psychiatry is also mentioned throughout the ACGME Milestones project. For example, the systems-based practice domain "community-based care" promotes familiarity with resources in the community, such as community support groups, as well as skills in coordination of care with community centers. The highest level of achievement for this milestone includes development and leadership of community programs. This milestone also recognizes the importance of the recovery model. References to the community also appear in the system-based practice domain of "resource management." For this milestone, residents must not only recognize health disparities but also "coordinat[e] patient access to community and system resources" (11).

The American Academic of Medical Colleges also recognizes the importance of community mental health care in its Medical Students' Objective Project under the "physicians must be dutiful" objective. This objective emphasizes understanding health disparities, knowledge of approaches to health care organization, and a dedication to provide care even to those who cannot pay for it and to advocate for a more equitable system of health care (12). All of these objectives may be achieved through community psychiatry clinical experiences.

FOSTERING EMPATHY

Positive educational experiences with public sector patients can foster empathy toward traditionally stigmatized populations. Studies from psychiatry clerkships indicate that increased exposure to psychiatric patients can lead to enhanced understanding of the social and biological factors of illness as well as the importance of patient narrative (13–15). In an editorial about her experience on an outreach team during residency, psychiatry resident Hermioni Lokko notes its impact on her empathy for the homeless, writing, "Going on homeless outreach as part of my community psychiatry rotation allowed me to see my homeless patients through a different lens as I spent more time in their world, reflecting on their strengths and their sources of hope" (16). It is true, as Kahlil Gibran seems to argue in the passage at the beginning of this chapter, that experience is the best teacher.

CASE STUDY: CONTINUED

With the consent of your center's chief executive officer, you decide to speak to the residency training director of one of the local psychiatry residency programs to determine if there is any interest in developing a partnership between your center and the department. To your delight, the residency training director already had identified community psychiatry as a relative weakness in his program and was happy to help foster a collaboration. He asks how you envision funding new rotations at your center.

PARTNERSHIPS

In order to be successful, partnerships between academia and the public sector must address the needs of the institutions involved. Those needs can be diverse. Medical schools have a mission to educate and to set standards for quality of medical care, but they also have a mission to foster research. State hospitals and community centers have a mission of service focused on access to care and stewardship of limited public dollars. Successful partnerships seek the common ground in these diverse missions. In addition, successful partnerships address the issue of financial sustainability of the training program, and they provide for a shared leadership structure to foster success.

Talbott et al. (4) outline four principles for the formation of a successful academic–public partnership. First, a common goal between the medical school and the community center or state hospital must be agreed upon, most likely rooted in their shared commitment to improving the lives of people who live with mental illness. Second, the ways in which academic and public sector can help meet each other's goals must be determined. For example, medical schools can benefit from the unique training and research opportunities offered in public settings, and public programs can benefit from the workforce that a medical school can offer. Third, public sector workforce development should be viewed as a primary goal of the partnership. Finally, the collaborations should include translational research programs that bring new solutions to the problems faced by public sector patients.

Faulkner et al. (17) outline a four-step process for development of a partnership. The first step is exploratory discussions, in which the institutions learn about respective philosophies and goals and use these to explore partnership possibilities. The second step is contract negotiations, in which specific objectives and obligations are delineated. Faulkner et al. encourage objectives to be overt. For example, the medical school might have the goal of funding new faculty positions or of offering more training opportunities, whereas the community center or hospital may be seeking to increase psychiatric coverage for services. Clarity of roles and authority should occur at this stage, as well as clarity about the financial relationship. Third, a contract is written and executed. It should include the specifics agreed upon in the negotiations as well as leadership structure and early termination procedures. Finally, ongoing monitoring and evaluation should occur. Regular feedback from all parties should lead to modifications in the relationship, as needed.

LEADERSHIP

Given the diverse interests and obligations of academic and public sector institutions, strong administrative leadership is required to ensure the success of joint educational projects. There are many competing interests that may leave both academic and public administrators wary of such collaborations. Chairs of psychiatry departments, for example, may fear that expansion of the residency training program using state dollars will leave the department vulnerable to changing political winds that might lead to withdrawal of support. Public sector administrators, on the other hand, might fear that the academic interest in research and training will overshadow delivering clinical care (4).

Talbott et al. (4) suggest formalizing a shared project leadership and support structure that can build trust for the long term. The leadership team might include the chair and residency training director from the psychiatry department and the chief executive officer (or hospital superintendent) and medical director from the public entity.

FINANCING

One of the major barriers to academic public partnerships is finding a viable and sustainable source of funding for the cost of resident and fellow rotations. Especially for academic departments of psychiatry, sustainable fiscal support that will allow long-term commitment to training in public settings is essential to the stability of residency training programs that have 4- or 5-year cycles. Typically, the community center or state hospital must pay the institution that sponsors the residency or fellowship positions for the time allocated to the public setting. In addition, from the perspective of a community center administrator, attending time spent in supervision is time away from seeing patients and so also has an associated cost that must be financed in some way.

One strategy to help pay for resident and fellow time is to bill public and commercial insurers for the services provided by the trainees under the supervision of the attending physician. Rules for doing this vary by insurer. For example, Medicare pays for services provided by a psychiatry resident only when an attending physician is physically present during the critical or key portions of the service. There is a primary care exception to the "critical or key" rule, and some psychiatry training settings may qualify for that exception if the setting provides comprehensive integrated care to the psychiatric patients—that is, if the setting functions as a health home to the patient (18). Medicaid rules may vary by state. They often follow Medicare rules but sometimes are more flexible, allowing, for example, the attending physician to simply be on site with the resident to consult and to co-sign medical record notations. Commercial insurance companies often follow Medicare billing rules, but contract terms are typically negotiable.

However, residents and fellows spend a significant portion of time in activities that are not billable. In addition, attending physicians are taken away from providing services themselves when supervising the clinical care of residents. Leaders in public sector training settings grapple with how to pay for these important activities. Throughout the years, many states have addressed this problem by allocating dollars to fund residency training positions and the associated faculty supervision time in state hospital and community centers using a variety of models.

In Ohio, for example, the state agreed to pay for faculty positions at a state-supported medical school to be placed in public mental health settings. A primary responsibility for these faculty was to develop residency training experiences in the community centers that met the needs of both the center and the medical school. From a workforce development perspective, the results were robust. More than half of residents who completed their psychiatric residencies took public psychiatry positions (19).

Many states, including Oregon, traditionally funded stipends for psychiatric residency positions within the state hospital system. Oregon later transferred stipends to Oregon Health Sciences University, where they were used to also create supervising faculty positions at the state hospital (6). Texas now uses similar historic funding of state hospital-based resident positions to fund resident positions in Texas state medical schools in return for clinical service in the state hospitals and community centers.

Public psychiatry fellowships have been funded in a number of ways. Columbia University uses a combination of dollars appropriated from the state with dollars paid by the community centers at which the fellows see patients (20). The University of California at San Francisco combines state support specifically for faculty and administration with local support in return for clinical care by the fellows (21). Yale University has a program completely funded by the state, whereas the University of San Diego's program is completely funded by the county. The University of Alabama started its program using a philanthropic grant (22).

CASE STUDY: CONTINUED

Both the medical school and your center agree to offer support to a training program. One of the stipulations of the funding by the community mental health center is that residents must see patients in order to help with the cost. With support and funding secured, you begin to consider what sorts of experiences might be best for the medical students and residents rotating through your community center. You begin by thinking about your own training experiences in community psychiatry and what had attracted you to community psychiatry as a career. You also think about what you learned in your own training about the factors that make for successful, engaging rotations. You speak with the residency training director to find out what rotations the residents in the program already had and his ideas about the community psychiatry rotation. He notes that the residents would benefit from greater familiarity with resources available in the community and learning more about systems-based practice and the recovery model. He also wants the residents to be exposed to a diverse patient population through their work at the center. Together, you begin to develop measurable objectives as a first step.

THE BASICS OF AN ENGAGING PROGRAM

One way to engage residents and fellows in public sector work is for trainees to learn the skills of effective community practice that are unique to the public clinical work. Those skills are classified into three areas. First, residents need to learn how to conceptualize biological and psychological dimensions of mental illness in their broad social and cultural context in the community. Second, residents need to understand their important consultation role in the community, educating primary care practitioners, other human services workers, advocates, and peer support groups about mental illness. Third, residents need to be exposed to the various administrative responsibilities that they will likely perform in a community center or state hospital, including medical administration (e.g., hiring and managing physicians), quality management (e.g., outcomes and productivity), and program development (23). The development of program goals, rotations, and didactics, as well as the recruitment of supervising faculty, should focus on developing these skills.

There is surprisingly little guidance in the literature on how to develop community-based experiences, but there are many descriptions of existing programs, a few of which are described later. There seem to be some common elements in successful rotations, including clear learning objectives for the rotations, strong clinical role models, trainee engagement in community-based treatment teams using a recovery-oriented model of care, and rigorous didactic programming. In addition, many programs emphasize education in health care systems and management because the community psychiatrist is often asked to take over leadership roles in community organizations.

Objectives

One of the first steps in considering a community psychiatry rotation is the establishment of clear and measurable objectives for the rotation. In considering the objectives, the needs of trainees and the psychiatry clerkship or residency training program should be considered, as well as what can be achieved by the community center (24, 25).

Objectives will be driven by the level of training of learners rotating through the center. For example, will medical students, junior-level or senior-level residents, or fellows rotate through the center? Or a mix of all? Trainees at various levels will have equally variable educational needs that should be encompassed by the objectives. For example, senior-level residents may be provided higher levels of responsibility compared with junior-level residents, including more autonomy in clinical decision-making but also more opportunities to learn about leadership and management. The length of the rotation may also dictate the objectives. Will the rotation be a certain morning each week for a semester or trimester? Or, instead, every day for a month?

Because psychiatry clerkships are under time constraints, community centers must think about what sorts of experiences can be achieved in a short period of time that remain cost-effective for the center with the least disruption in patient care. Some psychiatry clerkships designate a particular week or a morning per week to the rotation. For example, for short rotations that occur early on in medical training, it may make sense to have trainees get a broad overview of all the services provided by a local community center with opportunities to interact with the patients and with case workers rather than being solely assigned to a psychiatrist providing clinic-based psychopharmacology services.

The experience for all trainees, and especially medical students, who are new to community psychiatry should expose them to the unique aspects of community psychiatry, including mental health resources unique to the public sector and its diverse diagnostic and sociocultural populations. Community psychiatry provides an opportunity for learners at all levels to gain an appreciation for the challenges that patients face in the community and for their sources of resilience. Teaching about diagnosis and treatment of this patient population should also give special consideration to how learners may be coping with some of the challenges—including ethical challenges—of community work, such as less time working with patients, resource-poor settings, and patients facing a variety of psychosocial challenges (26).

One way to organize objectives for residents is around the ACGME Milestones Project, which can provide guidance regarding appropriate learning objectives for resident trainees. ACGME requires that medical specialties develop educational milestones with objective and measurable steps for each year in residency training (27). For example, for Level 2 (which is generally achieved by the end of postgraduate year 2 [PGY-2]) for the resource management milestone, a suggested competency is "recognizing disparities in healthcare at individual and community levels." Level 4 (generally achieved by the end of PGY-4) aims for a resident to "balance the best interests of the patient with the availability of resources" (11). Community rotation objectives can use the unique aspects of community psychiatry to reach these milestones.

Objectives, above all, should be specific. For example, the Oregon program developed objectives for community mental health training that include understanding the role of the psychiatrist in a community-based interdisciplinary treatment team, comfort in providing consultation to other agency workers or primary care providers, and the ability to perform case management services in the community (28).

Furthermore, trainees should be provided with the objectives at the beginning of the rotation, with discussion of expectations for the rotation. Trainees should be evaluated with regard to these objectives and also be given the opportunity to provide feedback to the rotation if the learning objectives are not being met by the educational activities.

Attending Physicians

Strong and committed leadership in the clinic is just as important to the success of public-academic collaborations as administrative leadership. The experience offered under an attending physician's guidance may greatly impact trainees' attitudes toward the training experience and toward psychiatry more generally. Therefore, it is important to recruit faculty with a positive regard both for public sector work and for the academic–public collaboration. Santos et al. (7) describe the need for faculty who are competent at clinical care in community-based systems of care and who are invested in mentoring in public settings. Attendings must be "willing to embrace and support the philosophy, spirit, and success of this collaboration" (7).

Trainees should have clear supervision from attending physicians throughout their clinical rotations. Along with providing guidance about clinical decision-making, supervision provides an opportunity to address trainee reactions to the differences in a community-based system of care versus other academic settings in which they train. These differences may include shorter appointment times or barriers that patients face in accessing care or resources. Attendings can model the ability to effectively work in complex community systems. Supervision also provides an opportunity to model the public psychiatrist role within the community, including administration, educational, and advocacy tasks, and to address any concerns residents have about a career in community psychiatry (15, 29).

As mentioned previously, community psychiatry rotations may present new challenges to students and residents. When first serving patients with severe mental illness who also endure various psychosocial challenges, such as poverty and homelessness, trainees need role models for dealing with the frustrations and challenges to empathy that arise when providing community-based care. The specific challenges may differ based on the level of training. For example, medical students may struggle with fear or uncertainty about working with psychiatric patients, worried that empathizing may lead to being consumed by these patients. For residents and fellows, this role modeling may be more focused on finding enhanced meaning in the work, preventing burnout, and working within the often resource-poor community setting and dealing with the stress of high patient volume.

If a lack of community resources is impacting care, it can be helpful for faculty to address this directly and discuss the ideal circumstances to which trainees aspire and reflect on how they cope with the current realities. It can be helpful for trainees to recognize that the attending also sees the challenges and the inequities.

The recruitment and development of senior faculty to meet all of these needs can be challenging in a public psychiatry setting. Graduating residents who do not enter private practice often prefer a position in the medical school rather than one at a state hospital or community mental health center, even if the medical school offers a lower salary. One strategy to address this is to hire attending physicians through the medical school with an academic appointment and rank and then place them in public settings through a contract between the medical school and the community center or state hospital. Migrating public sector employees into such positions might also foster engagement in the educational initiatives (4).

Rotation Sites and Experiences

Community centers offer a useful alternative to medical student clerkships in psychiatry that typically take place on inpatient units. Because patients on inpatient units are acutely ill, those experiences may have less applicability to the persistent psychiatric disorders that most trainees are likely to treat in their own practices. Community centers expose students to chronic mental illnesses when they are less acute and in the context of patients' social and cultural situations (30).

Unique training opportunities allow trainees to gain exposure in areas of psychiatry (and the community) that they may not have access to otherwise and that enhance understanding of the lived experience of the mentally ill in the community. In particular, trainees can gain experience with severe and persistent mentally ill populations, community case management, homeless and forensic populations, and advocacy work.

Severe and Persistent Mental Illness in the Community

Trainees often first encounter patients with severe and persistent mental illness in hospital settings when the patients are acutely psychotic or severely depressed. The focus of care is typically on the acute symptomatology, and the goal is to stabilize the patient and discharge as quickly as is prudent. On the other hand, rotations in a community center allow trainees an opportunity to work with these same patients when they are not acutely ill, to better understand the challenges they face on an everyday basis, and to experience the resiliency that they demonstrate in the face of psychiatric and social challenges.

In addition, contemporary psychiatrists, especially those working in the public sector, require training in the principles of the recovery movement, which stresses self-directed care over physician-directed care and also engagement in the community over symptom management (31). This model of care requires a different skill set of mental health workers, including psychiatrists, and offers novel training opportunities for resident and medical students (30). Seeing severely ill patients as part of a multidisciplinary team allows trainees the opportunity to experience the implementation of a person-centered treatment plan.

For example, on a month-long rotation during their second year, residents at the University of Texas Southwestern Medical Center rotate on the assertive community treatment team of the local community center. They serve on a multidisciplinary team that includes their attending psychiatrist, a psychiatric nurse, and case workers with specialties such as supported employment, substance use treatment, and community-based case management. In addition to performing office-based psychiatric evaluation and follow-up medication appointments, residents attend daily treatment team meetings. Residents also spend part of their time doing home visits with case managers, offering another opportunity for residents to see the social context for a patient's mental illness.

Community Case Management

Community-based case management seeks to help patients gain and retain independence in their activities of daily living. Case management takes place primarily in the field—in homes, in the offices of social service agencies, and even on the street. Its setting and tasks are less predictable than the work that occurs in a psychiatric hospital or clinic. It requires a perspective focused on each patient's role in the community rather than a diagnosis. It requires relentless will to do what it take to foster that independence, even in the face of persistent rejection, from both patients and service organizations (32).

Although trainees may work with social workers in the hospital and other clinic settings, community centers provide an opportunity for trainees to serve as a member of a multidisciplinary team with various members performing long-term case management tasks that enable patients to function better in their community. Depending on the team, students and residents might engage with community programs such as job training, disability benefits, and physical health care services. Homeless outreach teams, assertive community teams, and other specialized programs all typically offer some or all of these case management services.

For example, at the University of Texas Southwestern Medical Center, first-year residents rotate through the homeless outreach services offered by the local community mental health center during a month-long rotation. The experience includes traveling with the psychiatrist who works in different homeless shelters in the area, as well as going with a homeless outreach caseworker to visit patients without stable housing wherever they are staying in the community, including on the streets. This experience provides residents with an opportunity to learn more about the homeless shelters in the area and about the array of services offered by the local community center for persons experiencing homelessness.

Homelessness

Although trainees, particularly medical students, may interact with persons experiencing homelessness in the hospital and clinics, they often are unaware of the realities and hardships faced by those living without consistent housing. Community centers, which often have homeless outreach teams as well as clinics associated with homeless shelters, provide an opportunity for trainees to learn more about the lives of those experiencing homelessness, which can help trainees gain greater awareness of why individuals may be presenting the way they do to the clinic or the emergency room. Furthermore, a better understanding of resources available in the community can help trainees become better providers who can address more of their patients' needs when they present in other settings.

For example, the University of Florida developed a clerkship curriculum with sites that included an outpatient clinic in a homeless shelter and a primary care clinic with integrated mental health services; it also included an outreach team to people with mental illness or addiction who live on the streets. Medical students spent 2 weeks at each of the sites during their 6-week rotation in psychiatry (33).

A PGY-2 experience at Harvard University offered a 6-week outpatient experience caring for patients with severe mental illness complicated by addiction, chronic medical illness, and homelessness. The program was based at a homeless shelter. The residents had a caseload of three to five shelter patients. Residents were expected to serve as comprehensive case managers for patients by establishing rapport and then linking them with necessary medical, psychiatric, addiction, and social services using a patient-centered model of care. Residents also did outreach on the streets to identify new patients, and they participated in mental health court (34).

Forensic Populations

Exposure during training to patients with mental illness who have become involved with the criminal justice system may improve residents' understanding of the interface between the legal system and the public mental health system (35). Many community mental health centers have forensic teams and work with local court systems to provide services to patients on parole or probation or undergoing community competency restoration. Training in these venues offers residents the opportunity for a strong forensic experience as a result of the dramatic increase in forensic populations at state hospitals (36). Indeed, the exposure to forensic patients has been cited as a primary value of state hospital rotations (37).

For example, Yale University mandated a PGY-2 forensic psychiatry rotation of one half-day per week for 6 weeks. Half of the residents served in a court-ordered substance abuse treatment program, and the other half served in a jail diversion program for veterans. Supervision was provided by a board-certified forensic psychiatrist. In both settings, residents participated in evaluation and treatment planning, including assessing risks of diversion for criminally involved individuals with mental illness. They also learned about reporting requirements for criminally involved patients and how these requirements intersect with patient confidentiality (38, 39).

Advocacy

Community psychiatry offers an opportunity for other unique learning experiences, including experiential ones. Visits with state legislators and state-level policymakers and meetings with advocacy groups can also be included so that trainees learn more about the systems and policies that create public mental health systems and about how they can effect changes within those systems. For example, within the constraints of laws on lobbying by state employees, trainees may be encouraged to speak to local legislators about bills, providing education on how proposed laws might affect their practice of medicine or mentally ill patients.

CASE STUDY: CONTINUED

The residency training director notes that it would be helpful to include some readings and didactic training on public psychiatry in the curriculum for the residency and asks for your thoughts on what should be included. You begin to think about what topics might be helpful to include in this curriculum and about how best to incorporate the didactic training. For example, would it best occur while learners were on the rotation or would it be more helpful for it to occur during the residency's didactic afternoon (or a combination)? Furthermore, how can you ensure that the didactic material is appropriate to the needs of the learner as well as engaging?

Didactics

The development of a strong didactic component can sometimes be difficult to achieve in busy, service-based community center and state hospital settings because public programs may be reluctant to sacrifice direct care time for faculty or even for rotating residents. Furthermore, didactics require time for preparation—time that may be difficult for public psychiatrists to find, given clinical service requirements. It may therefore be important for academic–pubic partnerships to develop financing of, and contractual stipulations for, dedicated time for trainees and their faculty to engage in didactic training. Although formal classroom didactics can be helpful, programs with fewer residents may integrate didactics with clinical supervision time. However, the danger here is that one aspect will replace the other, leaving a gap in learning.

Other factors will drive the didactic component of rotations as well. Objectives will be important for determining how to approach didactic curriculum planning. What will be the goals of the curriculum? How much time has been allocated to formal learning, and when?

Public psychiatry experts have recommended areas that didactic training in community psychiatry should cover. Topics include a general history of community psychiatry; principles of public health, such as prevention strategies; financing structures of public mental health; government and private organizations and their influence on mental health care; the roles of various providers on a multidisciplinary team; and "service delivery strategies for a population with special needs such as, for example, impoverished and/or homeless populations, the chronic mentally ill, a specific ethnic group, the elderly, primary care medical patients, patients with 'dual-disorders,' or mentally ill prisoners" (23, p. 277). Consumer, supportive services, self-help, and advocacy organizations in the community, as well as the disability services and eligibility criteria, should also be discussed. A basic knowledge of community crisis care, as well as the challenges and clinical course of those with chronic and persistent mental illness in the community, can also be addressed (23).

Cultural psychiatry may also be addressed in the curriculum because residents may encounter communities of which they are unfamiliar during their community psychiatry rotations (40).

Evaluation

Evaluation is an important aspect of academic–community center partnerships; this includes evaluation of the trainee and evaluation of the attending physicians and of the rotation. Therefore, in establishing rotations through public sector systems, a method of evaluation for the trainees, the program, and program staff should be established. The program's educational objectives should guide evaluation, as stated previously. Trainees should be expected to make progress toward achieving the assigned objectives throughout the elective, and rotations and program staff should provide reasonable opportunities and support to trainees as they work toward their goals.

Trainee feedback about a rotation or clerkship, or a particular attending physician, should be anonymous, and rotation leadership should be open to using feedback to improve the rotation. Rotations must also be evaluated with respect to their contribution to residency program objectives. The rotation's clinical leadership should work with the clerkship or residency training directors to determine whether the rotation continues to fit the needs of the program.

PUBLIC PSYCHIATRY FELLOWSHIPS AND ALTERNATIVES

Public psychiatry fellowships have served as another strategy for offering graduating residents an opportunity to explore a career in the public sector as well as fostering workforce development. Although not offering board certification, public psychiatry fellowships do offer advanced training not only in clinical care but also in public mental health policy development and evaluation (22). The first academic medical center to create such a fellowship was Columbia University in association with the New York State Psychiatric Institute (41). In the past few years, typically approximately 15 departments of psychiatry have maintained programs (22).

Columbia University's program has been in continuous operation since 1981. Several factors have been cited for its success, including, in particular, its atypical consistent and generous funding stream from the state of New York. It also has a consistent faculty with years of experience in, and commitment to, public psychiatry (42). Columbia identified core elements for its program, and these were incorporated into guidelines promulgated by the American Association of Community Psychiatrists for developing and evaluating public psychiatry fellowships. The elements include a didactic curriculum; a primary field placement; faculty supervision and mentoring; teaching, presenting, and supervising; and research or a quality improvement project (30).

Public Psychiatry Tracks

Many graduating residents with an interest in public sector work are not attracted to public psychiatry fellowship because they lack a board certification process. An alternative way to explore public sector careers is a community psychiatry track during general psychiatry training. Community psychiatry tracks typically allow a resident to designate a percentage of time in fourth-year, or even throughout their 4 years of training, to rotations in public sector settings. Activities might include time in administrative psychiatry focusing on policy and/or advocacy or time spent on a forensic psychiatry team. From the community center or state hospital perspective, such a track brings a senior resident with a strong interest in the public sector. From the medical school's perspective, the track allows programs to focus limited community psychiatry training resources on those residents most likely to enter the public sector (40).

Fourth-Year Public Psychiatry Electives

Community mental health centers and state hospitals seeking to attract graduating residents into their clinics could consider offering fourth-year electives to allow residents to try out a possible post-residency position. Such electives can serve as a way to ensure a good match between the psychiatrist and the institution. For example, a resident might be offered an opportunity to work on an assertive community team for several months, spend a day in an outpatient clinic, or work in an acute crisis stabilization unit for the entire year (28).

CASE STUDY: CONCLUSION

As medical director of a community center, you have the exciting and potentially gratifying opportunity to foster resident and medical student education programs in your clinic and community—programs that can help train the next generation of public psychiatrists. The need is great. Finding psychiatrists for public service has long been difficult and seems to be getting increasingly difficult. Without these providers and the important work that they do, people languish on wait lists or, in despair, go without mental health care altogether.

There are many reasons for this shortage. One reason is relatively good news: Reduced stigma means more people are seeking mental health care (43). But the bad news is that there are not enough psychiatrists even for people who have commercial insurance to pay for the service (44). In the public sector, low salaries and difficult caseloads tend to dissuade all but the most committed from serving.

However, high-quality rotations with stimulating role models offer a potential path to establishing the next generation of leaders in public mental health. Rotations in unique, evidence-based programs such as assertive community treatment or homeless outreach teams offer trainees a firsthand perspective of their community that most in society choose to ignore.

In addition, your decision to engage the local medical school in a partnership will benefit the school by offering access to new training sites and areas for research. Your medical staff will benefit from the stimulation provided by the questions and enthusiasm of trainees. And your patients will benefit through increased access to care.

REFERENCES

1. Weitenkampf F. William Strang—Etcher. Arts Decoration. 1918 Feb;8(4):154–156.
2. Gibran K. The prophet. New York: Knopf; 1923.
3. Wilensky-Lanford B. Your children are not your children. CrossCurrents. 2015 Jun;65(2):239–253.
4. Talbott J, Bray J, Flaherty L, Robinowitz C, Taintor Z. State–university collaboration in psychiatry: The Pew Memorial Trust Program. Community Ment Health J. 1991 Dec;27(6):425–439.
5. Weintraub W, Hepburn B, Strahan S, Plaut S. Inspiration recruitment and the Maryland Plan: Overcoming the stigma of public psychiatry. Psychiatric Services. 1994 May;45(5):456–460.
6. Goetz R, Cutler DL, Pollack D, et al. A three-decade perspective on community and public psychiatry training in Oregon. Psychiatric Services. 1998 Sep 1;49(9):1208–1211.
7. Santos A, Ballenger J, Bevilacqua J, et al. A community-based public–academic liaison program. Am J Psychiatry. 151(8):1181–1187.
8. Ranz R, Deakins SM. Columbia University's Fellowship in Public Psychiatry. Psychiatry Services. 47:515.
9. Weinberg M, LeMelle S, Ranz J. Psychiatry residents' perception of public/community psychiatry fellowship training. Community Ment Health J. 2014 Jan;50(1):6–9.
10. ACGME program requirements for graduate medical education in psychiatry. 2017. Retrieved from https://medschool.ucsd.edu/som/psychiatry/education/Programs/residency/my-residency/Documents/9.0%20RRC%20from%20manual.pdf
11. ACGME Milestone Project. Retrieved from https://www.acgme.org/Portals/0/PDFs/Milestones/PsychiatryMilestones.pdf
12. Association of American Medical Colleges. Report I: Learning objectives for medical student education guidelines for medical schools. 1998. Retrieved from https://www.aamc.org/system/files/c/2/492708-learningobjectivesformedicalstudenteducation.pdf
13. Schatte D, Piemonte N, Clark M. "I started to feel like a 'real doctor'": Medical students' reflections on their psychiatry clerkship. Acad Psychiatry. 2015 Jun;39(3):267–274.
14. Pessar L, Pristach C, Leonard K. What troubles clerks in psychiatry? A strategy to explore the question. Acad Psychiatry. 2008 May;32(3):194–198.
15. Lyons Z, Janca A. Impact of a psychiatry clerkship on stigma, attitudes towards psychiatry, and psychiatry as a career choice. BMC Medical Educ. 2015 Mar 7;15(1):34.
16. Lokko H. Outside the hospital: Lessons learned from a community psychiatry rotation. Acad Psychiatry. 2016;40(5):859–860.
17. Faulkner LR, Eaton JS, Bloom JD, Cutler DL. The CMHC as a setting for residency education. Community Ment Health J. 1982;18(1):3–10.
18. Centers for Medicare and Medicaid and Services. Guidelines for teaching physicians, interns, and residents. 2018. Retrieved from https://www.cms.gov/outreach-and-education/medicare-learning-network-mln/mlnproducts/downloads/teaching-physicians-fact-sheet-icn006437.pdf
19. Svendsen D, Cutler D, Ronis R, et al. The professor of public psychiatry model in Ohio: The impact on training, program innovation, and the quality of mental health care. Community Ment Health J. 2005 Dec;41(6):775–784.
20. Le Melle S, Mangurian C, Ali OM, et al. Public–academic partnerships: Public psychiatry fellowships: A developing network of public–academic collaborations. Psychiatric Services. 2012 Sep 1;63(9):851–854.
21. Mangurian C, Shumway M, Dilley J. Mental health services research training for the next generation of leaders in the public health sector: A case study of the UCSF/SFGH Public Psychiatry Fellowship. Acad Psychiatry. 2014 Dec;38(6):690–692.
22. Steiner J, Giggie M, Koh S, Mangurian C, Ranz J. The evolution of public psychiatry fellowships. Acad Psychiatry. 2014 Dec;38(6):685–689.
23. Brown D, Goldman C, Thompson K, Cutler D. Training residents for community psychiatry practice: Guidelines for curriculum development. Community Ment Health J. 1993;277(3):271–283.

24. Brodkey A, Van Zandt K, Sierles F. Educational objectives for a junior psychiatry clerkship. Acad Psychiatry. 1997 Dec;21(4):179–204.

25. Burke M, Brodkey A. Trends in undergraduate medical education: Clinical clerkship learning objectives. Acad Psychiatry. 2006 Mar;30(2):158–165.

26. Stovall J, Fleisch S, McQuistion H, Hackman A, Harris T. Ethics and the treatment of the mentally ill, homeless person: A perspective on psychiatry resident training. Acad Psychiatry. 2016 Aug;40(4):612–616.

27. Hunt J, Thomas C. ACGME milestone development in general psychiatry: Patient care and medical knowledge. Acad Psychiatry. 2014 Jun;38(3):261–267.

28. Cutler D, Wilson W, Godard S, Pollack D. Collaboration for training. Admin Policy Mental Health Mental Health Services Res. 1993 Jul;20(6):449–458.

29. Lyons Z. Impact of the psychiatry clerkship on medical student attitudes towards psychiatry and to psychiatry as a career. Acad Psychiatry. 2014 Feb;38(1):35–42.

30. Sowers W, Pollack D, Everett A, et al. Progress in workforce development since 2000: Advanced training opportunities in public and community psychiatry. Psychiatric Services. 2011 Jul 1;62(7):782–788.

31. Cook JA, Russell C, Grey DD, Jonikas JA. Economic Grand Rounds: A self-directed care model for mental health recovery. Psychiatric Services. 2008 Jun 1;59(6):600–602.

32. Lerbæk B, Aagaard J, Andersen MB, Buus N. Assertive community treatment (ACT) case managers' professional identities: A focus group study. Int J Mental Health Nurs. 2016;25(6):579–587.

33. Christensen RC. Community psychiatry and medical student education. Psychiatric Services. 2005 May 1;56(5):608–609.

34. Shtasel D, Viron M, Freudenreich O. Community psychiatry: What should future psychiatrists learn? Harvard Rev Psychiatry. 2012 Dec;20(6):318–323.

35. Forman HL, Preven DW. Evidence for greater forensic education of all psychiatry residents. J Am Acad Psychiatry Law Online. 2016 Dec 1;44(4):422–424.

36. National Association of State Mental Health Program Directors. Forensic patients in state psychiatric hospitals: 1999–2016. 2017. Retrieved from https://www.nasmhpd.org/sites/default/files/TACPaper.10.Forensic-Patients-in-State-Hospitals_508C_v2.pdf

37. Talbott J, Faulkner L, Buckley P. State hospital–university collaborations: A 25-year follow-up. Acad Psychiatry. 2010 Mar;34(2):125–127.

38. Wasser T, Sun A, Chandra S, Michaelsen K. The benefits of required forensic clinical experiences in residency. Acad Psychiatry. 2019 Feb;43(1):76–81.

39. Michaelsen KC, Lewis AS, Morgan PT, McKee SA, Wasser TD. The barriers and benefits to developing forensic rotations for psychiatry residents. J Am Acad Psychiatry Law Online. 2018 Sep 1;46(3):322–328.

40. Rearden C, Factor R, Brenner C, Singh P, Spurgeon J. Community psychiatry tracks for residents: A review of four programs. Community Ment Health J. 2014 Jan;50(1):10–16.

41. Ranz J, Rosenheck S, Deakins S. Columbia University's fellowship in public psychiatry. Psychiatric Services. 1996;47:512–516.

42. Runnels P, Ronis R. Expanding the playing field: Public and community psychiatry fellowship and beyond. Community Ment Health J. 2014 Jan;50(1):1–5.

43. Cohen Veterans Network, National Council for Behavioral Health. America's mental health 2018. 2018. Retrieved from https://www.cohenveteransnetwork.org/wp-content/uploads/2018/10/Research-Summary-10-10-2018.pdf

44. Bishop TF, Press MJ, Keyhani S, Pincus HA. Acceptance of insurance by psychiatrists and the implications for access to mental health care. JAMA Psychiatry. 2014 Feb 1;71(2):176–181.

8

THE PUBLIC PSYCHIATRIST AS RESEARCHER

GOPALKUMAR RAKESH AND MARVIN SWARTZ

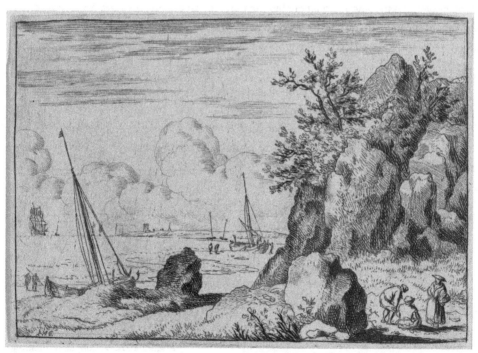

FIGURE 8.1 Allart van Everdingen, *Seascape with Three Figures to the Right*, c. 1645–1656, etching.

Allart van Everdingen (1621–1675) was a Dutch painter who lived in Amsterdam. Most of his works deal with landscapes. In the etching shown in Figure 8.1, he portrays the sea with a clouded sky.

CASE STUDY: INITIAL PRESENTATION

You are the medical director of a community mental health center that serves a large region of your state. You have a team of three other psychiatrists whom you manage, in addition to two social workers and a nurse practitioner. The nearest tertiary care center, a university-affiliated hospital, is 2 hours away. Your center provides medication management including depot injections to a large proportion of patients with schizophrenia. Your center also has a social worker who provides supported employment and some degree of guidance on vocational rehabilitation opportunities for these patients. You are approached by a faculty member from the university-affiliated medical center to plan a study comparing an experimental candidate drug to placebo for cognitive symptoms in schizophrenia. This is a multisite trial that aims to target patients with long duration of illness and severe cognitive deficits. Your center is of interest to the researcher because of the possibility of recruiting a large number of subjects eligible for the study. The candidate molecule and support staff for the study would be provided by a pharmaceutical company. It would also provide specialized teams to conduct the study and monitor for changes and side effects. You have questions about how patients would be randomized to the arms of the study and whether this would conflict with the therapeutic relationship the patients have with providers. You are also worried about the infrastructural changes this study would require, as well as potential conflicts of interest related to becoming a site for a pharmaceutical company-sponsored study.

QUESTIONS
1. What sorts of ethical issues are raised by this potential study with an academic institution and a pharmaceutical company?
2. What logistical issues must be considered to do the research in this setting?
3. What would be the next steps in developing the relationship?

PSYCHIATRY AND LITERATURE

My philosophy is really based on humility. I don't think we know enough to fix either diagnostics or therapeutics. The future of psychiatry is clinical neuroscience, based on a much deeper understanding of the brain.

——Thomas R. Insel

President and Co-Founder, Mindstrong

Director, National Institute of Mental Health (2002–2015)

In *Sybil*, the 1973 book by Flora Rheta Schreiber, the author portrays the protagonist as suffering from dissociative identity disorder, and interestingly, her parents do not align with her idea of reaching out to her psychiatrist. The story of Sybil provides the reader with a good description of the complexity of mental illness, particularly the interaction of trauma, genetic predisposition, and psychosocial issues in the presentation of mental illness. Case history illustrations of patients with "hysteria" by Charcot and, later, Freud align with the diagnosis of dissociative identity disorder as well. Dissociative identity disorder continues to engage students of clinical psychiatry, and research to elucidate the neurobiology of the disorder, especially at the interface between clinical psychiatry and neuroscience, is robust.

INTRODUCTION

Psychiatrists practicing in community settings are either in private practice or associated with a community hospital or clinic (American Psychiatric Association, 2018). A small proportion of community psychiatrists also work in, or consult to, federally qualified clinics, nursing homes, correctional settings, and other community mental health settings (Bishop, Seirup, Pincus, & Ross, 2016; Brenner et al., 2017). Practice in the community differs from an academic setting. Differences include greater collaboration with primary care physicians and other specialty providers; fewer avenues for patients to receive psychotherapeutic interventions; less exposure to complex treatment regimens; and, generally, fewer teaching and research opportunities unless the community clinic is closely affiliated with an academic medical center.

In the absence of any systematic estimates of the percentages of psychiatrists in academia versus community settings, it seems clear that there is an overall shortage of behavioral health providers (Hoge et al., 2013; Thomas, Ellis, Konrad, Holzer, & Morrissey, 2009). That means that psychiatrists in the community who engage in private practice or work as medical directors at community hospitals typically also devote a certain percentage of their time to administrative duties. The daily workload of patients plus administrative duties leaves little time to engage in research for the community psychiatrist.

Yet, the community setting offers numerous opportunities for research for those who wish to engage in it and can find the time. For example, community settings offer unique opportunities to conduct effectiveness research allowing real-world tests of findings from efficacy trials (Patsopoulos, 2011). In efficacy trials, research staff are employed to deliver interventions to highly selected patients, subject to rigorous inclusion and exclusion criteria. Often, such trials do not generalize to other real-world setting and patients. Effectiveness trials with the sort of broadly representative subjects offered by community centers are sorely needed to strengthen the evidence of intervention effectiveness. Multiple clinical trials involving psychotropic and psychotherapeutic interventions are designed as effectiveness studies. Several large-scale National Institute of Mental Health (NIMH)-funded clinical trials, such as Clinical Antipsychotic Trials of Intervention Effectiveness (CATIE), Recovery After an Initial Schizophrenia Episode (RAISE), and Sequenced Treatment Alternatives to Relieve Depression (STAR-D), conducted as collaborative efforts between academic medical centers and community mental health clinics, adopted modified methodological designs. These modified designs incorporated strategies to encompass clinical equipoise (meaning clinicians could be ethically neutral about study assignment) and rigorous randomization and blinding. Psychiatrists practicing in real-world community settings were instrumental to these trials.

In addition to efficacy trials, community settings provide rich opportunities for a range of other types of studies. Some areas of research that could engage patients in the community include health services utilization research; research at the interface of mental illness, violence, and suicide; community intervention and outreach studies; treatment of substance use disorders; and intervention trials with partnerships between university hospitals and community hospitals. This chapter reviews these as well as other areas of active community-based research, such as outpatient commitment studies—also called assisted outpatient treatment—and the relationship between violence and mental health. The chapter also summarizes how clinical trials relating to substance use disorders and health technology dissemination have changed the landscape of mental health research in the community. Studies in all of these areas are of the greatest practical importance to psychiatrists who practice in the community.

HISTORICAL CONTEXT OF COMMUNITY-BASED RESEARCH

The 1950s coincided with the beginning of the depopulation of state mental institutions— a policy referred to as deinstitutionalization—with the intent that community mental health clinics would provide ambulatory services to formerly hospitalized patients. The Community Mental Health Act proposed by President Kennedy in 1963 called for federal investment in research in mental illness as well as recommended strategies to enhance service delivery to catchment areas of 200,000 patients nationwide. However, federal funding of community mental health centers (CMHCs) between the 1950s and the 1980s never allowed for the number of centers intended. Although CMHCs delivered a variety of community-based services to patients with mental illness in an attempt to meet the needs of deinstitutionalized patients, declining funding and burgeoning need due to progressive waves of deinstitutionalization meant that clinics were unsuccessful in providing the range of services needed to serve seriously mentally ill patients living in the community, especially considering the need for safe and affordable housing and supports. The unmet need for appropriate "wrap-around" supportive services gradu-ally led to a phenomenon referred to as trans-institutionalization wherein seriously ill patients, unable to live independently without intensive support, found themselves in new institutions such as skilled nursing facilities, group homes, and other intermediate care facilities supported by Medicaid and Medicare. Even worse, some found themselves in jail for minor crimes—a trend that led to alarming rates of incarceration among people with severe mental illness. With growing recognition of the failure of the original CMHC model, policymakers proposed implementation of a new concept of the Community Support System project led by collaborations between NIMH and state mental health agencies. The program modified the original CMHC model by stipulating guidelines for providing care to patients with serious mental illness, including crisis stabilization, psychosocial rehabilitation, supportive living arrangements, integrated medical care, and case management services (Turner & Dean, 1978). In addition to that service array, under the Mental Health Planning Act of 1986, federal law also mandated that all states estab-lish case management for Medicaid patients in order to improve coverage of community mental health services. With decline in federal and state support of CMHCs, community mental health providers became increasingly reliant on insurance reimbursement rather than direct funding, largely in the form of Medicare and Medicaid reimbursement. By the late 1990s, private insurance and community mental health services moved toward aggressive cost containment in the form of behavioral health managed care. Under the ag-gressive application of managed care principles such as tight utilization review, it became essential to explore alternative models of community treatment approaches that did not involve extended periods of hospitalization.

ASSERTIVE COMMUNITY TREATMENT

The previously presented historical context is the background for one of the impor-tant success stories of academic–community research partnerships that emerged from the incentives to reduce hospital care: assertive community treatment (ACT). The first randomized controlled trial to evaluate the effectiveness of ACT, initially called the "training in community living model," was developed at the Mendota Mental Health Institute in Wisconsin (Stein, Test, & Marx, 1975). This seminal study compared patients who received wrap-around treatment in the community, sometimes referred to as a hospital without walls, with control patients who were treated in an inpatient setting. The initial phase of the study lasted 5 months, and the follow-up phase of the study extended for 2 years. The services provided to patients in the community included not just treatment but also psychosocial rehabilitation, which encompassed transitioning to gainful employment and leveraging available family support. This study showed the feasibility of ACT as an alternative to longer term hospital care as well as improved outcomes.

Throughout the years, researchers have studied the essential principles of ACT in community settings, such as considering the strengths of the patient, teaching the patient how best to cope with psychotic and other symptoms, avoidance of pathological dependency, and providing community-based rehabilitation and treatment. The initial studies provided the basic tenets of ACT: small caseloads at the ratio of one staff member to 10 patients, 24-hour crisis support, team-based approaches, careful monitoring of medications, individualized care, regular team meetings, and long-term community support in the form of a no-discharge policy.

A Cochrane systematic review (Marshall & Lockwood, 2000) compared the effectiveness of ACT with other standard methods of care using a pool of 75 studies based on study eligibility criteria. When comparing ACT versus standard community care, the authors found that those receiving ACT were more likely to remain in contact with services compared with people receiving standard community care (odds ratio [OR] = 0.51, confidence interval [CI] = 0.37–0.70). When comparing ACT versus hospital-based rehabilitative services, those receiving ACT were no more likely to remain in contact with services compared with those receiving hospital-based rehabilitation. People receiving ACT were significantly less likely to be admitted to the hospital compared with those receiving hospital-based rehabilitation (OR = 0.2, CI = 0.09–0.46). The meta-analysis also found that people receiving ACT consistently spend fewer days in the hospital compared with those receiving case management, although there was insufficient data to permit comparison of clinical or social outcomes.

Results from other clinical trials, namely the Dartmouth dual diagnosis study (McHugo, Drake, Teague, & Xie, 1999), Randomised Evaluation of Assertive Community Treatment (REACT; Killaspy et al., 2009), the UK700 study (Burns, 2002), and PRiSM (Thornicroft, Wykes, Holloway, Johnson, & Szmukler, 1998), have demonstrated less superiority of ACT versus other modalities of outreach and community-based treatments, such as other types of case management teams. However, ACT continues to be a dominant evidence-based, community-based service in the United States for seriously mentally ill patients living in the community (Burns, 2010).

OTHER NOTABLE CLINICAL TRIALS IN PUBLIC PSYCHIATRY

In addition to the research on ACT that was performed in community settings, several other well-known clinical trials provide examples of large-scale clinical studies that have benefited from collaborative efforts between university-affiliated academic centers and community mental health centers. The opportunity for meaningful clinical trials generalizable to clinical practice is most promising with pragmatic clinical trials, as showcased by the examples discussed in this section. Designing these trials requires consensus development, finesse, and sophistication built upon modified statistical techniques that take into account the pragmatic nature of the studies and use effectiveness measures, rather than efficacy, as outcomes. These studies demonstrate design approaches needed for success in public settings. They also demonstrate possible study designs as well as potential community-based collaborations.

PACE

The Personal Assessment and Crisis Evaluation (PACE) clinic in Melbourne, Australia, was one of the first clinics to utilize community recruitment strategies to identify young subjects at risk for psychosis. The clinic has been at the forefront of research to pinpoint biomarkers of psychosis and investigate new treatments for the same (Phillips et al., 2002). The clinic uses many strategies to increase collaboration, including holding educational sessions about prodromal symptoms and early psychosis, holding training sessions for non-mental health professionals (general practitioners, substance use counselors, school psychologists, and clergy) on screening for symptoms of early psychosis, and distributing newsletters and educational brochures that discuss symptoms and treatment options. In addition, most clinics have trained staff available to triage calls and perform evaluations of referrals (Phillips et al., 2002; Yung et al., 2007).

STAR-D

The STAR-D study used a novel method of randomization called equipoise stratified randomization (Lavori et al., 2001), which utilized an optimal combination of therapeutic orientation while keeping the randomization intact. This design is imperative when conducting trials at a community center that recruits subjects through physician–client relationships. A detailed description of equipoise stratified randomization is beyond the scope of the chapter, but briefly, the trial permits randomization within options encompassed by each level of the trial. Because of the way the trial is designed, subjects have the ability to refuse treatment options. This permits clinicians and subjects to choose a set of randomization options guided by patient preferences. The ethical basis for randomization relies on the assumption of clinical equipoise among treatment arms. This method of randomization allows for collaboration between patients and physicians and some degree of decisional autonomy for patients, making the trial pragmatic (Lavori et al., 2001).

IMPACT

The Improving Mood-Promoting Access to Collaborative Treatment (IMPACT) model for treating major depression focused on recruiting and identifying a sample of older adults with depression under real-world practice conditions. The study included interventions derived from evidence-based models for chronic illness care, including collaboration between psychiatrists and primary care physicians, development of a therapeutic alliance, and a personalized treatment plan. The treatment plan included patient preferences, proactive follow-up, and monitoring of outcomes by a depression care manager. Health maintenance organizations, Veterans Administration hospitals, university-affiliated primary care systems, and private practice groups were all recruitment sites for the trial. In addition to referrals from primary care providers and other medical staff at the recruitment sites, a depression screening process was implemented. This screening process was deemed to be generalizable to local practice conditions. Patients were randomized to an intervention comprising collaborative care between psychiatrists and primary care providers plus services from a new provider called a depression care specialist. The depression care specialists were nurses with and without mental health care experience (Unutzer et al., 2001, 2002).

CATIE

The purpose of the CATIE trial was to examine the comparative effectiveness of second-generation (atypical) antipsychotics versus a proxy exemplar for the general class of first-generation (typical) antipsychotics. CATIE was also designed as a pragmatic randomized controlled trial. The atypical antipsychotics chosen for comparison were olanzapine, risperidone, quetiapine, and ziprasidone. The typical antipsychotic chosen for comparison in the trial was perphenazine. Exclusion criteria were kept to a minimum. First-episode psychosis and treatment refractory schizophrenia were excluded with the rationale that the former group would be very responsive to most antipsychotics (making comparative effectiveness difficult to ascertain) and the latter group would be resistant to most antipsychotics such that it would be difficult to compare their relative effectiveness in treatment-resistant patients. Participants entering phase 2 of the study had the option to choose between two arms of the study. The first arm was clozapine versus another atypical antipsychotic that the participant had not previously been prescribed. The second arm was ziprasidone versus another atypical antipsychotic that the participant had not previously been prescribed. In phase 3, subjects and their clinicians were able to make an informed decision about an appropriate open-label treatment. When subjects entered phase 3, they were given details of the medications they received in phases 1 and 2 (Stroup et al., 2003).

RAISE

The RAISE Early Treatment Program trial engaged community treatment settings in a study of a specialized intervention—an array of recovery-oriented services—compared to usual care for first-episode psychosis delivered in a community mental health clinic (Kane et al., 2015). This study performed cluster randomization so that the intervention was site specific. Specific sites were designated to deliver the specialized intervention, NAVIGATE, whereas other sites were designated to deliver routine care. The NAVIGATE intervention was composed of a family education program, individual resiliency training, supported employment and education, and individualized medication treatment. Shared decision-making between patient and provider, weekly team meetings, and continuous assessment of physician and team functioning were all part of the NAVIGATE intervention as well (Kane et al., 2016).

CONSIDERATIONS IN PERFORMING COMMUNITY-BASED RESEARCH

In addition to providing examples of study designs, all of the historical examples discussed previously demonstrate the important value of community-based research for improving the lives of the people served in public settings, and therefore the reasons why a public psychiatrist should consider engaging with academia to foster research in clinical practice. However, there are practical considerations for the community psychiatrist who wants to do research.

Finding Opportunities

During the past few years, there has been a slowdown in central nervous system drug trials suitable for community settings due to lack of efficacious agents making it to the final rounds of testing. Another serious obstacle confronted by pharmaceutical companies is lack of relatively naive patients for conducting drug trials. Most drug trials are limited by the paucity of new-onset patients, leaving mostly potential subjects who are chronically ill and previously treated and who may or may not fulfill all criteria laid out for inclusion in a proposed random controlled trial (Tcheremissine, Rossman, Castro, & Gardner, 2014). However, there is certainly merit in conducting trials with such "real-world" patients who offer the opportunity for an effectiveness trial that takes into consideration their multiple comorbid conditions in addition to the condition targeted by the intervention drug in the clinical trial. Compared to an efficacy trial with extensive inclusion and exclusion criteria, an effectiveness trial has the advantage of broad inclusion and narrow exclusion criteria enhancing the generalizability of the trial. With a more robust drug development pipeline, collaborative efforts between pharmaceutical companies, private foundations, academic centers, and community mental health clinics could lead to the next generation of drug discovery in psychiatry. Pragmatic drug trials conducted with support from federal funding agencies such as the National Institutes of Health could establish a pipeline for continuous throughput studies for new candidate molecules.

There are instances of such partnerships among national agencies, private foundations, and academic centers that community centers could use as models (Brady & Potter, 2014). One example is the Alzheimer's Disease Neuroimaging Initiative (http://adni.loni.usc. edu), which is a joint venture involving the Foundation for NIH, National Institute of Aging, Alzheimer's Association, Canadian Institute for Health Research, Alzheimer's Drug Discovery Foundation, US Food and Drug Administration, and 13 pharmaceutical companies. Other examples of these partnerships include the Psychiatry Genomics Consortium (O'Donovan, 2015) for major depressive disorder (MDD), schizophrenia, post-traumatic stress disorder (PTSD), autism spectrum disorder, and attention-deficit/ hyperactivity disorder; One Mind for Research (https://onemind.org) for diseases such as Alzheimer's disease, PTSD, multiple sclerosis, and traumatic brain injury; Critical Path Institute Consortia: Coalition Against Major Diseases for MDD and multiple sclerosis; and Medical Research Council/AstraZeneca Mechanisms of Disease Initiative for anxiety disorders (Brady & Potter, 2014).

Design

Research studies usually originate in university-based or affiliated academic centers, and the researchers will recognize that community samples are needed to achieve an adequate sample or to identify patients who generalize to the population. Patient recruitment for these studies requires interfacing in the community with physicians who work with private practices or community clinics and hospitals. Research in the community requires researchers to develop collaborative relationships and practices between physicians in the community and the researchers. This need for collaborative relationships offers the opportunity for community psychiatrists to get involved in research.

The preferred design for such studies is a pragmatic randomized controlled trial. This design attempts to answer a question efficiently and by bridging routine clinical practice with the rigor of conducting a randomized controlled trial (Hotopf, Churchill, & Lewis, 1999). A pragmatic randomized controlled trial attempts to simulate the heterogeneity of patients encountered in common clinical practice. Exclusion criteria are kept to a minimum.

In community-based trials, great importance is placed on the process of randomization and allocation concealment. Pragmatic randomized controlled trials can use complex interventions and equipoise stratified randomization. Physician scientists often talk about clinical equipoise in a randomized controlled trial; however, a randomized controlled trial requires a null hypothesis, and usually clinical judgment cannot factor into random assignment. If clinical judgment influences treatment selection, it leads to negation of randomization. Hence, a treatment-based therapeutic relationship between a physician and a patient poses a conflict to discussing and recommending participation in a research study. A therapeutic orientation blurs the process of informed consent as well. In this regard, both physician investigators and patients are party to misconceptions about clinical trials (Miller & Rosenstein, 2003).

Studies such as IMPACT and STAR-D, discussed previously, were this sort of pragmatic trial that collaborated with providers in the community, and the design and preparation of these studies are good examples for the community psychiatrist seeking to pursue research. For the STAR-D study, there were a total of 14 regional centers overseeing care at 41 diverse primary care and specialty mental health care sites with academic affiliations and in both public and private sectors. Participating clinicians served as co-investigators rather than referring clinicians. Collaborators worked together to ensure that the trial was optimally designed to embed a randomized controlled trial within active clinical practices. For example, given that the design was a pragmatic randomized controlled trial, the study was predisposed to ethical risks of a blurring between clinical practice and research trial recruitment, as well as issues with informed consent (Goldstein et al., 2018). These were minimized by a randomization strategy that allowed patient preferences and minimal clinician choice and also by the use of specialized research staff to oversee patient recruitment. Before the trial started, a feasibility study or pilot study was conducted at three of the overseeing centers. As part of the feasibility study, investigators and clinical staff underwent a 2-day training program. These efforts to engage community clinicians and collaborate as a system led to acquiring a larger patient sample, so the trial was successful in recruiting approximately 4,000 patients.

Approvals

Before a proposed research study can start, a research proposal needs to be written and reviewed by a group of experts in order to address technical issues, feasibility, and ethical concerns. This group of experts comprises an institutional review board (IRB; Sugarman, 2000), and the community center at which the research is to occur should have one. The main function of an IRB is to review the research protocols and advise investigators and other research support staff about procedures for appropriate conduct of research. Even if the study is to be conducted in a community center, a trial that is a project of a medical school or university faculty will be subject to review of its protocol by the university's IRB. Typically, the collaborating community center's IRB relies heavily on the academic IRB for guiding its decision about project approval. If the trial involves a pharmaceutical company, the study would also be reviewed by the company's IRB.

Online resources are available to help community centers develop an IRB for trials (Office for Human Research Protections, n.d.). In addition to setting up IRBs, there are resources available online for registering IRBs and detailing IRB policies (Howard, Boyd, Nelson, & Godley, 2010). Research integrity officers are available at universities and private corporations that engage in research. For any clinical trial or research project that is done as a collaborative effort between a university academic center and a community hospital, the office of the research integrity officer would be a good resource to assist with training and certification requirements.

Interpreting Results

It is important for the public psychiatrist intent on engaging the local medical school or university in a research collaboration to have a good understanding of the concepts that are instrumental to the methodology, and therefore the results, of clinical trials. Even if not actively engaged in the research project design, understanding how to interpret the results of research studies and ensure that the findings are, in fact, evidence-based will be helpful in practice. Evidence-based medicine (EBM) is becoming increasingly pertinent to clinical practice, especially for pubic psychiatrists in leadership positions with responsibility for setting standards of care for medical staff. Apart from a few residency training programs, EBM is not required curriculum in clinical psychiatry residency training (Muzyk et al., 2017). Regardless of training, EBM can invoke anxiety for a practicing clinician expected to apply it to clinical practice and review available medical literature in order to do so (March et al., 2005).

When reading a research report, it is necessary to determine if the study is a randomized controlled trial, case–control study, or cohort study. The highest level of evidence is always provided by randomized controlled trials, and these are always prospective in nature. Cohort studies can be prospective or retrospective, and they measure whether the studied exposure leads to the condition or outcome of interest. As the name suggests, case–control studies compare subjects with the condition or exposure in question to control subjects. They can be prospective or retrospective in nature. Two other types of reports can be found in the research literature. Systematic reviews compile all of the studies that have been done on a particular topic, and meta-analyses examine whether all of the studies done on a particular topic collectively yield any quantifiable inferences.

Some key points to consider when reading a report on a randomized clinical trial include the nature of the patient sample recruited for the study, whether or not randomization was performed for the trial, and the nature of the study's blinding (Govani & Higgins, 2012; March et al., 2005). Although a randomized controlled trial has many other components, these three are the most crucial to understanding the trial methodology and results. To understand the nature of the patient sample recruited for the clinical trial, critically examine the inclusion and exclusion criteria. Do the exclusion criteria eliminate potential treatment complications or confounding factors from the study? Do the inclusion criteria identify patients who will generalize to the real world of clinical practice?

Randomization is a process intended to eliminate the effect of confounding variables. A confounding variable is any element that can affect the results of the study. In other words, randomization is a way to equally assign variations in the patient sample into the arms of the study. For example, if the study is comparing a trial of medication and a placebo, the study's process for randomization should ensure that comparable patients were assigned to the medications and placebo groups. Blinding encompasses whether or not the patients and investigators are aware of which of the arms of the study the subjects were assigned.

An important term to search for in the report of a randomized controlled trial is allocation concealment (Clark, Fairhurst, & Torgerson, 2016; Clark et al., 2013; Govani & Higgins, 2012), which refers to the process by which the investigator informs the trial's personnel about how to assign research subjects to study arms. A well-designed randomized controlled trial eliminates any possibility that study results are influenced by chance by using stringent procedures regarding the method of randomization, blinding, and allocation concealment. Most studies have dropouts, some of which may not be random or, in effect, be an outcome. When reviewing a study that has dropouts, determine whether investigators used recognized statistical methods to include the data from dropouts in the analyses. A commonly used method for doing this is intention-to-treat analysis (Govani & Higgins, 2012).

There are other important aspects of a well-designed research protocol, and in reports these are reflected in the terms relative risk, odds ratio, and effect size. Relative risk and odds ratio are related to exposure and outcome, respectively. Effect size helps describe the magnitude of the difference between intervention and comparator arms in a randomized controlled trial. Readers of any study should also examine the odds ratio and/or effect size in addition to the P values in order to make complete inference of results before deciding about translation of the results to clinical practice.

The descriptions of methods for analyses may also use terms such as dependent variable, independent variable, regression models, t-test, chi-square, analysis of variance, and P value. The clinician is concerned with P values when determining if an intervention arm (e.g., a new medication) performed better than the comparator arm. In reviewing a research report, it is important for the clinician to keep in mind that statistical significance may not always translate into clinical significance, so a positive outcome in a study may not translate into similar results in clinical practice (Guyatt, Rennie, Meade, & Cook, 2015).

Working with the Pharmaceutical Industry

Concerns about conflict of interest may leave community psychiatrists reluctant to engage with representatives of the pharmaceutical industry, let alone collaborate with the industry on research projects (Appelbaum & Gold, 2010; Freedman et al., 2009; Insel, 2010). Interactions with the pharmaceutical industry can happen in many ways, including visits with pharmaceutical drug representatives or educational liaisons, or meetings with personnel who manage research funding for studies conducted by pharmaceutical companies.

Psychiatrists who engage with industry on research studies may also deliver talks on the new medications that they have studied, often with continuing medical education credit. Although psychiatrists and other providers are required to disclose involvement with the pharmaceutical industry, this does not eliminate potential bias that may exist during the conduct of research study or when delivering a talk funded by the industry (Appelbaum & Gold, 2010; Freedman et al., 2009). A sunshine act passed into law by Congress in 2013 requires that companies make available data regarding payments to physicians. Physicians are also asked to be transparent about these payments through adequate disclosures about them when authoring research papers or providing presentations.

Nonetheless, the chance remains for bias when the psychiatrist engaged in industry-sponsored research or presentations prescribes or recommends a medication. One way to protect against this bias is through a firm knowledge of evidence-based medicine, including focusing on research findings that are presented in a nonpartisan manner. In addition, consulting with peers and discussing the available evidence may help identify biases. For research studies conducted in collaboration with the pharmaceutical industry, a review of a proposed protocol by independent, non-industry experts can help ensure rigorous, unbiased design.

OTHER COMMUNITY RESEARCH POSSIBILITIES

In addition to the types of studies described previously, there are many other potential ways for the community psychiatrist to engage in meaningful research.

A VIGNETTE

You are the chief medical officer at a state hospital, and you are approached by a nonprofit organization seeking to conduct a study to determine if involuntary outpatient commitment provides any long-term benefit to patients. The organization and its investigators would like your hospital to be a recruitment site for a grant they plan to submit to fund this study. In addition to patient recruitment, they would like you to be involved in patient follow-up. As a long-term goal of the grant proposal, they would like you to develop an outpatient clinic to follow up patients discharged from your facility to the community who will receive involuntary outpatient commitments.

Community-Based Health Services Research

The previous vignette offers a good example of health services research. Involuntary outpatient commitment is a civil court procedure wherein a patient with mental illness can be mandated to adhere to an outpatient treatment regimen. It is usually enforced by law enforcement transporting a nonadherent patient to the treatment facility for clinical re-evaluation. Forty-seven states and the District of Columbia have statutes permitting some form of outpatient commitment. Laws enacted in several states—Kendra's Law in New York, Laura's Law in California, and Kevin's Law in Michigan—have adopted a preventative form of the procedure, referred to as assisted outpatient treatment. Use of these laws has been controversial because of its perceived coerciveness and so the process has received intense scrutiny concerning its effectiveness. A recent Cochrane review concluded that there were no significant differences in service use, social functioning, or quality of life for subjects receiving mandated outpatient treatment as opposed to standard care, although such systematic reviews are largely limited to evidence from randomized controlled trials and neglect considerable evidence from other studies. The review did find that patients who received mandated outpatient treatment were less likely to be victims of violent or nonviolent crime (Kisely, Campbell, & O'Reilly, 2017). Primary outcomes considered in the systematic review included admission to hospital and mean number of days spent in hospital every month as measures of health service contact and utilization. Imprisonment, police contact, and arrests were considered to be measures of social functioning.

The methodology and results of a randomized controlled trial performed in North Carolina that compared outpatient commitment to standard care offer good examples of some of the methodology issues to be considered when performing health services research (Swartz, Swanson, Hiday, et al., 2001). The study randomized patients into two groups. However, subjects with a baseline history of serious violence were not randomized but instead were followed as a naturalistic comparison group. This design was the result of concerns voiced by clinicians about their potential liability in releasing violent patients who might then ber randomized to the standard care group and therefore released from their court orders (Swartz, Swanson, Wagner, Burns, & Hiday, 2001). When analyzed strictly within study groups, the investigators found no significant difference in adherence between the two groups. When subjects with a baseline history of serious violence were included in the analysis and outpatient commitment intervention was redefined as receiving at least 6 months of court-ordered treatment, subjects with the sustained intervention had a higher likelihood of treatment adherence and fewer negative outcomes.

The investigators encountered several other practical problems impacting this randomized controlled trial. A large proportion of outpatient commitment orders were not renewed in the community after an initial period of 90 days, based on the judgment of the clinicians and the court. Because many of the favorable outcomes were contingent on a longer period of commitment, critics argued that many findings of benefit could be classified as post hoc. This was necessarily a result of the pragmatic design of the study, in which commitment order renewal decisions were beyond the control of the study. Despite these caveats, repeated measures multivariable analyses of rehospitalization in successive months demonstrated that the outpatient commitment group indeed had significantly fewer hospital relapses (Swartz et al., 1999). The study also highlighted that sustained outpatient commitment was effective for individuals with non-affective psychotic disorders, reducing hospital readmissions approximately 72% and requiring 28 fewer hospital days.

Health services research is significantly different from a clinical trial involving a psychotropic drug or intervention. In addition to using sophisticated statistical modeling, investigators involved in studies such as the one discussed previously must give adequate thought to the design of the study to ensure pragmatic approximation of real-world situations and careful interpretation of results from the trial. While examining questions such as the one detailed previously, it may also be essential to accommodate large-scale and quasi-experimental naturalistic studies with multivariable statistical controls rather than try to design an ideal randomized controlled trial (Swanson & Swartz, 2014).

Community-Based Research on Violence and Mental Illness

With the many recent, highly publicized shooting incidents, prediction of gun violence in the community continues to be an active area of research and therefore is another area in which psychiatrists in the community can contribute. Two seminal studies have shown a modest predisposition to violence among patients with mental illness, especially when in the presence of comorbid antisocial personality traits and substance use (Swanson, 1994; Swanson, McGinty, Fazel, & Mays, 2015). The Epidemiologic Catchment Area (ECA) study used trained lay interviews of nearly 10,000 people in the community and showed a statistically significant, but fairly modest, positive association between violence and mental illness. The 12-month prevalence of either minor or serious violence among people with schizophrenia, bipolar disorder, or major depression was approximately 12% overall, of which 7% had no substance abuse comorbidity. The ECA study debunked stigmatizing claims about mental illness having a significant relationship to violence because the study showed younger age and history of substance use disorder to be predictive of violent behavior regardless of the presence or absence of mental illness. Whereas ECA was a community-based epidemiological study, the design of the MacArthur Violence Risk Assessment Study included the participation of community psychiatrists in the research. It engaged three community mental health inpatient facilities and a general hospital in identifying patients who were then followed for 1 year after discharge from the inpatient units. The study found that in the absence of comorbid substance use, patients were at no greater risk for violence compared to individuals without mental illness.

Other studies have reported similar findings, including the Dunedin study (Arseneault, Moffitt, Caspi, Taylor, & Silva, 2000) and studies from Europe (Hodgins, Mednick, Brennan, Schulsinger, & Engberg, 1996; Tiihonen, Isohanni, Rasanen, Koiranen, & Moring, 1997) and Australia. The CATIE trial demonstrated a higher predisposition to violence among patients with schizophrenia, especially in the context of childhood antisocial traits and criminal behavior prior to onset of psychotic illness. A meta-analysis found a higher risk for violent behavior among women with a diagnosis of schizophrenia than men with the diagnosis. Again, risk was accentuated by a comorbid diagnosis of substance use. The degree of risk for violent behavior was the same for substance use disorder regardless of the presence or absence of comorbid psychosis (Fazel, Gulati, Linsell, Geddes, & Grann, 2009).

The medical records of community mental health centers offer another source for research studies. For example, a recent report using such medical records studied the relationship between mental illness and the use of guns in nonviolent crimes in two Florida counties. The study relied on the de-identified records of people served in the community mental health system for the counties. It found that 49% of arrests due to crimes involving guns were of people with a previous criminal record. Ten percent of the arrests involved people with both mental health issues and a criminal record, and only 3% of the arrests involved people with mental health issues but no prior record. In the same study, only 10% of suicides by firearm involved people known to the public mental health system, whereas 54% involved people who had a history of previous short-term involuntary holds apparently without subsequent public sector mental health care (Swanson et al., 2016).

Community-Based Research on Substance Use Disorders

The most common substance use disorders in community settings involve alcohol, cannabis, and pain reliever drugs including opiates (Substance Abuse and Mental Health Services Administration, 2015). Medication-assisted treatment (MAT), which combines psychopharmacological agents with psychosocial interventions, is an emerging evidence-based approach to public sector patients with substance use disorders (Aaronson, Adelstein, & Csernansky, 2018; Ma et al., 2018; Robertson et al., 2018). Specific substance use disorders for which MATs have shown greatest benefit include alcohol use disorder and opiate use disorder (Aaronson et al., 2018; Ma et al., 2018). Psychopharmacological agents to treat alcohol use disorder include naltrexone, disulfiram, and acamprosate. For opiate use disorder, treatment consists of opiate replacement therapies such as methadone or buprenorphine given in conjunction with psychosocial interventions.

Opiate replacement therapies such as suboxone and naltrexone can be dispensed by primary care providers in the community, but it is typically done with minimal support from psychosocial interventions (Rosenblatt, Andrilla, Catlin, & Larson, 2015). There is also a shortage of providers to prescribe suboxone and deliver psychosocial interventions for patients in the community (Rosenblatt et al., 2015), partly because physicians need a waiver to prescribe suboxone and those who practice in the community face other barriers to prescribing suboxone (Andrilla, Coulthard, & Larson, 2017).

In addition to the health services research opportunities related to increasing access to MAT in the community and to overcoming treatment barriers, patients at community mental health clinics, public health clinics such as federally qualified health centers, incarcerated at local jails or in prisons, and even state hospital patients with substance use disorders all offer potential study populations for emerging candidate molecules that might address craving and prevent relapse in these disorders—mainly alcohol use disorder and opiate use disorder—as well as studies on associated psychosocial interventions. New agents continue to be tested for effectiveness in substance use disorders, and collaborative efforts between academic centers and community mental health clinics can target this patient population. This patient population also affords an opportunity for trials comparing other stand-alone psychosocial interventions, such as therapeutic communities; ACT targeting patients with dual diagnoses encompassing concomitantly occurring mood, anxiety, or psychotic illnesses; and substance use disorders.

Community-Based Health Technology Research

Mobile technologies, smartphone applications, and telehealth services have great potential to change the face of mental health care delivery in the community. Smartphone applications have revolutionized data collection strategies and opened up windows for digital phenotyping, helping to potentially prevent relapse in illnesses such as schizophrenia and to detect depressive disorder and suicide in the community (Torous, 2018). Smartphone applications have also decreased communication gaps between mental health providers and patients, allowing real-time symptom reporting (Kuhn et al., 2016; Owen et al., 2015; Tiet et al., 2018). Telehealth services provide venues for psychiatry care and psychotherapeutic interventions in areas with poor access to these services on-site.

Many community-based research opportunities exist to assess the effectiveness of these mobile applications, including standardizing them for pilot and validation studies. Although most mobile applications involve active data collection using application interfaces, a proportion utilize passive data collection for predictive purposes. Such use of data analytics would be an avenue for partnership between treatment settings in the community and companies that specialize in predictive analytics capitalizing on these potential massive data sets. The focus of these studies could even be as simple as utilizing vital sign data collected using Fitbits for prediction of relapse for depressive and psychotic symptoms. Pertinent issues that need to be focused on include ethical issues and informed consent in these clinical trials (Torous, 2018).

CASE STUDY: CONCLUSION

Prior to venturing into the sort of human research that is envisioned in this case study, an optimal understanding of ethical and logistical requirements is key. Ethical issues include determining a procedure for informed consent and educating research associates about this procedure. It is important to avoid coercion of any nature and to inform research participants that their decision regarding research participation will not influence treatment. Sufficient attention to ethical concerns also mandates training all staff involved in the project about the protocols. The Collaborative Institutional Training Initiative (CITI Program) is an online collection of resources that can facilitate training for those who wish to engage in research. The website offers courses in bioethics, biosafety, good clinical practice, responsible conduct of research, clinical trial billing competence, and clinical trial design (CITI Program, 2018). Similarly, the National Institutes of Health (2018) also offers a clinical research training program available online.

The study proposed in this case would also require IRB approval. Because this is a clinical trial associated with an academic university center, it would be reviewed by the university IRB in addition to the CMHC's IRB. Also, because this is a trial to be conducted by a pharmaceutical company, the study would be reviewed by the company's IRB or by a commercial IRB.

If the relationship proposed in the case study is not a comfortable one for the CMHC but the center still wishes to engage in research, another approach that the center might take is to perform community-based participatory research (CBPR). CBPR is different from typical research projects using sites in the community for patient recruitment in that, by using a CBPR, community members, organizational representatives, and investigators collaborate in all aspects of the research process (Israel, Schulz, Parker, & Becker, 2001). Partners contribute their expertise, share responsibilities, and take ownership together. Examples of such partners are FHI360, RTI International, and RAND Corporation.

Through this community partnership process, CBPR can also ensure that talent is recruited and trained from the community to continue changes, interventions, and processes that result from the partnership research venture. Such partnerships between the community and established research centers have also been instrumental in growing research ventures that target marginalized and vulnerable populations (Carey et al., 2005; De Marco et al., 2014). A notable example is the collaboration between a church in rural North Carolina and an African American population at the North Carolina Translational and Clinical Sciences Institute and the University of North Carolina. CBPR was used to propagate a research project (Harvest for Hope Project) that resulted in healthier dietary practices and increased exercise among members of the rural community (De Marco et al., 2014).

Regardless of the format for research study, it is important that public sector providers find ways to make research studies acceptable in their settings. Studies such as STAR-D,

RAISE, and CATIE took advantage of the collaboration between community sites for patient recruitment and academic centers in a manner similar to that proposed in the case study. These collaborations yielded valuable insights into interventions for MDD, schizophrenia, and early psychosis—insights that improved understanding of mental illness and its treatment—and the knowledge gained from the research can therefore enhance the health and well-being of the entire community. Likewise, epidemiological studies and field trials performed with community collaborators served to refine the criteria for both the *Diagnostic and Statistical Manual of Mental Disorders* and the *International Classification of Diseases* manuals. With the multiple advancements the field makes every day, the psychiatrist in the community needs to be equipped to take on multiple roles in addition to being a clinician and administrator.

REFERENCES

Aaronson, A., Adelstein, J., & Csernansky, J. G. (2018). Medication-assisted treatment for alcohol use disorder: Hope for incarcerated patients and for our communities. *Am J Psychiatry*, 175(7), 596–597. doi:10.1176/appi.ajp.2018.18040445

American Psychiatric Association. (2018). *Choosing a career in psychiatry*. Retrieved from https://www.psychiatry.org/residents-medical-students/medical-students/choosing-a-career-in-psychiatry

Andrilla, C. H. A., Coulthard, C., & Larson, E. H. (2017). Barriers rural physicians face prescribing buprenorphine for opioid use disorder. *Ann Fam Med*, 15(4), 359–362. doi:10.1370/afm.2099

Appelbaum, P. S., & Gold, A. (2010). Psychiatrists' relationships with industry: The principal-agent problem. *Harv Rev Psychiatry*, 18(5), 255–265. doi:10.3109/10673229.2010.507038

Arseneault, L., Moffitt, T. E., Caspi, A., Taylor, P. J., & Silva, P. A. (2000). Mental disorders and violence in a total birth cohort: Results from the Dunedin Study. *Arch Gen Psychiatry*, 57(10), 979–986.

Bishop, T. F., Seirup, J. K., Pincus, H. A., & Ross, J. S. (2016). Population of US practicing psychiatrists declined, 2003–13, which may help explain poor access to mental health care. *Health Aff*, 35(7), 1271–1277. doi:10.1377/hlthaff.2015.1643

Brady, L. S., & Potter, W. Z. (2014). Public–private partnerships to revitalize psychiatric drug discovery. *Expert Opin Drug Discov*, 9(1), 1–8. doi:10.1517/17460441.2014.867944

Brenner, A. M., Balon, R., Coverdale, J. H., Beresin, E. V., Guerrero, A. P., Louie, A. K., & Roberts, L. W. (2017). Psychiatry workforce and psychiatry recruitment: Two intertwined challenges. *Acad Psychiatry*, 41(2), 202–206. doi:10.1007/s40596-017-0679-3

Burns, T. (2002). The UK700 trial of intensive case management: An overview and discussion. *World Psychiatry*, 1(3), 175–178.

Burns, T. (2010). The rise and fall of assertive community treatment? *Int Rev Psychiatry*, 22(2), 130–137. doi:10.3109/09540261003661841

Carey, T. S., Howard, D. L., Goldmon, M., Roberson, J. T., Godley, P. A., & Ammerman, A. (2005). Developing effective interuniversity partnerships and community-based research to address health disparities. *Acad Med*, 80(11), 1039–1045.

CITI Program. (2018). *Collaborative Institutional Training Initiative*. Retrieved from https://about.citiprogram.org/en/homepage

Clark, L., Fairhurst, C., & Torgerson, D. J. (2016). Allocation concealment in randomised controlled trials: Are we getting better? *BMJ*, 355, i5663. doi:10.1136/bmj.i5663

Clark, L., Schmidt, U., Tharmanathan, P., Adamson, J., Hewitt, C., & Torgerson, D. (2013). Allocation concealment: A methodological review. *J Eval Clin Pract*, 19(4), 708–712. doi:10.1111/jep.12032

De Marco, M., Kearney, W., Smith, T., Jones, C., Kearney-Powell, A., & Ammerman, A. (2014). Growing partners: Building a community–academic partnership to address health disparities in rural North Carolina. *Prog Community Health Partnersh, 8*(2), 181–186. doi:10.1353/cpr.2014.0021

Fazel, S., Gulati, G., Linsell, L., Geddes, J. R., & Grann, M. (2009). Schizophrenia and violence: Systematic review and meta-analysis. *PLoS Med, 6*(8), e1000120. doi:10.1371/journal.pmed.1000120

Freedman, R., Lewis, D. A., Michels, R., Pine, D. S., Schultz, S. K., Tamminga, C. A., . . . Yager, J. (2009). Conflict of interest—An issue for every psychiatrist. *Am J Psychiatry, 166*(3), 274. doi:10.1176/appi.ajp.2009.09010093

Goldstein, C. E., Weijer, C., Brehaut, J. C., Fergusson, D. A., Grimshaw, J. M., Horn, A. R., & Taljaard, M. (2018). Ethical issues in pragmatic randomized controlled trials: A review of the recent literature identifies gaps in ethical argumentation. *BMC Med Ethics, 19*(1), 14. doi:10.1186/s12910-018-0253-x

Govani, S. M., & Higgins, P. D. (2012). How to read a clinical trial paper: A lesson in basic trial statistics. *Gastroenterol Hepatol, 8*(4), 241–248.

Guyatt, G., Rennie, D., Meade, M. O., & Cook, D. J. (2015). *Users' guides to the medical literature: A manual for evidence-based clinical practice* (3rd ed.). New York, NY: McGraw-Hill.

Hodgins, S., Mednick, S. A., Brennan, P. A., Schulsinger, F., & Engberg, M. (1996). Mental disorder and crime: Evidence from a Danish birth cohort. *Arch Gen Psychiatry, 53*(6), 489–496.

Hoge, M. A., Stuart, G. W., Morris, J., Flaherty, M. T., Paris, M., Jr., & Goplerud, E. (2013). Mental health and addiction workforce development: Federal leadership is needed to address the growing crisis. *Health Aff, 32*(11), 2005–2012. doi:10.1377/hlthaff.2013.0541

Hotopf, M., Churchill, R., & Lewis, G. (1999). Pragmatic randomised controlled trials in psychiatry. *Br J Psychiatry, 175,* 217–223.

Howard, D. L., Boyd, C. L., Nelson, D. K., & Godley, P. (2010). Getting from A to IRB: Developing an institutional review board at a historically Black university. *J Empir Res Hum Res Ethics, 5*(1), 75–81. doi:10.1525/jer.2010.5.1.75

Insel, T. R. (2010). Psychiatrists' relationships with pharmaceutical companies: Part of the problem or part of the solution? *JAMA, 303*(12), 1192–1193. doi:10.1001/jama.2010.317

Israel, B. A., Schulz, A. J., Parker, E. A., & Becker, A. B. (2001). Community-based participatory research: Policy recommendations for promoting a partnership approach in health research. *Educ Health, 14*(2), 182–197. doi:10.1080/13576280110051055

Kane, J. M., Robinson, D. G., Schooler, N. R., Mueser, K. T., Penn, D. L., Rosenheck, R. A., . . . Heinssen, R. K. (2016). Comprehensive versus usual community care for first-episode psychosis: 2-Year outcomes from the NIMH RAISE early treatment program. *Am J Psychiatry, 173*(4), 362–372. doi:10.1176/appi.ajp.2015.15050632

Kane, J. M., Schooler, N. R., Marcy, P., Correll, C. U., Brunette, M. F., Mueser, K. T., . . . Robinson, D. G. (2015). The RAISE early treatment program for first-episode psychosis: Background, rationale, and study design. *J Clin Psychiatry, 76*(3), 240–246. doi:10.4088/JCP.14m09289

Killaspy, H., Kingett, S., Bebbington, P., Blizard, R., Johnson, S., Nolan, F., . . . King, M. (2009). Randomised Evaluation of Assertive Community Treatment: 3-Year outcomes. *Br J Psychiatry, 195*(1), 81–82. doi:10.1192/bjp.bp.108.059303

Kisely, S. R., Campbell, L. A., & O'Reilly, R. (2017). Compulsory community and involuntary outpatient treatment for people with severe mental disorders. *Cochrane Database Syst Rev, 2017*(3), CD004408. doi:10.1002/14651858.CD004408.pub5

Kuhn, E., Weiss, B. J., Taylor, K. L., Hoffman, J. E., Ramsey, K. M., Manber, R., . . . Trockel, M. (2016). CBT-I Coach: A description and clinician perceptions of a mobile app for cognitive behavioral therapy for insomnia. *J Clin Sleep Med, 12*(4), 597–606. doi:10.5664/jcsm.5700

Lavori, P. W., Rush, A. J., Wisniewski, S. R., Alpert, J., Fava, M., Kupfer, D. J., . . . Trivedi, M. (2001). Strengthening clinical effectiveness trials: Equipoise-stratified randomization. *Biol Psychiatry, 50*(10), 792–801.

Ma, J., Bao, Y. P., Wang, R. J., Su, M. F., Liu, M. X., Li, J. Q., . . . Lu, L. (2018). Effects of medication-assisted treatment on mortality among opioids users: A systematic review and meta-analysis. *Mol Psychiatry*. doi:10.1038/s41380-018-0094-5

March, J. S., Silva, S. G., Compton, S., Shapiro, M., Califf, R., & Krishnan, R. (2005). The case for practical clinical trials in psychiatry. *Am J Psychiatry, 162*(5), 836–846. doi:10.1176/appi.ajp.162.5.836

Marshall, M., & Lockwood, A. (2000). Assertive community treatment for people with severe mental disorders. *Cochrane Database Syst Rev, 2000*(2), CD001089. doi:10.1002/14651858.CD001089

McHugo, G. J., Drake, R. E., Teague, G. B., & Xie, H. (1999). Fidelity to assertive community treatment and client outcomes in the New Hampshire dual disorders study. *Psychiatr Serv, 50*(6), 818–824. doi:10.1176/ps.50.6.818

Miller, F. G., & Rosenstein, D. L. (2003). The therapeutic orientation to clinical trials. *N Engl J Med, 348*(14), 1383–1386. doi:10.1056/NEJMsb030228

Muzyk, A. J., Gagliardi, J. P., Rakesh, G., Jiroutek, M. R., Radhakrishnan, R., Pae, C. U., . . . Szabo, S. T. (2017). Development of a diverse learning experience for diverse psychiatry resident needs: A four-year biological psychiatry curriculum incorporating principles of neurobiology, psychopharmacology, and evidence-based practice. *Psychiatry Investig, 14*(3), 289–297. doi:10.4306/pi.2017.14.3.289

National Institutes of Health. (2018). *Clinical research training.* Retrieved from https://crt.nihtraining.com

O'Donovan, M. C. (2015). What have we learned from the Psychiatric Genomics Consortium. *World Psychiatry, 14*(3), 291–293. doi:10.1002/wps.20270

Office for Human Research Protections, US Department of Health and Human Services. (n.d.). *Office for Human Research Protections (OHRP) database for registered IORGs & IRBs.* Retrieved from https://ohrp.cit.nih.gov/search/irbsearch.aspx

Owen, J. E., Jaworski, B. K., Kuhn, E., Makin-Byrd, K. N., Ramsey, K. M., & Hoffman, J. E. (2015). mHealth in the wild: Using novel data to examine the reach, use, and impact of PTSD Coach. *JMIR Ment Health, 2*(1), e7. doi:10.2196/mental.3935

Patsopoulos, N. A. (2011). A pragmatic view on pragmatic trials. *Dialogues Clin Neurosci, 13*(2), 217–224.

Phillips, L. J., Leicester, S. B., O'Dwyer, L. E., Francey, S. M., Koutsogiannis, J., Abdel-Baki, A., . . . McGorry, P. D. (2002). The PACE Clinic: Identification and management of young people at "ultra" high risk of psychosis. *J Psychiatr Pract, 8*(5), 255–269.

Robertson, A. G., Easter, M. M., Lin, H., Frisman, L. K., Swanson, J. W., & Swartz, M. S. (2018). Medication-assisted treatment for alcohol-dependent adults with serious mental illness and criminal justice involvement: Effects on treatment utilization and outcomes. *Am J Psychiatry, 175*(7), 665–673. doi:10.1176/appi.ajp.2018.17060688

Rosenblatt, R. A., Andrilla, C. H., Catlin, M., & Larson, E. H. (2015). Geographic and specialty distribution of US physicians trained to treat opioid use disorder. *Ann Fam Med, 13*(1), 23–26. doi:10.1370/afm.1735

Stein, L. I., Test, M. A., & Marx, A. J. (1975). Alternative to the hospital: A controlled study. *Am J Psychiatry, 132*(5), 517–522. doi:10.1176/ajp.132.5.517

Stroup, T. S., McEvoy, J. P., Swartz, M. S., Byerly, M. J., Glick, I. D., Canive, J. M., . . . Lieberman, J. A. (2003). The National Institute of Mental Health Clinical Antipsychotic Trials of Intervention Effectiveness (CATIE) project: Schizophrenia trial design and protocol development. *Schizophr Bull, 29*(1), 15–31.

Substance Abuse and Mental Health Services Administration. (2015). *Behavioral health trends in the United States: Results from the 2014 National Survey on Drug Use and Health.* Retrieved from https://www.samhsa.gov/data/sites/default/files/NSDUH-FRR1-2014/NSDUH-FRR1-2014.pdf

Sugarman, J. (2000). The role of institutional support in protecting human research subjects. *Acad Med, 75*(7), 687–692.

Swanson, J. W. (1994). Mental disorder, substance abuse, and community violence: An epidemiological approach. In S. H. Monahan (Ed.), *Violence and mental disorder* (pp. 101–136). Chicago, IL: University of Chicago Press.

Swanson, J. W., Easter, M. M., Robertson, A. G., Swartz, M. S., Alanis-Hirsch, K., Moseley, D., . . . Petrila, J. (2016). Gun violence, mental illness, and laws that prohibit gun possession: Evidence from two Florida counties. *Health Aff, 35*(6), 1067–1075. doi:10.1377/hlthaff.2016.0017

Swanson, J. W., McGinty, E. E., Fazel, S., & Mays, V. M. (2015). Mental illness and reduction of gun violence and suicide: Bringing epidemiologic research to policy. *Ann Epidemiol, 25*(5), 366–376. doi:10.1016/j.annepidem.2014.03.004

Swanson, J. W., & Swartz, M. S. (2014). Why the evidence for outpatient commitment is good enough. *Psychiatr Serv, 65*(6), 808–811. doi:10.1176/appi.ps.201300424

Swartz, M. S., Swanson, J. W., Hiday, V. A., Wagner, H. R., Burns, B. J., & Borum, R. (2001). A randomized controlled trial of outpatient commitment in North Carolina. *Psychiatr Serv, 52*(3), 325–329. doi:10.1176/appi.ps.52.3.325

Swartz, M. S., Swanson, J. W., Wagner, H. R., Burns, B. J., & Hiday, V. A. (2001). Effects of involuntary outpatient commitment and depot antipsychotics on treatment adherence in persons with severe mental illness. *J Nerv Ment Dis, 189*(9), 583–592.

Swartz, M. S., Swanson, J. W., Wagner, H. R., Burns, B. J., Hiday, V. A., & Borum, R. (1999). Can involuntary outpatient commitment reduce hospital recidivism? Findings from a randomized trial with severely mentally ill individuals. *Am J Psychiatry, 156*(12), 1968–1975. doi:10.1176/ajp.156.12.1968

Tcheremissine, O. V., Rossman, W. E., Castro, M. A., & Gardner, D. R. (2014). Conducting clinical research in community mental health settings: Opportunities and challenges. *World J Psychiatry, 4*(3), 49–55. doi:10.5498/wjp.v4.i3.49

Thomas, K. C., Ellis, A. R., Konrad, T. R., Holzer, C. E., & Morrissey, J. P. (2009). County-level estimates of mental health professional shortage in the United States. *Psychiatr Serv, 60*(10), 1323–1328. doi:10.1176/ps.2009.60.10.1323

Thornicroft, G., Wykes, T., Holloway, F., Johnson, S., & Szmukler, G. (1998). From efficacy to effectiveness in community mental health services: PRiSM psychosis study. *Br J Psychiatry, 173*, 423–427.

Tiet, Q. Q., Duong, H., Davis, L., French, R., Smith, C. L., Leyva, Y. E., & Rosen, C. (2018). PTSD coach mobile application with brief telephone support: A pilot study. *Psychol Serv, 16*(2), 227–232. doi:10.1037/ser0000245

Tiihonen, J., Isohanni, M., Rasanen, P., Koiranen, M., & Moring, J. (1997). Specific major mental disorders and criminality: A 26-year prospective study of the 1966 northern Finland birth cohort. *Am J Psychiatry, 154*(6), 840–845. doi:10.1176/ajp.154.6.840

Torous, J. B. (2018). Focusing on the future of mobile mental health and smartphone interventions. *Psychiatr Serv, 69*(9), 945. doi:10.1176/appi.ps.201800308

Turner, J. C., & Dean, B. (1978). New NIMH program promotes community support systems. *Innovations, 5*(1), 16–17.

Unutzer, J., Katon, W., Callahan, C. M., Williams, J. W., Jr., Hunkeler, E., Harpole, L., . . . Langston, C.; for the IMPACT Investigators. (2002). Collaborative care management of late-life depression in the primary care setting: A randomized controlled trial. *JAMA, 288*(22), 2836–2845.

Unutzer, J., Katon, W., Williams, J. W., Jr., Callahan, C. M., Harpole, L., Hunkeler, E. M., . . . Langston, C. A. (2001). Improving primary care for depression in late life: The design of a multicenter randomized trial. *Med Care, 39*(8), 785–799.

Yung, A. R., McGorry, P. D., Francey, S. M., Nelson, B., Baker, K., Phillips, L. J., . . . Amminger, G. P. (2007). PACE: A specialised service for young people at risk of psychotic disorders. *Med J Aust, 187*(7 Suppl), S43–S46.

///9/// THE PUBLIC PSYCHIATRIST AS ADVOCATE

EBONY DIX AND AYANA JORDAN

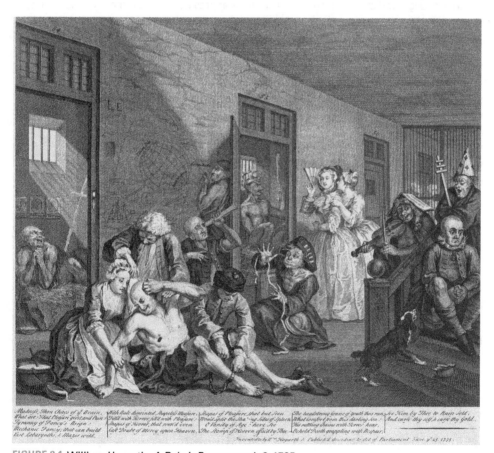

FIGURE 9.1 William Hogarth, *A Rake's Progress: pl. 8*, 1735.

William Hogarth (1697–1764) was an English artist famous for his serial engravings offering a satirical approach to English customs of his day. A Rake's Progress is one of his most famous such series. In eight plates it portrays the life of a man who has squandered his inheritance. Plate 8 is entitled "Bedlam." Hogarth's use of the infamous mental hospital in this series reflects the common belief in his society that madness was a result of moral weakness.

CASE STUDY: INITIAL PRESENTATION

Mrs. J is a 35-year-old married, Caucasian stay-at-home mother of four. She has a history of major depressive disorder, generalized anxiety disorder, attention-deficit/hyperactivity disorder, obesity, and migraine headaches. She is presenting for a routine outpatient psychiatry follow-up visit at the public hospital clinic where you serve. She tells you that she has been having very high levels of anxiety related to a physical complaint she believes has been overlooked by her primary care provider. Specifically, she reports having a lump in her axilla that has been getting larger and has not been addressed. She tearfully describes feeling helpless and ignored by physicians, alluding that her provider seemed more concerned with her anxiety rather than her physical complaint. She tells you that her anxiety has been negatively impacting her sleep, appetite, energy levels, and frequency of migraines. Although she denies any suicidal ideation, intentions, or plans, you are concerned about her level of emotional distress as well as her strong family history of breast cancer. Mrs. J accepts your offer to perform a physical examination so that you can document any findings, which may help expedite the appropriate referrals.

QUESTIONS
1. How might you help this patient access the appropriate care she needs in a timely manner?
2. How could you help a patient with limited health care literacy navigate a complex referral system?
3. Are there ways you can help educate your colleagues in other fields about a mutual patient's mental health condition?

PSYCHIATRY AND LITERATURE

Memorial of Miss Dix
January 11, 1847

Excerpted from Dorothea Dix's memorial to the Senate and House of Representatives of the State of Illinois, 15th assembly, 1st session (Dix, 1847)

But, gentlemen, I do not come to move your *benevolent feelings*, so much as to present *just claims.* I do not ask of you the performance of *generous acts* from yourselves and constituents, but respectfully urge you to fulfill a*bsolute obligations*: the obligations of man, favored with competence and sound reason, to his fellow-man, rendered helpless and dependent through infirmities to which *all* are exposed, and from which none are too rich to be exempt, or too poor to escape.

INTRODUCTION

Mental health advocacy is an integral part of the psychiatrist's professional role, yet it is a challenging pursuit that most psychiatrists feel ill-equipped to pursue or accomplish, despite completing years of training. Advocacy has a rich yet complicated history that has been influenced by diverse individuals who are well known for their contributions to the field of psychiatry and mental health policy. Mental health advocacy is indeed multifaceted and continuously evolving, which makes it particularly difficult to pragmatically teach and effectively implement instruction in this area. To better understand the role of the psychiatrist as a patient advocate, one must first be familiar with the various definitions and interpretations of the terms "mental health" and "advocacy," how they have changed over time, and their implications for the community psychiatrist whose duties extend beyond the individual patient. Next, one must consider the philosophical and historical background of mental health advocacy that has not only influenced many contemporary policies but also can serve as inspiration for the future. Finally, one must consider how and where to learn public policy and advocacy skills. For example, varying national and local mental health organizations provide education on how best to advocate, and there are educational and training initiatives implemented by some medical schools and residency programs. Although these initiatives are far from perfect, they are a good starting point for teaching and developing public policy and advocacy skills to the future community psychiatrist.

DEFINITIONS

Mental Illness

Throughout the course of history, the concept of mental illness has had many interpretations, dating back to ancient medical, religious, and philosophical texts. Mental illness has been conceptualized in many ways, including, but not limited to, divine punishment or demonic possession in Biblical times and an imbalance of the humors by Hippocrates and Galen, a perturbation of the mind by Cicero, a disease of the soul by Plato, and even an aberration from normal human nature by Aristotle in ancient philosophy (Ahonen, 2019). Regardless of the interpretation, one common theme that has been consistent throughout the ages is that mental illness is a malady that interferes with an individual's ability to conform to social norms.

The terms mental illness and mental health are often used interchangeably, but these terms confer different meanings. *Mental illness* has been defined by the National Alliance on Mental Illness (NAMI, 2019a) as a condition that may be due to multiple factors that affect one's thinking, feeling, mood, and ability to relate to others and function on a daily basis. The American Psychiatric Association (APA, 2015) defines mental illness as a condition that may encompass a combination of changes in emotion, thinking, and behavior that are associated with distress and impaired functioning in a variety of domains of daily life.

Mental Health

By contrast, *mental health* has been defined by the World Health Organization (WHO, 2003, 2013) as "a state of well-being in which the individual realizes his or her own potential, can cope with the normal stresses of life, can work productively and fruitfully, and is able to make a contribution to his or her community." This "state of well-being" might be interpreted as synonymous with good physical health, and perhaps the two should be fully integrated when considering overall general health. However, in many areas of the world, mental health is not regarded with the same importance as physical health. In fact, the dichotomy remains, hence the need for advocacy to not only advance understanding about mental health conditions but also improve detection, prevention, and treatment methods. Complicating matters further is the need for mental health advocacy for specific populations (i.e., low income, homeless, underrepresented minority groups, immigrants, older adults, intellectually and developmentally disabled, and incarcerated), given their challenges accessing overall health care.

Advocacy

The term *advocacy* typically refers to support for a cause, policy, or individual ("Advocacy," 2019). When considering the agents for advocacy, one often thinks of political groups or legislators. However, in the context of health care, who embodies a patient advocate is variably understood. Patient advocates may include, but are not limited to, medical students, nurses, social workers, therapists or physicians, local coalitions, or national organizations.

In the global medical community, there is no consensus regarding what constitutes the duties of a physician patient advocate. Physicians as patient advocates may listen and intervene on behalf of a patient who may be unable to access information and services, express their views and concerns, defend and promote their rights and responsibilities, or explore choices and options (Lustig, 2012). The Royal College of Physicians and Surgeons of Canada defines the role of the physician as health advocate as one in which "physicians contribute their expertise and influence as they work with communities or patient populations to improve health" (Frank, Snell, & Sherbino, 2015).

WHO (2003, 2013) defines mental health advocacy as a variety of actions aimed at changing the major structural and attitudinal barriers to achieving positive mental health outcomes. Specifically, in its 2003 Mental Health Policy and Service Guidance Package, WHO states, "Advocacy is an important means of raising awareness on mental health issues and ensuring that mental health is on the national agenda of governments. Advocacy can lead to improvements in policy, legislation and service development." In addition, WHO suggests that the concept of advocacy began with the intention "to promote the human rights of persons with mental disorders and to reduce stigma and discrimination," and it has broadened in scope to include prevention, less severe mental disorders, and the mental health of the general population (WHO, 2003, 2013).

The American Medical Association (AMA) and other professional organizations have included language in their policies regarding the psychiatrist's obligation toward professional advocacy (Thompson, 2019). The education and training of physicians would be incomplete without the teaching of classical and humanistic concepts that aim to develop and mold the physician into an advocate *for* the patient, *with* the patient, and their communities (To & Sharma, 2015). Some psychiatry residency training programs have expanded their curricula to include advocacy teaching. The implementation of advocacy-based education, however, does not come without its challenges, which are further explored later in this chapter.

ADVOCACY IN HISTORICAL CONTEXT

The act of caring for the sick has been considered one of the most honorable and noble deeds that mankind has been able to accomplish. In fact, caring for the sick has been historically documented by world religions and cultures as an act of religious duty, divine commands, or moral obligation. Even in atheism, aspects of one of the oldest moral precepts, the Golden

Rule ("Do unto others as you would have them done unto you"), have guided many acts of kindness, altruism, and empathy when caring for the sick (Kalman, 2010).

However, people with mental illness have not always been subject to such care, as illustrated by the case study. Instead, historical attitudes toward mental illness as a moral failure or defect or malady of the humors have led individuals with mental illness to be cast to the margins of society, ignored, stigmatized, and even dehumanized. Unfortunately, some of the earliest treatment methods aimed to correct or eliminate mental illness were techniques that are considered inhumane today. These treatments included trephination (drilling a hole or removing part of the skull to release demons or evil spirits), bloodletting (medical procedure for removing blood for a therapeutic purpose), isolation, confinement to asylums, and lobotomies (Ahonen, 2019; Caruso & Sheehan, 2017). Although there were some who at least intended these approaches to be effective treatments, others were more inclined to treat people with mental illness like criminals, warranting isolation in order to protect the rest of society (Ahonen, 2019).

Even though stigma persists today, the progress in treatment methods and growth of awareness about mental illness, mostly dating to the 18th and 19th centuries, could not have been achieved without a few acts of bravery. The French physician Phillippe Pinel (1745–1826), who has been referred to as the "father of modern psychiatry," played an early role in mental health advocacy (Weiner, 1992). He authored several works based on his observations while working in asylums in France that promoted the humane treatment of individuals with mental illness. In one of his most well-known writings, *Memoirs on Madness* written in 1794, Pinel described how the treatment of mentally ill men at the Bicêtre Hospice was conducted in a cruel and harsh way, not always resulting in therapeutic outcomes (Weiner, 1992). He described an alternative approach, treating mentally ill patients in a "psychologically sensitive manner," with "an intelligent mixture of affability and firmness . . . in a well-timed manner . . . using only innocent repressive means, never blows or harsh treatment" and while "respecting human rights" (Weiner, 1992, p. 730). He argued that treating the mentally ill with empathy benefited not only the patient but also society as a whole (Weiner, 1992).

Benjamin Rush (1745–1813), an American politician and physician considered by many as the "father of American psychiatry," was one of the first physicians to approach mental illness as a disease (Levin, 2019; Farr, 1944) rather than a result of demonic possession. Rush argued that there was a medical basis to mental illness and advocated for compassionate care of individuals, organizing efforts to abolish the inhumane conditions for the mentally ill in American hospitals. In 1812, he published *Medical Inquires and Observations Upon the Diseases of the Mind*, which was the first American textbook on psychiatry that approached mental illness in a systematic way (Levin, 2019; Farr, 1944).

Although his contribution to the field of psychiatry cannot be refuted, some of Rush's ideas relating to the human condition and disease were flawed and controversial. Rush proposed a "disease theory of race," in which blackness was a form of leprosy that could be contracted like any other disease (Willoughby, 2017). He further proposed that "with proper treatment," Blacks could be cured and become white (Omi and Winant, 1986).

Dorothea Lynde Dix (1802–1887) was probably one of the most influential mental health advocates in history. She was a teacher, nurse, and humanitarian crusader who defied the boundaries frequently placed on Victorian women to advocate for mental health reform in the United States and abroad. Her work set the stage for others to also lobby for social reform. She observed firsthand the downstream effects of stigma on mental illness that led to patients essentially becoming imprisoned in asylums. One of her most well-known manuscripts, the Massachusetts *Memorial* written in 1843, depicts a graphic and powerful testimony of the mistreatment of mentally ill individuals that she witnessed (Dix, 1843a). Her use of rhetoric enabled her to not only effectively communicate her moral outrage but also appeal to her audience's intellect and emotions. During a 40-year period, she subsequently "reformed the moral sensibility of her time by persuading state legislatures, the federal government, the British Parliament, and even the pope to establish mental hospitals for the poor" (Brown, 1998, p. xi). An excerpt from her *Memorial* to the Legislature of Massachusetts, 1843 (Dix,1843a) reads,

> If my pictures are displeasing, coarse, and severe, my subjects, it must be recollected, offer no tranquil, refined, or composing features. The condition of human beings, reduced to the extremest [sic] states of degradation and misery, cannot be exhibited in softened language, or adorn a polished page.
>
> I proceed Gentlemen, briefly to call your attention to the *present* state of Insane Persons confined within this Commonwealth, in *cages, closets, stalls, pens! Chained, naked, beaten with rods, and lashed into obedience.*
>
> . . I state cold, *severe facts. . . .*
>
> Gentlemen, I commit to you this sacred cause. Your action upon this subject will affect the present and future condition of hundreds and of thousands.

Clifford Whittingham Beers (1876–1943), a Yale University alumnus, psychiatrist, and former patient who struggled with mental illness and was institutionalized during his twenties, was the founder of the Mental Hygiene Movement (March & Oppenheimer, 2014; Mental Health America [MHA], 2019). This movement aimed to improve stigma, prevention, and the treatment of mental illness. Following his release from the hospital, he wrote a book about his experiences titled *A Mind That Found Itself,* published in 1908

(MHA, 2019). That same year, Beers founded the Connecticut Society for Mental Hygiene, which became the National Committee for Mental Hygiene in 1909 (MHA, 2019).

In contrast to the asylum-based care, the Mental Hygiene Movement of the early 20th century promulgated the movement to community-based care for mental illness (MHA, 2019). Over the course of several years, as asylums were phased out, wards within general hospitals and outpatient clinics began to open, eventually leading to the deinstitutionalization movement of the mid-1950s and 1960s. The Community Mental Health Centers Act of 1963, which favored the treatment of individuals with mental illness in the least restrictive environment, authorized grants for the construction of community mental health centers. In 1965, the Medicaid Act passed by Congress helped expand access to mental health care. Legislative and policy changes continued to flourish from the 1970s onward, including the development of several advocacy organizations.

Beers' National Committee for Mental Hygiene founded in 1909, which became MHA in 2006, is a community-based, nonprofit organization whose main goal is to promote mental health as an important part of general well-being (MHA, 2019). Specifically, the organization aims to improve stigma, methods of prevention and early detection, access to interventions, and integrated care and treatment (Nguyen, Hellebuyck, Halpern, & Fritze, 2017; MHA, 2019). MHA has consistently demonstrated this through its legislative advocacy for the inclusion of mental health services in Medicare in the 1960s and the Mental Health Parity Act in 1996, which later led to the passing of the Mental Health Parity and Addiction Equity Act of 2008 (MHA, 2019).

CASE STUDY: CONTINUED

Based on the findings from the physical exam, you order imaging and place an urgent consultation request to a primary care colleague. Mrs. J returns to your clinic for follow-up approximately 3 weeks later and shares that she has learned that she has breast cancer. She expresses both gratitude for your diligence in getting her access to the care she needs and also how sad and anxious she is about the diagnosis. She shares her worries about the cancer treatment and prognosis because she was unable to grasp all of the information conveyed to her during her oncology appointment. She has an upcoming appointment with a breast surgeon and wonders if surgery is the appropriate course of action because she fears that "the cancer will spread when it's cut open."

QUESTIONS
1. How can you help your patient better understand her condition?
2. How can you help your patient communicate her concerns with her other medical providers despite her poor health care literacy?

ADVOCACY ROLES

Psychiatrists within the community can play a vital role as patient advocate because they are well positioned as witnesses to the mental health issues rooted in poverty, racism, and structural inequities. Community psychiatrists are privy not only to the immediate contributors to mental health disorders but also to their social, structural, and systemic antecedents (Kirmayer, Kronick, & Rousseau, 2018). In order to succeed as a mental health advocate, the physician must engage in interdisciplinary partnerships and promote activities that address these biological and behavioral bases of mental illness and substance abuse, as well as the social, environmental, cultural, economic, and political factors impacting mental health and recovery (Kirmayer et al., 2018). This frequently entails collaborating with other health care providers, members of the general public, nongovernmental organizations, and policymakers.

Role in Disparities Advocacy

Those with a substance use history may be especially stigmatized by members of their family, community, and even other medical providers due to a lack of knowledge and understanding of addiction.

A VIGNETTE: STIGMA

Ms. C is a 45-year-old female with a history of diabetes mellitus type 2; hypertension; hyperlipidemia; obesity; chronic obstructive pulmonary disease; insomnia; major depressive disorder, recurrent, severe, without psychotic features in partial remission; and opioid use disorder on maintenance therapy in a controlled environment. She comes to your office for a routine follow-up visit. She established care with your practice 6 months ago after moving to the area, and you have taken over treatment of her depression as well as her opioid use disorder through the comprehensive medication-assisted treatment program at your practice. She has been compliant with all appointments and medications. She has maintained a total of 18 consecutive months of sobriety from illicit substances since the initiation of medication-assisted treatment for opioid use disorder. During the visit, the patient shares that she is very frustrated with the primary care provider to whom you referred her because the provider is unwilling to take her on as a patient due to her addiction history. You are surprised to hear this and advise the patient that you will look into this further. You contact the primary care provider to clarify the reason for the declined referral. The primary care provider tells you that the practice "doesn't treat those kinds of patients."

In the context of community psychiatry, advocacy aims to protect the rights of vulnerable groups in society (Box 9.1) from stigma, discrimination, and other impediments to achieving positive mental health outcomes. Bearing witness to the disparities that exist within a patient population can be a source of inspiration and empowerment for the community psychiatrist to engage in advocacy efforts. Once an area of need is identified, the physician must find the right avenues to navigate in order for his or her voice to be heard. There are many different ways in which a psychiatrist can engage in advocacy, including raising awareness, dissemination of information, education, mutual help, training, counseling, mediating, defending, and denouncing (WHO, 2003; NAMI, 2018, Fadus, 2019). However, putting these advocacy efforts into practice is often difficult because the psychiatrist is often faced with several challenges, including learning how to navigate the proper channels to advocate for patients as well as learning to strike a balance between supporting the patient wishes and what the physician believes is best for patients (Schwartz, 2002). In addition, physicians will want to be mindful about managing the balance between going above and beyond the call of duty for patients and reaching the point of physician burnout.

BOX 9.1
POTENTIAL VULNERABLE POPULATIONS

- Children and adolescents
- Older adults (aged 65 years or older)
- Intellectually and developmentally disabled
- Immigrants and other underrepresented ethnic, racial, and geographic minority groups (i.e., rural, ingenious peoples, and refugees)
- Lesbian, gay, bisexual, transgender, questioning (LGBTQ)
- Low-income/indigent/homeless
- Uninsured
- Veterans
- Convicted felons (incarcerated, pre- or post-prison)
- People with substance use disorders
- Chronically ill
- Terminally ill
- Physically disabled
- Victims of sexual assault/abuse/trauma
- People with HIV/AIDS

Role in Prevention

A VIGNETTE: SECONDARY PREVENTION

TJ is a 17-year-old Hispanic, transgender female, high school senior who you treat in your clinic for attention–deficit/hyperactivity disorder and post-traumatic stress disorder (PTSD). She presents for a routine appointment accompanied by her grandmother, who is also her legal guardian. TJ tells you about a recent panic attack she had at school, leading to a visit to the nurse's office. She states that it took approximately 30 minutes for the panic attack to abate, and because of this she missed the end of her fifth period class and a portion of the sixth period class. She states that the panic attacks have been happening a few times per week, and she attributes them to being bullied at school by someone who triggers her PTSD, leading to flashbacks. She expresses concern about missing several classes and assignments each week because of the need to go to the nurse's office so frequently. She has tried to explain the situation to her teachers, but they have not been responsive. This is, in turn, causing her additional anxiety because she is in her final year of high school and fears that she may not graduate on time because of the missed assignments.

You offer to write a letter to the school principal to advocate on her behalf, specifically for her to be allowed to have breaks during the day to go to the nurse's office where she can safely regroup after a panic attack. In addition to writing a letter, you follow up with a phone call and speak to the principal directly, explaining TJ's underlying PTSD diagnosis and urging the principal to consider your request for accommodations for your patient. You emphasize to the principal that your efforts are not only to assuage a pre-existing issue but also to reduce her risk of developing depression and suicidality.

Despite all of the policies and movements toward improving detection, prevention, and treatment of mental illness, there is more work to be done, and this cannot be emphasized more poignantly than by a brief overview of the current data related to the incidence and prevalence of mental illness. In 1992, Congress established the Substance Abuse and Mental Health Services Administration (SAMHSA), an agency within the US Department of Health and Human Services, whose major role is to enhance the dissemination of information, services, and research related to mental illness and substance use disorders (SAMHSA, 2019). SAMHSA estimates that nearly 20% of adults in the United States experience some form of mental illness in a given year, and 60% of those received no mental health treatment in the previous year. The prevalence is higher among women and non-White compared with White adults. Of the nearly 44 million American adults who experience mental illness in a given year, approximately 10 million have a co-occurring substance use disorder (NAMI, 2019a). Twenty percent of children and teens between the ages of 13 and 18 years also live with a mental health condition, and suicide is estimated to be the third leading cause of death among individuals between the ages of 10 and 24 years (NAMI, 2019b). Lesbian, gay, bisexual, transgender, and questioning (LGBTQ) youth are two or three times more likely to attempt suicide compared with heterosexual youth (NAMI, 2019b). More than $190 billion dollars in lost earnings per year is secondary to serious mental illness (NAMI, 2019b). These are just some of the staggering statistics that highlight the scope and impact of mental illness on society and the need for continued primary prevention efforts.

Primary prevention in mental health has its roots in the Mental Hygiene Movement of the early 20th century. Prevention of mental illness, in addition to the promotion of mental health, ultimately reduces the health, social, and economic burdens of mental disorders (Shea & Shern, 2011). The ultimate goal of the community psychiatrist is to see the primary prevention prioritized within the community (Shea & Shern 2011; Caplan & Caplan, 2000). Needs of a population may vary from location to location; therefore, there is no one approach that a physician can take to identify and meet those needs. Given that clinical and systemic challenges will occur, a team-based approach is recommended. Through collaborative efforts with colleagues within the community and across other medical subspecialties, as well as with nonclinician stakeholders, the community psychiatrist may help decrease the prevalence of existing cases (secondary prevention) and rates of residual disability (tertiary prevention).

First, the psychiatrist may wish to help identify members of the community who are at greatest risk or who are most vulnerable, such as children, adolescents, immigrants, or older adults. Many of these individuals do not receive mental health treatment until they are in crisis (Derr, 2016; Nguyen et al., 2017; NAMI, 2018). This may happen for obvious reasons, including financial hardship, lack of insurance coverage, stigma, discrimination, or disability, and for less obvious reasons such as peer rejection, limited social support, poor nutrition, and geographic isolation (NAMI, 2018; WHO, 2018; Nguyen et al., 2017). Next, the psychiatrist may wish to consult with other stakeholders, such as school personnel or agencies, who might help identify individuals at risk and may also be able to help facilitate interventions using evidence-based strategies (Table 9.1).

Finally, the psychiatrist will want to engage identified individuals in need of treatment, which may require the involvement of an interdisciplinary team of therapists, social workers, dieticians, physical or occupational therapists, and agencies such as the local branch of the US Department of Health and Human Resources. Sometimes treatment entails addressing social and family-related determinants (Box 9.2), which can ultimately reduce risk and improve quality of life (WHO, 2004).

TABLE 9.1 Evidence-Based Interventions in the Primary Prevention of Mental Disorders

Mental Health Condition	Interventions
Conduct disorders/aggression/violence	Classroom behavior management, parent–child interactive therapy, and child social skills
Depression	Strengthening protective factors, anxiety detection and prevention, and challenging negative thinking styles
Anxiety disorders	Reducing trauma re-exposure, enhancing resilience, and debriefing after traumatic events
Eating disorders	Improving knowledge about eating problems and dieting behavior, and targeting self-esteem
Substance use disorders	Regulatory interventions; media, school, and community interventions
Psychotic disorders	Improving mental health literacy and awareness, encouraging young people to seek help at the onset of symptoms, and screening high-risk individuals for prodromal symptoms
Suicide	Hotlines, early intervention in primary care settings, and reducing access to lethal means

Source: World Health Organization Department of Mental Health and Substance Abuse; in collaboration with the Prevention Research Centre of the Universities of Nijmegen and Maastricht. *Prevention of mental disorders: Effective interventions and policy options: Summary report.* Geneva, Switzerland: World Health Organization; 2004.

BOX 9.2
FACTORS TO ADDRESS DURING TREATMENT IN PRIMARY PREVENTION

- Economic insecurity
- Family discord
- Work-related stress/Unemployment
- Poor nutrition
- Access to education
- Unsecure Housing
- Improve social support/strengthening of community networks
- Harm reduction strategies for substance abuse
- Promoting a healthy life style to enhance resilience
- Addressing child abuse, elder abuse, and neglect
- Healthy aging
- Support for refugees

Role in Community Awareness

A VIGNETTE: COMMUNITY EDUCATION

Mr. H is an 85-year-old married, retired, African American male veteran with major depressive disorder, in sustained remission, who recently established care in your clinic for increased depressive symptoms following the death of his brother-in-law John. He explains to you that John died of Alzheimer's disease and although the family had expected that he was near death, they were not emotionally prepared for the loss. Mr. H shares that John and he were not only family but also best friends, having served in Korea together. Upon returning home from the war, John introduced Mr. H to his sister Jane, and the rest is history. He states that it was love at first site, and they have been married for more than 60 years. He shares that his sadness is magnified by the fact that his wife also has Alzheimer's disease, and he is very worried she will soon meet the same demise. He says, "You know doc, many of us in my community are struggling. Everyone we know is either dead or in a nursing home. It's getting really lonely." You provide a supportive presence and extend your condolences for his loss. You inquire about your new patient's current support system, such as family, friends, or a religious community. He says that he is very active at his church. He attends every Sunday, and lately he has been attending more frequently to serve as a pall-bearer for funerals. He expresses his sadness about the many recent losses in his parish that have left many members of his church widowed.

Caregiver burden is undoubtedly a risk factor for depression (Omranifard, Haghighizadeh, & Akouchekian, 2018; Geng et al, 2018; National Alliance for Caregiving, 2016). Addressing this population could have a profound impact on overall health and quality of life for individuals, families, and communities. The community psychiatrist's role as an advocate for mental health care, including primary prevention, often involves educating members of the general community on this, and other, mental health issues. This may include giving educational talks in schools, places of worship, community centers, primary care clinics, local organizations, and to special interest groups. The relationship between the psychiatrist and the community fosters mutual learning and engagement in discourse. This enables the psychiatrist to gain a better understanding of the community in which he or she serves, thereby providing more culturally competent care. Community members may learn things about mental health that they had not previously understood and that may help them care for loved ones with mental illness or detect warning signs in members of their community. Once the relationship has been established, many opportunities for collaboration may be possible. The psychiatrist might learn about a need in the community he or she had not been previously aware of, such as the need for a caregiver support group for those caring for spouses with dementia, as in the previous vignette. In addition, physicians forming partnerships with communities may be a source of empowerment and can promote individual patients to advocate for themselves.

Speaking at a local place of worship about mental health awareness, especially in a community of minority elderly individuals who are struggling with grief, can be a very meaningful gesture and form of advocacy that requires little time and effort. The acknowledgment of such a need and willingness of a physician to provide education and support can help those who may otherwise feel marginalized or silenced because of their age or ethnicity to be more willing to seek or engage in mental health treatment. Educating the older people within a community can also help raise awareness about mental health issues that might occur in the community's younger population, creating another avenue for primary prevention efforts. Additional work can be done by educating faith leaders and providing them with resources for screening and identifying mental health issues and help to facilitate referrals for professional treatment in their communities. The APA website (https://www.psychiatry.org/faith) has several online resources for faith leaders about mental health that psychiatrists can share with places of worship in their communities.

Role in Social Justice/Legislative Advocacy

A VIGNETTE: ADDRESSING BARRIERS TO CARE

Ms. S is a 25-year-old divorced, Caucasian female, mother of one, with depression, anxiety, and opioid use disorder, presenting for enrollment in your office-based medication-assisted treatment (MAT) with buprenorphine–naloxone. She arrives after just having completed inpatient detoxification, but she tells you that she was just informed that she may not be allowed to start MAT because of her legal circumstances. She is enrolled in her local county's drug court program, and she explains that the judge in her county is against anyone in the program being on this medication. She asks you for your help in the matter because she is currently unsure about what she should do to control her cravings and maintain her sobriety, and she has had success with MAT in the past. You are familiar with this stance as common among judges in your state, and you suspect that it may be due to stigma related to opioid addiction and lack of understanding about treatment. You offer to compose a letter to the judge on her behalf, advocating for her to receive MAT, which at your particular institution is well structured and highly regarded within the medical community. In your letter to the judge, you describe some of the requirements of treatment, such as once weekly appointments, the option of group or individual therapy, and attendance at a minimum of three 12-step meetings each week. You assure the judge that in addition to the random urine drug tests (UDTs) mandated by the court, your patient will undergo regular UDTs and pill or film counts at your office. You also provide the judge with some data regarding the efficacy of this treatment and how it significantly reduces the risk of relapse and subsequent death from overdose. The judge accepts your letter and allows your patient to participate in treatment. One year later, the patient has maintained sobriety without any relapses, has regained custody of her son, and is working toward rebuilding her life.

The patient in the vignette is one of thousands of people throughout the country facing the same problem: They have a need for mental health or substance abuse treatment, but barriers limit their access to appropriate, evidence-based care. These barriers, often legally or socially sanctioned, may ultimately exacerbate other co-occurring mental health conditions, perpetuate the substance abuse epidemic, and subsequently result in many unintentional overdose deaths.

Therefore, the role of the community psychiatrist as social justice advocate is of great importance, as well as professionally pragmatic. Active participation in governmental advocacy and public engagement enable policymakers and the public to better understand topics related to psychiatry, which will subsequently benefit patients, society, and the profession (Thompson, 2019). Psychiatrists provide a valuable role in educating policymakers, courts, and government officials about the relevant clinical and scientific aspects of mental health legislation and local policies, such as the court policy in the previous vignette (Piel, 2018). Given the unique skill set and expertise of psychiatrists, especially those with additional subspecialty training, it is critical that community psychiatrists offer education to policymakers and legislators on topics such as criminal justice reform, the opioid epidemic, and improving school violence risk assessment (Thompson, 2019).

Although providing education is typically acceptable, community psychiatrists must keep in mind that even when intended as pragmatic and altruistic, engaging in organized lobbying might have the potential for institutional reprimands. Physicians must be mindful of their affiliated institutions and the policies regarding their engagement in certain politically related activities. In addition, a psychiatrist might be interested in promoting social justice reform or legislative initiatives that may not be fully supported by the physician's affiliated institution. Keen awareness of these limitations is paramount so as to not jeopardize one's employment status or create undue conflict. Finally, although advocacy is considered a noble effort, there are times when a psychiatrist must remain objective—for example, when serving as an expert witness or evaluator for a case in litigation.

CASE STUDY: CONTINUED

Your patient, Mrs. J, returns for routine follow-up several weeks into her chemotherapy treatment. She is status post radical mastectomy and radiation treatment. She shares with you that she was recently hospitalized for medical complications related to her cancer treatment, which include upper extremity lymphedema, a lower extremity deep vein thrombosis, and anemia requiring a blood transfusion. Since getting out of the hospital, she has been feeling very fatigued and she has had several falls due to feeling weak. Her primary provider has recommended she use a quad cane inside her home, but Mrs. J cannot afford to purchase one. Her husband is the breadwinner for her and their four young children, and money is very tight. She is unable to look for work because of her weakness, fatigue, and chronic nausea from chemotherapy.

QUESTIONS

1. How might you be able to advocate for your patient who has financial barriers to care?
2. What are some ways that you can assist your patient in obtaining access to resources in her community (e.g., breast cancer support groups or nonprofit agencies that provide goods and services to cancer patients who have low income)?

ADVOCACY RESOURCES

Learning how to advocate for patients requires not only inspiration and grit, as exemplified by the historic bravery of people such as Dix, Pinel, and Beers, but also formal training. Psychiatrists as patient advocates require the development of multiple specific, complex skills, such as writing, legislative and media outreach, public speaking, and coalition-building (Kennedy, Vance, Pinals, & Tally, 2018). Community psychiatrists have several places to turn in order to learn more about how to be an effective advocate. In addition, some residency training programs include such training.

Participation in National and Regional Organizations

The easiest place to begin to learn about how to participate in advocacy and public policy may be through national organizations such as the AMA or the APA. Many national organizations such as these facilitate dialogue between psychiatrists and legislators, and some actively participate in influencing state and federal affairs. These groups provide advice to federal entities such as Congress and the White House on issues pertaining to the field of psychiatry. The APA plays an active role in influencing state and federal policy through its Department of Government Relations, Political Action Committee, and Council on Advocacy and Government Relations (http://www.psychiatry.org/psychiatrists/advocacy). Furthermore, the APA is actively involved in lobbying for mental health-related issues and electing members to government positions who support the field of psychiatry. Specific endeavors include coalition efforts, health care reform, the opioid epidemic, patient safety, mental health parity, and suicide prevention. Trainees may join the state or regional branches of these organizations, and even their local state medical societies, as a way to get more involved on the local and national levels.

CASE STUDY: CONTINUED

Mrs. J arrives for a follow-up visit 2 weeks after completing chemotherapy. She reports that she was able to obtain a quad cane through a donation from a local nonprofit agency, and she has not had any additional falls. She shares that she continues to struggle with "brain fog" after completing chemotherapy, making it difficult for her to concentrate or think clearly at times. She finds it very difficult to follow what her doctors are telling her during visits, and she is having difficulty helping her children with their homework after school. Despite the antidepressant medication that you have prescribed, she continues to report feeling overwhelmed and depressed at times. When probing further, you discover that she has been struggling with her appearance since her mastectomy, with hair loss post chemotherapy. In addition, she is having marital conflicts. You tell her that you wonder if she might benefit from psychotherapy, and although she agrees, she requests to be seen by a female provider only.

QUESTIONS
1. How might you be able to address some of the psychosocial issues your patient is facing? Are there any outside organizations or supports that you might try to engage?
2. How can you help educate your patient (and possibly her husband) about cognitive and mood changes that often occur in cancer patients receiving chemotherapy? How might you be able to help facilitate better communication between your patient and her other providers?

Resources Online

Many sources for education on effective advocacy are available online. For online mental health advocacy resources and some basic advocacy pearls, refer to Tables 9.2 and 9.3, respectively. In addition, several organizations have online resources available for learning about public policy and health care advocacy in general (Box 9.3).

TABLE 9.2 Mental Health Advocacy Resources

Organization	Website
American Psychiatric Association (APA)	https://www.psychiatry.org
American Academy of Child and Adolescent Psychiatry (AACAP)	https://www.aacap.org
Substance Abuse and Mental Health Services Administration (SAMHSA)	https://www.samhsa.gov
National Alliance on Mental Illness (NAMI)	https://www.nami.org
National Association for Behavioral Healthcare (NABH)	https://www.nabh.org
National Council for Behavioral Health	https://www.thenationalcouncil.org
Mental Health America (MHA)	https://www.mentalhealthamerica.net
National Institute of Mental Health (NIMH)	https://www.nimh.nih.gov
Parity Implementation Coalition	https://www.parityispersonal.org

Advocacy Education in Medical Education

The APA released a resource document in 2018 highlighting the importance of advocacy as a professional obligation that is not unique to the field of psychiatry (Kennedy et al., 2018). The resource document proposes that training in advocacy become formalized because it is not currently taught in a systematic manner.

Curricula in medical schools and psychiatry residency training programs are now incorporating advocacy-based education. The APA resource document provides a review of survey data collected on several psychiatry residency programs that developed advocacy curricula and examined some of the advantages and disadvantages of various training models (Kennedy et al., 2018). The role of the physician as a patient advocate has become an integral part of competency-based education frameworks in medical schools and residency training programs, such as the University of California, San Francisco; the University of Illinois College of Medicine at Peoria; Vanderbilt University; and the University of Texas Southwestern (Kennedy et al., 2018). One example is the Global Health Working Group at Yale University School of Medicine, which developed a training module called Advocacy and Activism that consists of a 4-week period of formal didactic teaching and skills-based training that concludes with the development and presentation of advocacy projects (Peluso, Seavey, Gonsalves, & Friedland, 2013).

Another approach to advocacy education as a part of formal medical education is to invoke Accreditation Council for Graduate Medical Education (ACGME) standards. ACGME requires psychiatric residencies to help trainees develop and achieve competency in six core domains throughout the course of training (Box 9.4).

TABLE 9.3 Advocacy Pearls

Identify a cause	Identify a topic or cause about which you are passionate.
Get involved	Become a member or join a listserv of a local or national professional organization or interest group.
	This is an excellent place to start if you do not have a specific area of interest.
Find support	Find like-minded individuals with whom you can collaborate.
	Tap into resources within your institution or community.
	Many national organizations have local or state chapters as well as online resources.
Know your elected officials	Federal: Members of Congress and US Representatives
	State: Governors and legislators
	Local: Mayors, county executives, other government officials
	https://www.usa.gov/elected-officials
Do your research	Learn about what matters most to the legislators and policymakers in your area.
	Legislators are often motivated most by a personal, relevant, compelling story that demonstrates an economic and social impact that is supported by data.
Know your audience	Congressional office staff
	Personal staff
	Chief of staff or administrative assistant
	Legislative director
	Legislative assistants
	Legislative correspondents
	Press secretary
	Caseworkers
	Personal secretary/executive secretary
	Office manager
	Receptionist
	Committee staff
	Staff director
	Counsel
	Professional staff/policy analysts
	Press secretary
	Administrative assistant
	District office staff

TABLE 9.3 (Continued)

Methods of communication	In-person visit
	Letter writing/email
	Phone call to office (Washington, DC, or district)
	Social media
How to address correspondence	To a Senator
	The Honorable (full name)
	United States Senate
	Washington, DC 20510
	Dear Senator (last name):
	To a Representative
	The Honorable (full name)
	United States House of Representatives
	Washington, DC 20515
	Dear Representative (last name):
Planning the meeting	Schedule far in advance, and reconfirm as time nears.
	Clarify directions and office logistics ahead of time.
	Know your audience and with whom you will be talking.
	Clearly identify who you are and what you want to discuss.
	Review key points.
	Anticipate questions.
	Be polite and gracious to everyone.
	Be flexible to changes.
Meeting etiquette	Be prepared:
	Be on time (early).
	Bring business cards.
	Review key points.
	Anticipate questions.
	Be polite:
	Wait quietly.
	Turn cell phone off.
	Treat all staff with respect.
	Be concise:
	Prepare what you will say in advance.
	Review key points.
	Anticipate questions.

TABLE 9.3 (Continued)

During the meeting	Introduce yourself and have a good handshake.
	Establish rapport and listen.
	Be specific, succinct, and organized.
	Remember your goal/objective; have a clear task.
	Provide a reason for action.
	Do not use acronyms.
	Do not be technical.
	Personalize your points (all politics are local).
	Backup the points with supporting materials.
	Do not make up answers; offer to follow up with the information at a later time.
	Identify point of contact for follow-up.
Ending the meeting	Leave something behind (business card).
	Offer yourself as a resource.
	Thank legislator/staff for their time.
	Do not linger.
	Follow up with a timely thank-you.

Sources: American Association for Geriatric Psychiatry. *Legislative and regulatory agenda*. 2011–2012. Retrieved from https://www.aagponline.org/clientuploads/LegislativeAgenda2011FINAL.pdf; and National Council for Behavioral Health. *A handbook for advocates*. 2017. Retrieved from https://www.thenationalcouncil.org/wp-content/uploads/2017/07/AdvocateHandbook-v9.pdf.

Milestones within the core competency domains are used as a framework to formally evaluate residents and fellows as they progress through training. The milestones help guide the professional growth and development of trainees and their respective ACGME-accredited residency or fellowship programs. Box 9.5 identifies the relevant ACGME psychiatry milestones that have advocacy embedded into specific subcompetency domains at

---

BOX 9.3

NATIONAL ORGANIZATIONS WITH HEALTH CARE POLICY AND ADVOCACY RESOURCES

- The Joint Commission: https://www.jointcommission.org
- Agency for Healthcare Research and Quality (AHRQ): https://www.ahrq.gov
- World Health Organization (WHO): https://www.who.int
- Centers for Medicare and Medicaid Services (CMS): https://www.cms.gov
- Association of American Medical Colleges (AAMC): https://www.aamc.org
- American Medical Association (AMA): https://www.ama-assn.org

THE SIX ACGME CORE COMPETENCIES

- Patient care (PC)
- Medical knowledge (MK)
- Systems-based practice (SBP)
- Practice-based learning and improvement (PBLI)
- Professionalism (PROF)
- Interpersonal and communication skills (ICS)

Source: Edgar L, Roberts S, Holmboe E. Milestones 2.0: A step forward. *J Grad Med Educ.* 2018;10(3):367–369.

PSYCHIATRY MILESTONES THAT HIGHLIGHT THE IMPORTANCE OF ADVOCACY

MK3. Clinical Neuroscience

   5.4/D Integrates knowledge of neurobiology into advocacy for psychiatric patient care and stigma reduction

MK6. Practice of Psychiatry

   4.2/C Describes professional advocacy*

   *Advocacy includes efforts to promote the wellbeing and interests of patients and their families, the mental health care system, and the profession of psychiatry. While advocacy can include work on behalf of specific individuals, it is usually focused on broader system issues, such as access to mental health care services or public awareness of mental health issues. The focus on larger societal problems typically involves work with policy makers (state and federal legislators) and peer or professional organizations (American Psychiatric Association, National Alliance on Mental Illness, etc).

   5.2/C: Proposes advocacy activities, policy development, or scholarly contributions related to professional standards

SBP2. Resource Management

   5.2/A Advocates for improved access to and additional resources within systems of care

PROF2. Accountability to self, patients, colleagues, and the profession

   5.3/B Participates in the professional community (e.g., professional societies, patient advocacy groups, community service organizations)

Source: Accreditation Council for Graduate Medical Education (ACGME) and American Board of Psychiatry and Neurology (ABPN). *The Psychiatry Milestone Project*. Chicago, IL/Deerfield IL: ACGME/ABPN; July 2015.

various milestone levels. Although not included as one of the six core competencies, advocacy is one of the critical ways to translate insights about the social determinants of health care into structurally competent practice (Kirmayer et al., 2018; Metzl & Hansen, 2018).

CASE STUDY: CONCLUSION

As a community psychiatrist, advocacy for patients with mental illness and for the overall mental health of the general population is an integral part of your role. Community psychiatrists should strive to mirror the dedication and perseverance that enabled our mental health advocacy predecessors during the 18th and 19th centuries to achieve so much with far fewer resources. In the spirit of their tradition, the community psychiatrist should feel empowered and well-equipped in the role of patient advocate, in promotion of real change. At times, this may present as a challenge because of the obstacles that must be overcome. However, unlike many patients, community psychiatrists are in the unique position to form stakeholder partnerships and to receive support from local and national organizations to help achieve advocacy goals.

There are many ways that you can serve to advocate for individuals such as Mrs. J, for other patients similar to her, and for the community at large. Endeavors can vary and may include individual efforts such as writing a letter on behalf of a patient to schools, judges, or local governmental officials, or efforts might require an action with more complexity, such as lobbying Congress for health and public policy reform. Regardless of the level of effort or skill involved, all acts of advocacy have the potential to lead to long-standing results, which can benefit both individual patients and society as a whole. Advocacy through raising awareness and outreach within a community benefits not only the individuals of that community but also the physician. This enables the community psychiatrist to gain insight about the cultures, beliefs, values, and perspectives of a community and gain empathic awareness that can empower the psychiatrist to pursue additional advocacy efforts.

However, effective advocacy requires learning a special skill set. The community psychiatrist may obtain those skills through work with local and national associations or through online resources. But incorporating advocacy-based education into medical school and residency training curricula ensures the development of essential skills needed for the community psychiatrist to expand advocacy efforts from individual patient-centered work to partnerships with communities, organizations, policymakers, and legislatures. Community psychiatrists can also advocate for their patients by supporting education on advocacy as a key structural competency. Advocacy training helps future psychiatrists have the skills needed to overcome obstacles to access and quality of care. Advocacy training also helps trainees expand their ability to conceptualize how institutional and systemic factors lead to health care disparities. Through the incorporation of different learning techniques, coupled with the online resources available from federal and state organizations (see Box 9.3) and some general advocacy tips and techniques (see Table 9.3), trainees can learn how to practically apply the theoretical information and effectively put the learned skills into practice.

REFERENCES

Advocacy. *Oxford Learner's Dictionary*. Oxford University Press. 2019. Retrieved February 20, 2019, from https://www.oxfordlearnersdictionaries.com/us/definition/english/advocacy?q=advocacy

Accreditation Council for Graduate Medical Education (ACGME) and American Board of Psychiatry and Neurology (ABPN). *The Psychiatry Milestone Project*. Chicago, IL/Deerfield, IL: ACGME/ABPN; July 2015. Retrieved from https://www.acgme.org/Portals/0/PDFs/Milestones/PsychiatryMilestones.pdf?ver=2015-11-06-120520-753

Ahonen M. Ancient philosophers on mental illness. *Hist Psychiatry*. 2019;30(1):3–18.

American Association for Geriatric Psychiatry. *Legislative and regulatory agenda*. 2011–2012. Retrieved from https://www.aagponline.org/clientuploads/LegislativeAgenda2011FINAL.pdf

American Psychiatric Association. *Understanding mental disorders: Your guide to DSM-5*. Arlington, VA: American Psychiatric Publishing; 2015.

Brown TJ. *Dorothea Dix: New England reformer*. Cambridge, MA. Harvard University Press; 1998.

Caplan G, Caplan R. Principles of community psychiatry. *Community Ment Health J*. 2000;36(1):7–24.

Caruso JP, Sheehan JP. Psychosurgery, ethics, and media: A history of Walter Freeman and the lobotomy. *Neurosurg Focus*. 2017;43(3):1–8.

Derr AS. Mental health service use among immigrants in the United States: A systematic review. *Psychiatric Services*. 2016;67(3):265–274.

Dix D. *Memorial to the Legislature of Massachusetts*. Boston, MA: Munroe & Francis; 1843a.

Dix D. Memorial to the Senate and House of Representatives of the State of Illinois, 15th assembly, 1st session. Excerpted from *Memorial of Miss Dix: Springfield, Illinois, January 11, 1847*. Retrieved from https://archive.org/details/0335336.nlm.nih.gov

Edgar L, Roberts S, Holmboe E. Milestones 2.0: A step forward. *J Grad Med Educ*. 2018;10(3):367–369.

Fadus, M. Mental health disparities and medical student education: Teaching in psychiatry for LGBTQ care, communication, and advocacy. *Acad Psychiatry*. 2019;43(3):306–331. https://doi.org/10.1007/s40596-019-01024-y

Farr CB. Benjamin Rush and American psychiatry. *Am J Psychiatry*. 1944. Published online April 1, 2006. Retrieved from https://ajp.psychiatryonline.org/doi/pdf/10.1176/ajp.100.6.2-2

Frank JR, Snell L, Sherbino J, eds. *Can Meds 2015 Physician Competency Framework*. Ottawa, Ontario, Canada: Royal College of Physicians and Surgeons of Canada; 2015.

Geng H, Chuang D, Yang F, Yang Y, Liu W, Liu L, Tian H. Prevalence and determinants of depression in caregivers of cancer patients: A systematic review and meta-analysis. *Medicine*. 2018;97(39):1–8.

Kalman I. The true meaning of the Golden Rule: Love your bullies. *Psychology Today*. 2010. Retrieved from https://www.psychologytoday.com/blog/resilience-bullying/201002/the-true-meaning-the-golden-rule-love-your-bullies?eml

Kennedy KG, Vance MC, Pinals DA, Tally R. *Resource document: Advocacy teaching in psychiatry residency training programs*. 2018. Retrieved from https://www.psychiatry.org/psychiatrists/search-directories-databases/library-and-archive/resource-documents

Kirmayer LJ, Kronick R, Rousseau C. Advocacy as key to structural competency in psychiatry. *JAMA Psychiatry*. 2018;75(2):119–120.

Levin A. The life of Benjamin Rush reflects troubled age in U.S. medical history. *Psychiatric News*. January 29, 2019. Retrieved from https://doi.org/10.1176/appi.pn.2019.2a23

Lustig S. *Advocacy strategies for health and mental health professionals*. New York, NY: Springer; 2012.

March D, Oppenheimer GM. Social disorder and diagnostic order: The US mental hygiene movement, the Midtown Manhattan study and the development of psychiatric epidemiology in the 20th century. *Int J Epidemiol*. 2014;43(1):i29–i42.

Mental Health America. *Celebrate 100 years of the mental health movement*. Retrieved February 20, 2019, from http://www.nmha.org/go/history

Metzl JM, Hansen H. Structural competency and psychiatry. *JAMA Psychiatry*. 2018;75(2):115–116.

National Alliance for Caregiving. *On pins and needles: Caregivers of adults with mental illness.* 2016. Retrieved from https://www.nami.org/getattachment/Get-Involved/NAMI-National-Convention/2015-Convention-Presentation-Slides-and-Resources/B-5-Findings-from-a-National-Survey-of-Family-Caregivers-of-Adults-with-Mental-Illness.pdf

National Alliance on Mental Illness. *Engagement: A new standard for mental health care.* Arlington, VA: National Alliance on Mental Illness; 2016. Retrieved February 23, 2019, from https://www.nami.org/About-NAMI/Publications-Reports/Public-Policy-Reports/Engagement-A-New-Standard-for-Mental-Health-Care/NAMI_Engagement_Web.pdf. Accessed February 23, 2019.

National Alliance on Mental Illness. *Navigating a mental health crisis: A NAMI resource guide for those experiencing a mental health emergency.* Arlington, VA: National Alliance on Mental Illness; 2018. Retrieved from https://www.nami.org/About-NAMI/Publications-Reports/Guides/Navigating-a-Mental-Health-Crisis

National Alliance on Mental Illness. *About NAMI.* 2019a. Retrieved from https://www.nami.org/About-NAMI

National Alliance on Mental Illness. *Mental health facts.* 2019b. Retrieved February 23, 2019, from https://www.nami.org/learn-more/fact-sheet-library.

National Council for Behavioral Health. *A handbook for advocates.* 2017. Retrieved May 10, 2019, from https://www.thenationalcouncil.org/wp-content/uploads/2017/07/AdvocateHandbook-v9.pdf

Nguyen T, Hellebuyck M, Halpern M, Fritze D. *The state of mental health in America 2018.* Alexandria, VA: Mental Health America; 2017. Retrieved from www.mentalhealthamerica.net/sites/default/files/2017%20MH%20in%20America%20Full.pdf

Omi, M, Winant H. *Racial formation in the United States: From the 1960s to the 1980s.* New York, NY: Routledge & Kegan Paul; 1986.

Omranifard V, Haghighizadeh E, Akouchekian S. Depression in main caregivers of dementia patients: Prevalence and predictors. *Adv Biomed Res.* 2018;7(34):1–14.

Peluso MJ, Seavey B, Gonsalves G, Friedland G. An inter-professional "advocacy and activism in global health": Module for the training of physician-advocates. *Global Health Promotion.* 2013;20(2):70–73.

Piel J. Legislative advocacy and forensic psychiatry training. *J Am Acad Psychiatry Law.* 2018;46:147–154.

Schwartz L. Is there an advocate in the house? The role of health care professionals in patient advocacy. *J Med Ethics.* 2002;28:37–40.

Shea P, Shern D. *Primary prevention in behavioral health: Investing in our nation's future.* Alexandria, VA: National Association of State Mental Health Program Directors; 2011.

Substance Abuse and Mental Health Services Administration. *About us.* 2019. Retrieved February 23, 2019, from https://www.samhsa.gov/about-us.

Thompson C. A seat at the table. *J Am Acad Psychiatry Law.* 2019;47(1):1–10.

To MJ, Sharma M. Training tomorrow's physician-advocates. *Medical Educ.* 2015;49:748–754.

Weiner DB. Phillippe Pinel's "Memoir on Madness" of December 11, 1794: A fundamental text on modern psychiatry. *Am J Psychiatry.*1992;149:725–732.

Willoughby CD. "His Native, Hot Country": Racial science and environment in antebellum American medical thought. *J Hist Med Allied Sci.* 2017;72(3):328–351.

World Health Organization. *Advocacy for mental health: Mental health policy and service guidance package.* Geneva, Switzerland: World Health Organization; 2003. Retrieved February 17, 2019, from https://ebookcentral.proquest.com/lib/yale-ebooks/reader.action?docID=284613

World Health Organization, Department of Mental Health and Substance Abuse; in collaboration with the Prevention Research Centre of the Universities of Nijmegen and Maastricht. *Prevention of mental disorders: Effective interventions and policy options.* Geneva, Switzerland: World Health Organization; 2004. Retrieved from https://www.who.int/mental_health/suicide-prevention/national_strategies_2019/en

World Health Organization. *Mental health action plan 2013–2020*. Geneva, Switzerland: World Health Organization; 2013. Retrieved May 5, 2019, from https://www.thenationalcouncil.org

World Health Organization. *National suicide prevention strategies: Progress, examples and indicators*. Geneva, Switzerland: World Health Organization; 2018. Retrieved from https://www.who.int/mental_health/suicide-prevention/national_strategies_2019/en

BACK TO THE FUTURE OF COMMUNITY PSYCHIATRY

DAVID SAUNDERS AND KENNETH MINKOFF

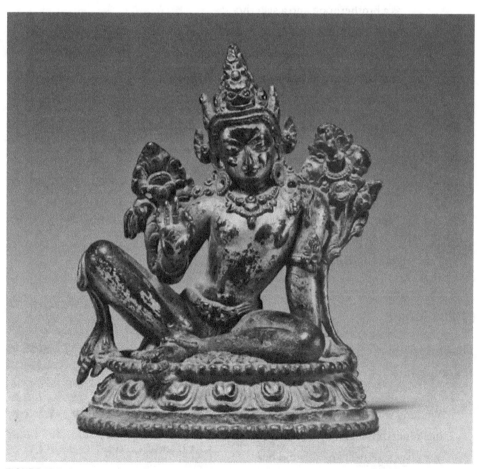

FIGURE 10.1 Seated Bodhisattva Maitreya (The Buddha of the Future), c. 1250–1350, sculpture.

Maitreya is known as the bodhisattva of loving-kindness and is thought to become the next Buddha, succeeding the current Buddha Sakyamuni. The sculpture shown in Figure 10.1, from the Kathmandu Valley in modern-day Nepal, depicts Maitreya posing with the Vitarka mudra (gesture), which represents the transmission of the teachings of the Buddha (Buswell, 2004).

PSYCHIATRY AND LITERATURE

When Death Comes
by Mary Oliver

I want to step through the door full of curiosity, wondering:
what is it going to be like, that cottage of darkness?

And therefore I look upon everything
as a brotherhood and a sisterhood,
and I look upon time as no more than an idea,
and I consider eternity as another possibility,

and I think of each life as a flower, as common
as a field daisy, and as singular,

and each name a comfortable music in the mouth,
tending, as all music does, toward silence,

and each body a lion of courage, and something
precious to the earth.

When it's over, I want to say all my life
I was a bride married to amazement.
I was the bridegroom, taking the world into my arms.

INTRODUCTION

The original vision of the "community psychiatry" movement was built on a foundation of strong values:

- Working with individuals and families who are most in need and least able to pay, including those with the most serious mental health and substance use conditions, as well as significant health and human service needs of all kinds
- Working in interdisciplinary teams, including with community members, to provide services

- Engaging patients/clients—and their families and support networks—as partners in change
- Inspiring people with significant challenges to succeed in their natural community settings and to engage natural community supports for both prevention and intervention
- Working not only with individual clients and families but also with challenging and at-risk community populations and helping them collectively achieve more fulfilling lives
- Transforming and empowering the communities in which people live, leveraging the strengths and resources of the whole community for the purposes of preventing trauma and illness, and promoting health and wellness

As a trainee, I (D. Saunders) was inspired by these values to put my energy and passion to work by meeting the needs of people—children especially—who were underserved. I wanted to put myself on the other side of the spectrum from those who practice psychiatry in exclusive cash-only practices serving only people who can afford to pay out of pocket. I was hopeful that my training program at Yale University, long recognized for its leadership in community psychiatry, would provide me with many opportunities to learn how to implement these values in my work. I knew that during the past several decades, the original champions of community psychiatry have tried to maintain these core values, even as the behavioral health system has changed substantially. I welcomed the opportunity to work in community settings in which I could see these values in operation and practice the kind of value-based care that I could embrace with heart and soul.

I quickly discovered, however, as I'm sure many readers have, that my early exposure to community psychiatry—in my case, working at a community mental health center in New Haven, Connecticut—was often more stressful than inspiring.

Here's an example: I have been called out from my busy schedule of back-to-back medication visits to address the needs of, let's say, Robert, an intoxicated and suicidal patient who is disturbing the waiting area of our community mental health center by refusing to accept an escort to the emergency room, requiring the intervention of five police officers. Despite the fact that I know I "should" feel like this situation is exactly what I wanted to be able to manage as a community psychiatrist, I feel myself getting angry at this patient who has dared to upset the delicate milieu of the center—as if his behavior was an act of deliberate, willful malice rather than, say, the result of many years of sexual and physical trauma, poverty, homelessness, and a dearth of hope—the victim of a system that has forsaken him. I sense myself becoming even more upset because, of course, I have to document this incident immediately, then see my already overbooked list of patients later into the evening. I then face harsh internal recriminations from my always-alert superego as I try to remind myself that it was precisely this type of patient who motivated me to practice community psychiatry in the first place. Which, of course, is followed by renewed anger that I will miss my son's soccer game that night because of Robert's actions. I know on some level that I do this work because it is "good for me and good for my patients"—that it is work that presents challenges I presumably welcome—but in the moment, this feels way less than inspiring, and certainly not fun. "Maybe," I say to myself, "I should just find easier work."

But meanwhile, I also realize that the challenge I am facing goes beyond my own individual abilities and values. These types of situations do not take place in isolation, nor are they uncommon. In the same way that Robert's actions were partially determined by forces beyond his control, I too live and work within a system that is affected by system-level forces beyond *my* control. Indeed, the field of community psychiatry has seen developments during the past several decades that have dramatically altered the way in which we deliver care, challenging our continued adherence to the values listed at the beginning of this chapter. Here are a few examples:

- In response to the noble effort of deinstitutionalization, we began to narrow the definition of whom we would serve and widen the definition of whom we would reject.
- As we became dependent on—or even addicted to—Medicaid and third-party fee-for-service funding to survive, we became more focused on the product of delivering billable units rather than caring for people, populations, or communities.
- As the structure of service became increasingly more mechanized, psychiatrists increasingly assumed the narrow role of "medication prescribers" (a.k.a., "docs in a box") rather than clinical leaders, population health specialists, and community interventionists.

All of these dynamics affect the context in which I work, as well as the context in which I respond to the crisis involving Robert, fueling the questions swirling around in my head: Should we consider this man as one of our "priority" clients, or extrude him because he may be "just" an alcoholic? Should my direct involvement in his care during the crisis be a priority, or should I prioritize accumulating "billable units" of medication visits to meet my "productivity" requirements (which, admittedly, help keep the community health center financially solvent)? Do I have a role in clinical leadership of my team in thinking about how to address the needs of this man, or do I limit myself to discussing his medications (which, of course, are only a small part of what he needs)? Clearly, it is not enough that I think about how to implement "values" on an individual level; I also have to think about whether I can have an influence on the system in which I work and the system in which my patients or clients live. This is daunting but exciting at the same time. These challenges embody the attraction of community psychiatry and are the essence of what we want to address in this chapter.

Facing "difficult" patients in dire need of care while embedded in a challenging system that may be misaligned with what both I and my patients need, I have found as a resident and early career psychiatrist that living up to the values that inspire me often proves more elusive in times of stress than I care to admit. I have had many inspiring mentors on faculty, but I have quickly realized that I have to face very difficult day-to-day situations on my own, without as much direct assistance as I would have wanted or suspected. I have worried a lot that I would "never make it," and I still do. But I haven't given up, either on myself or on my chosen field. Since my first exposure to these challenges, I have worked hard to make progress, and "stay in the game," although I realize I still have a long way to go. I chose to write this chapter because I felt that I wanted to share my experiences with others who were possibly interested in the path of community psychiatry. With the wisdom of my mentor and co-author, I want to show you how to make progress and, most important, to encourage you not to give up when things are difficult. In fact, I would like you to realize, as I have come to learn, that the difficulty itself is what makes community psychiatry so appealing— it challenges our professional growth emotionally and intellectually in the deepest possible way. Continuing to learn how to meet these challenges in the service of my own values is far more rewarding than just massaging neurotransmitters. I want to share this excitement with you; community psychiatry still has the passion of a movement, and the energy of young psychiatrists like me (and you) is what brings this movement "Back to the Future."

What do we mean by Back to the Future? It means that in my journey, I am not alone. During the past several years, a movement within the field of community psychiatry has emerged, imbued with energy, idealism, and youth, moving forward into the future with renewed connection to the old ideals. While young psychiatrists (such as myself) do not always live up to these ideals, as in the previous example, a number of historical developments have provided a ripe breeding ground for us to join a cohort of community psychiatrists who are willing to unite and embrace the vision of the original community psychiatrists, despite the difficulties put upon us by systemic forces.

Among the contributing forces and ideologies are

- a renewed focus in all of medicine on the importance of social justice, social determinants of health, and the need to address health disparities among disadvantaged populations;

- Triple Aim (improving patient experience of care, improving the health of populations, and reducing the per capita cost of health care) as a driver of health system improvement;
- customer-oriented care and customer-focused quality improvement beginning to emerge in health and behavioral health systems;
- alternative payment models that move away from focusing on "billable units" alone to valuing attention to complex populations;
- awareness of the impact of trauma on populations, driven by research on adverse childhood experiences, leading to investment in upstream prevention through building resiliency; and
- attention to the complexity of overlapping health, behavioral health, and human service needs, which brings renewed importance to the need for community-oriented psychiatric leadership to manage services, programs, systems, and populations.

Young psychiatrists like myself are now once again attracted to the values that spawned the community psychiatry movement. The chapter title—Back to the Future—acknowledges the fact that the young and energetic community psychiatrists of the future are returning full circle to share the values of the founders of the movement.

On my journey, I have been blessed with great teachers, at Yale and elsewhere. In fact, one of the attractions of this particular project has been the opportunity for further learning from the editors and other authors to help me continue to grow. Along with my co-author, I hope to share this learning with you in this chapter.

Through case examples, personal reflection, and discussion, we will elaborate on this Back to the Future vision for community psychiatry. The fundamental question we will tackle is "How do you implement the highest values of community psychiatry in your own work, and how, as a psychiatrist on an interdisciplinary team, do you inspire others to do the same?" We address this question on two levels, each of which hearkens to the original vision of the community psychiatry movement:

- How do you embody and implement these values with challenging and so-called "difficult" or "resistant" clients, both adults and children?
- How do you embody and implement these values with particular challenging "high cost, poor outcome" populations in your community, both high-risk adults and high-risk children and families?

We employ case examples of real people (with poetic license, of course) that I (and probably you) have encountered, to ensure that this abstract discussion of values can be understood in terms of the concrete day-to-day challenges facing younger (and older) community psychiatrists. The cases each evoke a "difficult" client, and a "high cost, poor outcome community," so as to emphasize two of the foundational principles of community psychiatry: working with challenging or "difficult" patients and working with "at-risk" communities. Although the case examples differ slightly—one is a 25-year-old who is in and out of jail and the other is a 13-year-old Mexican immigrant—they share common solutions to the two questions proposed previously: How do you embody and implement these values with "difficult" clients, and how do you embody and implement these values in high cost, poor outcome populations? Although there are a variety of solutions to these challenges, we propose two in particular: (1) an attitude of "welcoming" and "customer service" for the difficult patient and (2) developing novel solutions that meet the *needs* of at-risk populations rather than solutions that merely fit nicely into what we currently offer.

A desire to serve "difficult" clients and high-risk populations was present when the movement was borne, and it will undergird the movement in the future, as young psychiatrists such as myself embark on our careers with the Back to the Future vision in mind. Our goal is to motivate other aspiring community psychiatrists to adopt these values, and we hope the personal reflections, discussion, and proposed solutions will help.

CASE STUDIES: INITIAL PRESENTATION

Mario is a 25-year-old unmarried man who is referred to your community mental health center by his probation officer. He had been treated briefly at your center approximately 18 months ago and was diagnosed with atypical bipolar disorder and substance use disorder (alcohol, marijuana, methamphetamine, and opioids). He had been prescribed medication and assigned to a clinician, but he did not follow through with his appointments and was eventually discharged from the clinic after only a few months in care. The recent history obtained from his probation officer indicates that he was arrested after police were called to respond to an altercation involving Mario at a local bar. They noticed Mario was behaving strangely and considered bringing him for psychiatric evaluation, but he pushed one of the police officers, so he was arrested. He has been released on bail supplied by his parents, even though he does not live with them consistently. He has been directed to get help at your clinic and told that it will be beneficial in his eventual court disposition if he is receiving treatment. He has no steady job, and he "couch surfs" for places to sleep. If he has any further legal infractions—even minor—he will be arrested.

When he arrives in the clinic waiting room, he appears somewhat disheveled and "high," smelling faintly of alcohol. He is given paperwork to fill out and gets angry at the receptionist for expecting him to complete so many forms. The other patients in the waiting room are visibly anxious.

As the available psychiatrist in the clinic, you are contacted to address the situation. One of the staff members who had tried to work with him previously says to you as you prepare to respond: "This guy doesn't belong here. He's not really mentally ill. He's antisocial, dangerous, and addicted to drugs—I think you should send him away and we should let his probation officer know that we can't help him until he's sober."

Carlo is a 13-year-old, Spanish-only speaking boy who immigrated from Mexico 14 months ago to escape violence stemming from his father's former involvement in the local drug cartel. Carlo lives with his father, mother, and 7-year-old sister Ella in a studio apartment in the local Mexican neighborhood. Carlo reads and writes at a third-grade level, several years behind his peers. He has also been diagnosed with "disruptive mood dysregulation disorder" by a psychologic evaluation in the school and has been suspended several times for hitting classmates. He was referred to your clinic by the school for psychiatric treatment and assistance with behavior issues. His continued ability to attend school is dependent, to some extent, on his and his family's ability to participate in the recommended treatment.

Reports sent from the school along with the referral indicate that, in addition, Carlo's sister Ella has fetal alcohol syndrome and is intellectually disabled, requiring special education. She requires near 24-hour care at home and school, which is provided (amazingly) by Carlo's mother, Isabelle, age 27 years. Carlo's father (Juan) is 32 years old and has multiple substance use disorders (alcohol, methamphetamine, and cocaine) but is only actively using alcohol at present. He was involved in several gun fights in his hometown, sustaining multiple gunshot wounds, including one during a shooting incident that occurred during an attack while he was at home. His own father (Carlo's grandfather) was in the local drug cartel, and Juan was physically and sexually abused as a child. He is currently employed as a construction worker, getting paid in cash, under the table, and goes to the bar after work every day, having limited involvement in childcare. When he is home, particularly when he is intoxicated, he is physically and emotionally abusive toward his wife and emotionally abusive toward his children. He has threatened Carlo with physical harm but has not actually hurt him (as far as we know). Carlo's mother, Isabelle, is reported to have possible major depressive disorder and post-traumatic stress disorder (from intimate partner and drug cartel violence at her home) as well as an alcohol use disorder. She has never received any mental health or substance use disorder treatment. She has continued to drink since immigrating and has occasionally gone to the bar with Carlo, leaving the children home alone (with Carlo watching Ella) for several hours.

In recent months, a neighbor called child welfare after hearing screams from the apartment upon the father's return home from the bar. Child welfare has determined that the children are not at *immediate* risk and are therefore currently not candidates for removal from the home. Child welfare has also indicated (along with the school) that it expects the family to seek services from the clinic.

Today was Carlo's intake appointment. His mother got off of work at the local Wendy's for 2 hours to attend the appointment, traveling by bus. She arrives 90 minutes late with Carlo and Emma, 15 minutes before the closing of the clinic that day. She is overwhelmed, has limited English, and no one she knows has ever received psychiatric care before. The normal intake process is lengthy, comprising paperwork completion and signatures, an initial clinician interview, and a brief meeting with the "intake psychiatrist." The clinic is not staffed with child and adolescent psychiatrists, and there is only one psychiatrist who speaks Spanish, but that person is not present. In this instance, you are the psychiatrist on call for all intakes, including adolescents. Although you have previously treated many youths, you hardly consider yourself an expert in the needs of immigrant refugee teenagers and their families.

QUESTIONS

1. What are some values that are required of the community psychiatrist in everyday practice?
2. What factors in everyday practice hamper the psychiatrist in holding to those values?
3. What are some strategies to address the impediments to holding fast to the values?

WELCOMING AND CUSTOMER SERVICE

Welcoming Mario

Mario would clearly be labeled by most psychiatrists, and by most community mental health centers, as a "difficult patient." So would Robert, in the opening scenario. As you can determine from the case example, neither Mario nor Robert are particularly "welcome," in that state, at that moment. Would they be welcomed by you? Would they be welcomed by me?

Perhaps the signature feature of being a community psychiatrist is a desire to treat what are usually known as "the most difficult patients"—the so-called "intractable," "treatment-resistant" individuals who present a panoply of psychiatric, substance use, cognitive, medical, social, legal, and cultural challenges. In short, the people no one else will serve. In this way, we as community psychiatrists not only embrace a *willingness* to treat the most difficult patients but also are inspired by a calling to serve them. Ideally, we continuously channel the words and inspiration of Mary Oliver:

> I think of each life as a flower, as common
> as a field daisy, and as singular,
> and each name a comfortable music in the mouth,
> tending, as all music dose, toward silence,
> and each body a lion of courage, and something
> precious to the earth.

But that's not always so easy. Following this logic, if I am truly inspired to serve people such as Mario and Robert, it should be easy for me to welcome them and be inspired by the opportunity to serve them. But as I noted in the introduction, that's not always how it works. As a young psychiatrist, I have found that on most days, my "natural" reaction to someone such as Mario is negative. I am still inspired by the *thought* of working with very difficult patients, but in the moment, I would rather that Mario went away, and a more "sympathetic" or "easier to deal with" patient came in his place. Over time, I've begun to learn strategies for how to address this conflict, both internally and with my team. These are the strategies I want to share with you here.

First, I've learned that simply "beating myself up" for not living up to the Platonic ideal of a community psychiatrist is not an effective strategy. Guilt will only get me so far. If my only approach to working with people such as Mario is to force myself to suffer because of guilt and shame, I'm going to burn out pretty quickly.

But what's the alternative? Working with a variety of mentors in the community psychiatry field (and being supported by my co-author in putting this into words for the readers of this chapter), I've come to realize that I first need a different approach in my own mind, and then I need a different set of tools or skills to apply. So here's the approach:

People such as Mario are not the "difficult patients," they're the "fun" patients. My goal is not to "suffer" working with people like Mario. My goal is to enjoy it!

Consider the following analogy, which also relates to other branches of medicine: When you are a young surgeon, you may aspire to do brain surgery, but you may still be at the stage of your career where being left alone to do anything more complicated than an appendectomy would be terrifying. That doesn't mean you won't enjoy brain surgery; it just means that you have not yet acquired the tools to really enjoy doing what inspires you.

This is no less true in community psychiatry. I have realized that the problem is the way we have created an inaccurate context. This is the context that we as members of the Back to the Future movement have to challenge. In community psychiatry, we have permitted the development of a cultural context in which we indirectly externalize the responsibility for developing the tools we need to both succeed and have fun working with people who have enormous challenges. In short, we blame the patients, or we blame the lack of resources, or we blame the regulations, or we blame the funding streams. In fact, all of those are challenges, but if we acquire the necessary skills and take the time to learn how to use them, then we can overcome those challenges and not only serve people who are challenging but also have fun doing it.

So to reframe the situation: Mario is someone who does not appear to be fun to deal with in the moment, but he could be, if I have the right tools and skills in my mental pocket. My job is to learn those skills. Furthermore, I know I will not learn them unless I practice (and Mario clearly represents a wonderful teaching opportunity). I also know that I will not get it right the first time; I will have to keep practicing. But if I have the right support and guidance, I can acquire these skills, and not only be a more artful community psychiatrist but also come ever closer to my personal ideals.

In short, any psychiatrist can learn to work with "easy" patients, but community psychiatrists can pride themselves on having fun working with folks who others find challenging and difficult. We are the brain surgeons of psychiatry. But even brain surgeons were early career physicians once and required expert teaching, which calls to mind the role of mentorship.

Now, not everyone reading this chapter will have access to the kind of mentors and supports that I have been blessed with, and you may need. I am hopeful that this chapter will provide you some mentorship by proxy and encourage you to reach out (even beyond the walls of where you work) to find the tools and learning to help you achieve your goals. What are the tools? We propose two: welcoming and customer service.

"Welcoming," in this sense, as Cline and Minkoff (2012) state, refers to

deliberate attention, at every level of organization structure, process, program, and practice, to ensure that those most in need and that those most likely to be 'misfits' in other settings are not only tolerated and accepted but also accepted and proactively welcomed for care—and inspired with the hope and promise of recovery—wherever, whenever, and however they present.

"Customer service" means the capacity of a community psychiatric organization to be responsive to people and families—"customers"—who have serious needs that would not be treated or helped otherwise, and create a culture in which every staff person (including the psychiatrist) has the tools they need to know how to be welcoming to those most in need (Cline & Minkoff, 2012). Customer service is not just about being nice out of guilt. Customer service involves not only learning very specific scripts and skills to engage the so-called "easy customers" but also the specific application of those skills to the people who are perceived as difficult and challenging.

What is the role that welcoming and customer service plays in the delivery of compassionate, effective community psychiatric care? The previous scenarios present opportunities for a community psychiatrist such as myself to demonstrate the welcoming and customer service that can positively impact the life of a patient who otherwise would have fallen through the cracks. Each situation presents two specific challenges. First, how do I demonstrate welcoming and customer service, and how can I have fun showing the positive impact of "applied welcoming" or "applied customer service" to the management of these situations? Second, how can I as a community psychiatrist leader (even as a young psychiatrist on a team, let alone as a team leader or medical director) harness a welcoming and customer service-oriented approach to build a culture on my team or in my program or agency that is able to consistently and systematically address the needs of such patients?

Customer service teaches us that "welcoming" is not about how you feel; it's about what you do. You may be angry and upset that the person you are seeing has disrupted the flow of your day, but you apply a set of tools and strategies that help you behave in a welcoming way. When you become good at this, you learn that this approach not only helps the patient but also helps you. Amazingly, you become less frustrated when you fully commit to acting less frustrated. You actually start to have fun because you are welcoming the person the way they are. You apply new skills and learn as you go, which will lead to better results.

Let us consider Mario. A welcoming psychiatrist models the type of customer service orientation that is most effective, simultaneously addressing Mario's needs and demonstrating the effectiveness of welcoming for onlooking staff members, community members, and fellow patients. Of course, this is easier said than done! When Mario enters the clinic and it is evident that he is in crisis, he is likely to have encountered several individuals—such as a receptionist or case manager—who may have already been "less than welcoming," before being seen by me, the psychiatrist. By the time I see him, I will likely be arriving on the scene to attempt to address the imminent needs of a patient who may be feeling scared, disempowered, and disrespected. In addition, my own "inner voices" are carrying on a dialogue that is not at all welcoming: A host of feelings and thoughts consciously and unconsciously swirl in my head in such situations—intense anger, panic, compassion, fear, love, and everything in between. "Mario interrupted my session with an equally sick but more compliant patient who finds herself in a life situation no less dire, but who is *not* behaving this way." I am frustrated with the other staff who may be behaving in ways that make things more difficult for both Mario and me. At my worst, I am thinking: "Mario got drunk and messed up, now he's here bothering us. The receptionist has made things worse, and I wish the police had picked him up and brought him to jail. There's no hope for him anyway." Clearly, I don't want to act in accordance with these feelings, and I want to learn a different approach. So the challenge is set: How do I enact the type of welcoming and customer service orientation that Mario requires and that I desire to provide?

Here are some examples. I am not very good at this yet, but it works better for me the more I try. Upon meeting Mario, I immediately recognize that he is frightened and feeling out of control. I sit down calmly, look Mario in the eyes, and say, "I don't know what happened, but it seems that you're in a serious crisis right now. I'd love to sit down and talk about what's going on." I may even thank Mario for trusting the clinic enough to visit during a time of crisis: "I want to let you know that we're grateful you came in during such a difficult time. Thank you for your trust." I will treat Mario like a partner, in need of hope: "Let's talk about how we can get through this difficult time together."

The first time I tried doing this, I felt awkward. Like a fraud. But much to my surprise, it worked better than the alternative (even when I did it imperfectly). Mario calms down, looks at me a bit warily, and agrees to talk. I am able to take him to a room and spend time listening to his view of the situation. We develop an initial partnership in which I can offer to connect him to services to help figure out how to reduce his legal jeopardy and start getting his life in better shape, so that he can find a job and a place to live, without being hassled by the police. He does not yet view himself as having a problem with alcohol, nor does he have an immediate desire to get sober, but that's something we can work on together if he agrees that we will be useful, helpful, and hopeful partners instead of just another bunch of professionals who are trying to make his life more difficult. The welcoming, customer service-oriented approach provides the best chance to help Mario feel safe, seen, and capable of beginning the road to recovery. Despite my ambivalences about feeling welcoming and devoted to customer service, I have come to learn that striving for these ideals in times of stress embodies what it means to be a community psychiatrist. And most important, when it's all over with Mario, and he calms down and agrees to sit down with a crisis worker for a more thorough discussion, and to come back for further care, I realize that even though my adrenaline has been pumping, and I was feeling anxious the whole time, I actually had fun using all my emotional and cognitive tools to engage Mario successfully. I am making progress!

And I am not acting in isolation. On a more systematic level, as the community *psychiatrist*, I am in a position to create a culture that lives and breathes the values of customer service and welcoming. I am virtually obligated to do so, if I want my team and program to be successful and therapeutic—if I want us all to work together supporting each other rather than splitting over whether people such as Mario should even be seen. I work within an ecosystem, with other professionals, and an audience to boot. From the receptionist and security personnel to nurses, case managers, therapists, psychologists, and potentially other psychiatrists, welcoming ultimately can only be effectively delivered as a team. It is clear to me that my organization is only as welcoming as its least welcoming member, so it is incumbent on me, as the community psychiatrist leader, to cultivate an atmosphere in which the highest possible standard for welcoming clients is met by each and every staff member. From the moment a so-called "misfit" walks in the door to the day they are discharged from the clinic, welcoming is a critical trait of every person with whom a client interacts. Furthermore, it is as important at the beginning as it is at the end: Welcoming is not simply a strategy to get patients to enter the clinic but, rather, a way of life for an organization that seeks to treat those who fall through the cracks in the mental health system—those who are desperate for help and hope.

So how do I embody welcoming for the staff as the leader of the community health center? Modeling is of course important, but it's not the only strategy. After the situation with Mario, it would be helpful for me to debrief with the "team" involved at the front door. My job is not to make people feel bad—quite the contrary. I have to welcome everyone on the team into the conversation and assume everyone did the best they could in the moment but that everyone (including, and especially, me) could do better, and we can all learn from the experience. The goal is to talk it through. What did you think about what happened? Did you think that welcoming Mario was the right approach? What are the pros and cons? What can we do better as a team? What skills should we learn and practice? What policies or procedures would help us to do better?

I can facilitate these discussions even without having a formal leadership role, and in so doing, I have found that I can have a positive impact. There is so much more that I will be able to do as I grow in my career and am able to take on more leadership responsibilities, but just the same, I am starting to move from feeling that I am helpless in my context to believing that I can have fun helping all of us have fun *together* working with the people who are most challenging and who need us the most.

Welcoming Carlo and His Family

The situation with Carlo and his family is in many ways even more challenging than that of Mario, even though the family is not presenting with an acute behavioral disturbance. Specifically, in addition to the fact that Carlo is in the care of two individuals who both have substance use disorders and significant trauma and are only coming for help because they are essentially being coerced by external systems, the family speaks little, if any, English, is struggling with parenting a different child with fetal alcohol spectrum disorder, has significant transportation barriers, and, perhaps most important, has committed the cardinal sin of showing up for an appointment 90 minutes late and right at closing time.

It is so tempting, and would be so easy, for us all to decide that even talking to the mother and Carlo would be "inappropriate" and to send her away. One of our staff might say, "We can't reward her for being late; she needs to learn her lesson." We might also say that we can't help her because we don't have time to complete the registration paperwork in order to bill her visit, that our Spanish-speaking therapist is now busy, or that we don't have a trained interpreter available. After all, it's not our fault that she didn't show up on time when all of that was available.

And were we to send her away, we would not be doing anything out of the ordinary. As I pointed out previously, there is often a tremendous disconnect between our stated values in community psychiatry and the way our underresourced and stressed systems actually operate vis-à-vis "customer service," particularly with the types of clients who are "messy" and "challenging"—the ones who are simultaneously the most stressful to care for and the most in need. *Any* community clinic is unlikely to accept a first-time patient who arrives an hour and a half late and just minutes before closing. *Any* clinic is likely to provide instructions to the receptionist that it is very important to tell such clients they cannot show up so late and expect to be seen today. (This is not to pick on receptionists— they are no more at fault than unwelcoming doctors or other clinicians. All staff are pro- grammed by the "system"—receptionists just happen to be at the entrance.) We have all encountered these situations before; such a patient is usually robotically and reflexively told: "You'll have to come during regular clinic hours, like everyone else" or "We are about to close. If you are in a crisis, the nearest ER is across the street, so why don't you go there? Otherwise, we will reschedule your intake for 3 weeks from now."

And just like with Mario, if I am the community psychiatrist on call when this situa- tion happens, I have the same set of mixed feelings. I would like to be responsive to Carlo and his family, but I also want to leave on time, I don't want to struggle with talking to someone who doesn't speak English very well, and I don't feel terribly competent with either adolescents or substance-using parents. The easiest thing for me to do is to use my authority to support the decision to send them away.

But once again, as an early career community psychiatrist, I have to realize that Carlo and his family represent a wonderful "practice opportunity" for people and families who are most in need. Furthermore, I know that part of my passion for community psychi- atry lies in wanting to help children and families, and I am planning to apply for a child psychiatry fellowship. In my personal life, I am passionate about the plight of immigrants fleeing gang warfare and violence in their home countries and believe strongly that these immigrant families (especially the children) are deserving of a welcoming response by our whole nation. So, it feels particularly difficult for me to resolve in my own mind that it would be okay just to be irritated with this family for coming late and that this family who has been through so much should just be sent away because they are being "inconvenient."

Clearly, Carlo and his family are precisely the people who need me the most—and the exact clients who inspire me to work in the field of community psychiatry in the first place. If I am truly committed to welcoming and customer service, I need to develop a set of skills for myself, as well as support my team members to build a culture in which it would be natural to welcome Carlo's mother, Carlo, and Ella with open arms and warm hearts, especially when they have shown up 90 minutes late.

A welcoming clinic would take a completely different approach than what I just described. A family such as this is viewed not only as a priority but also as fun! During my time living in Nepal, I came across some timeless Tibetan wisdom that invites us to view challenges and difficult circumstances in life as "wish-fulfilling gems"—that is, precious jewels that are to be cherished, as opposed to enemies that ought to be feared or hated. Analogously, Carlo and his family can be viewed as a wish-fulfilling jewel and cherished as something that all of us (including me) can grow from individually and as a clinic.

So where do we begin? The starting place is to move beyond our own feelings to thinking about what it's like for Carlo and his family to be showing up. Rather than focusing on how we experience them in *our* world, let's ask how they experience *us* in *their* world. In our world, we (and other staff members) are likely subject to the same dialogue of "inner voices" that Mario provoked: anger at Carlo and his family for arriving late, compassion for their situation, fear for what these children are bound to encounter as their lives move forward in a system stacked against them, and guilt for not feeling able to serve them adequately in the moment.

If we stay caught up in ourselves, then we are more concerned about what will make *us* less stressed than what would be most helpful to Carlo's family. Let's think for a moment about what this all looks like in their world. First, think about this young mother. She does not speak English well and has no idea what mental health treatment consists of. She is an immigrant who is so terrified about what might happen to Carlo (and the whole family) if she does not abide by the mandate to show up at our clinic that she manages to get time off work (not easy at all) to schlep her two kids, on multiple buses, to come to our building, which is itself a strange and scary place. All she knows is that if she doesn't show up, Carlo may be kicked out of school or, worse yet, she may lose custody of her children or even be deported. She is distressed that she is running late, but she has very little control over when she can get time off from work. She has no idea that our clinic is going to close soon after she arrives, and even if she did, what could she do differently?

Stopping to empathize with the family's situation and world view, and to recognize their strengths, is one of the "tools" I mentioned previously. Speaking just for myself, if I take a moment to apply my own empathic capacity to this situation, it only takes a few seconds before I can start to feel less irritated and more compassionate. And, of course, I learned a lot in Nepal about Buddhist teachings on universal compassion for all sentient beings. Immediately, I begin to calm down.

What other tools are at my disposal? Part of learning about "welcoming" is to shift from thinking about all the things we can't do in the limited amount of time available at the end of the day ("We can't complete the paperwork!" "We can't complete the assessment form!" "We can't diagnose and bill!") and think instead about what we *can* do. What tools can I use to have Carlo, his mother, and his sister feel really happy that they took the trouble to show up today? What tools can I use to make it more likely that they will feel some hope that we can help them and that they will be inclined to come back? Is it possible that I can apply these tools in 15–30 minutes? Well, maybe not the first time that I try, but this is a great opportunity to practice!

So, when the staff contacts me to say they are sending this family away ("Just checking with you Dr. Saunders, to make sure that it's OK. . . . but just so you know, it's standard procedure"), I say "no." I say,

> Look guys, I know you have to leave soon, but let's remember the effort this family took to get here, and see if we can take a few minutes to help them feel happy that they came. If any of you needs to leave right away, please go ahead, but I plan to stay a few minutes to talk to them. Can anyone join me? If there's anyone around who speaks Spanish who can stay for a while, that would be super helpful as well.

Then, I go take the family into an office and sit down with them calmly. I don't want this to take long, but I don't want to act like I'm in a hurry either. I start with a warm greeting and offer them a drink or a snack. Then, I acknowledge that they came late, and unfortunately that means that many of the people who were here to help them today have left, but I want them to know, on behalf of the entire clinic, that we are very glad they came. We have read the referrals and we know that the whole family needs a lot of help, and they deserve to get the best possible help. We are so impressed that Mom got the kids here today, and we want to make sure we let everyone who sent her know that she came. Finally, I want to let her know that although we have not had time to learn all the details of the situation, the family is in the right place and we have the tools to help them. This takes approximately 5 minutes.

Then, I ask if there is anything that is on their minds that they need to tell us today and if there is anything we need to do about scheduling future appointments that may make it easier for her to get to us on time. I make sure to look Carlo in the eyes and let him know how important it was that he supported his mother by coming in with her today—she would have been very worried had he not come along. I would also take time to connect with Ella in whatever way worked for her. And then I would ask the family if perhaps we could arrange for them to get transportation back home, given the lateness of the hour.

By the time they leave, 30 minutes later, they are smiling and happy. I am smiling and happy too. What might have been miserable turned into a feel-good moment for all of us. This is the power of prioritizing welcoming and hope even when nothing else seems to be possible, and purposely learning and practicing the tools to succeed. I hope these kinds of tools are useful to you, the reader, in your own work.

Furthermore, just like with Mario, it will be possible to debrief with staff (not now, but tomorrow, perhaps) and determine how to work as a team to help us all understand how to improve our ability to be welcoming in these situations, even while acknowledging the limitations of the clinic (e.g., the clinic hours) and paperwork requirements.

In the debrief, we can think about what a "welcoming receptionist" would do when people such as this family show up late for their intake. A welcoming receptionist thanks them for coming in when they could, letting Carlo's mother know he is grateful that she took time off work to visit and that he is impressed that she was able to bring along two children. He invites the family to sit down in the lobby to catch their breath and reassures them that the clinic is more than happy to see them today. Carlo and his family would be offered some water to drink and perhaps a snack. They are treated like partners, working together with the clinic to get through trying times. The receptionist becomes an important part of a *team* of individuals that is committed to the cause of serving such people— whom other clinics would dub "difficult patients"—so is therefore ready for such a situation, and even excited about being able to make a contribution. The receptionist has had debriefings with staff members after encounters with similar clients and feels heard by other staff members, so he is prepared and motivated to act in a welcoming manner that has become increasingly natural for him over time.

And what would a welcoming clinician or case manager do? A welcoming case manager offers similar courtesies of rest, refreshment, and, most important, empathy and hope. And the task is made easier by the work of the receptionist—by the fact she is not working in isolation. The social worker takes a few minutes to listen to why it was so important for the family to come in today. There is not enough time to get a deeper understanding of all of the family's concerns that may be contributing to Carlo's problems (mental health issues, housing, trauma, substance use disorders, domestic violence, immigration, language, school, etc.), but the social worker has the time to convey how much she really wants to get to know Carlo and the family when they return. The case manager views Carlo and his family as part of a broader system, embodying the welcoming attitude of seeing the family as a *whole unit, held together by love and strength*, not just a repository of pathology. She does this not only because the receptionist did it first, or because the staff had a debriefing about a similar situation, or because she views the patient as a "wish-fulfilling jewel." She does it because it works—for her *and* for the family. Without this type of approach to treatment, not only will Carlo and his family suffer (as they may never even return, with potentially devastating consequences) but also she will suffer, feeling increasingly frustrated and burnt out rather than inspired, energized, and helpful.

As a psychiatrist, and perhaps an informal leader of the team, I can not only model the customer service and welcoming for others, turning this difficult situation into a fun teaching opportunity, but also, as discussed previously, facilitate discussion and debriefing with staff members about what has happened and about their ambivalences and conflicting feelings. In so doing, I not only prepare all of us on the team to be able to address similar encounters in the future but also help us to combat the helplessness that can seep into the DNA of our clinic when encountering such situations routinely. We need to take the time to build a positive culture and toolkit for ourselves so we can have more success, and have more fun, addressing the needs of the challenging youth and families we all came to serve.

Of course, welcoming and customer service orientation do not come naturally to most of us; even the most devoted community psychiatrists require mentorship and supervision to help them wrestle with the internal struggles and realities that are part and parcel of the profession. If you are like me, you have to bring these issues time and again to your supervisors and mentors so that you can learn from such challenging experiences. Mentors and supervisors are a part of the psychiatric ecosystem, and I bring these challenges to them because I want to learn how to serve patients such as Mario and Carlo with the welcoming and customer service they deserve. Furthermore, I do it because I want to feel good about myself and the work I do, embodying welcoming and customer service for those I work with along the way.

These case examples, then, display the welcoming and customer service that are critical to the future of community psychiatry. As an aspiring community psychiatrist, I face existential crises on a regular basis (okay maybe that's a little dramatic, but I do believe it) as I regularly strive for (and regularly fall short of) achievement of these ideals and mastery of the tools that would help me to do so. However, perseverance, seeking mentorship, striving to improve and better myself are of paramount importance because welcoming and customer service are the mother's milk of community psychiatry: Without them, patients and providers suffer and burn out, and the ecosystem threatens to collapse.

ENGAGING POPULATIONS IN NEED

The ideals of the "future" of community psychiatry go beyond just working with challenging individuals and families. Here, we discuss Mario and Carlo from a population-level perspective to address the next key value of community psychiatry: engaging populations in need. Each case highlights a different population in need: Mario represents persons with mental illness (usually with co-occurring substance use disorders) in the criminal justice system, and Carlo's situation represents the population of multiproblem immigrant families who, in addition, suffer from the cultural challenges facing undocumented immigrants and belong to cultural/linguistic minorities. These illustrative case examples lead to presentation of a general approach to "system improvement" for designing and implementing welcoming best practice services at your organization for identified populations in need in your community.

Engaging People with Mental Illness in the Criminal Justice System

Let's start with Mario. You'll recall that Mario was referred to your clinic by a probation officer for psychiatric treatment in the context of an altercation at a bar. He was behaving strangely and drinking at the bar, so patrons called the police. When they arrived, he attempted to fight them and was arrested. He was released from jail on the condition that he would seek mental health treatment, and he risks returning to jail if he does not follow through on the court orders. In the beginning of this chapter, we discussed the strategies for welcoming and engaging Mario as an individual, and how I (as the community psychiatrist "on the scene") can work to apply more successful (and inspiring) clinical approaches in my own work and in the work of my team members.

But now we want to take on a greater challenge. Unfortunately, individuals such as Mario are not rare. In any setting serving individuals with serious mental illness, a high percentage (usually cited as 30–50%) will have a co-occurring substance use disorder (which may or may not be in remission at any point in time), and a similarly high percentage (usually cited as approximately one-third) will have past or present criminal justice involvement (Cline & Minkoff, 2012). From the perspective of community psychiatry, persons with serious mental illness clearly represent a population in need: high volume, underserved, poor outcomes. In my vision of myself as a community psychiatrist, I realize it is not enough to challenge myself *individually* to provide better service to the individuals I personally encounter. In order to have an impact, I must learn how to help my whole *agency* do a better job to serve this population.

Sounds challenging, right? Imagine 20 Marios walking into my clinic every day. What can I do, as a newbie community psychiatrist, to improve my organization's response? What tools can I learn to get better at having a population-level impact for my agency? How can I help my agency meet the needs of this population by routinely offering not only the welcoming and customer service that they deserve but also a full array of best practice interventions?

The scary part of being a young community psychiatrist is that there is so much to learn. The wonderful part of being a young community psychiatrist, however, is that you can make a difference, even while you are still learning. If you seek out strategies for helping your entire program or agency better meet the demands of high-need populations, you can make a difference. The need is so great that any steps of progress are valuable on a large scale. In your role as a clinical leader (even if you are just a young psychiatrist), you can learn the organizational skills to design interventions that are based on what a population *needs* rather than fitting the patients to what your "system" can currently offer.

What's your first step? First, make the assumption that there may already be "system" or "population" approaches that can help the population you are concerned about. Your job is to review the literature to identify them. If you can't find them yourself, ask mentors or experts in the field. There is much more known about effective practices, and how to implement them, than those practices are actually implemented in real-world provider agencies. If you ask for help (e.g., on the American Academy of Community Psychiatry listserv), people will help you. That's been my experience.

For example, in the literature on implementing services for individuals with co-occurring disorders (COD), there is discussion of approaches for implementing integrated services and systems, referencing an approach known as Comprehensive, Continuous Integrated System of Care (CCISC; Minkoff & Cline, 2004, 2005; Substance Abuse and Mental Health Services Administration, 2002). According to this approach, any program or agency can take specific steps to use the organizational technique of "continuous quality improvement" (CQI) to redesign itself to be a "co-occurring program," capable of routinely providing integrated best practice interventions within base resources to the individuals with COD who show up for treatment on a regular basis.

Furthermore, CCISC has a toolkit (ZiaPartners, 2016) and a "12 Steps of Implementation" process that can be undertaken by any agency that uses evidence-based organizational change strategies to support step-by-step implementation of best practices—such as welcoming, integrated screening, engagement in integrated hopeful strength-based relationships, and individualized integrated stage-matched, skill-based interventions for each co-occurring condition—so that any "Mario" being served can get connected to services that help him (or her) make progress toward attaining a meaningful and successful life.

Here's another example, for individuals such as Mario who are involved in the criminal justice system (including those with COD): the Group for Advancement of Psychiatry, Committee on Psychiatry and Community published a manual in 2016 titled *People with Mental Illness in the Criminal Justice System: Answering a Cry for Help. A Practice Manual for Psychiatrists and Other Practitioners*. Within this manual, there are a series of step-by-step tools and recommendations that can help any psychiatrist answer the following questions: What can I do in my own work? What can I do in my own organization? and What can I do in my own community? The latter two questions are directly relevant to the issue of helping populations in need at the organization or community level.

What's your second step? Take time to learn the techniques of organizational change. The simplest strategies to master relate to customer-oriented continuous quality improvement (COCQI), which describes how to use the FOCUS-PDCA process, a management method developed in the health care industry used to improve processes. FOCUS stands for *find* a process to improve (e.g., organizational response to individuals with COD who are also involved in the criminal justice system; CJS); *organize* a team to improve the process; *collect* information on the process to identify a baseline; *understand* the contributors to the current results at a level of detail; *select* some things to improve; and then engage in *plan–do–check–act* cycles with your team to make step-by-step progress in identifying and embedding new practices that are designed to serve the population of interest, rather than have the population be a "misfit" for what is currently offered. (We return to the COCQI and the FOCUS-PDCA process later in our discussion of how to engage Carlo and his family.)

The third step is to become a change agent. This is not easy—in fact, one of the reasons I decided to write this chapter is so I can improve at this skill. I'm great at reading and studying but not so great at taking the risk of putting my ideas into action. I suspect that's true for most everyone. We all want to see things change, but we are not very good at what is called the "Serenity Prayer of System Change" from Minkoff and Cline (2016):

> The serenity to accept the things you cannot change (which is everyone else)
> The courage to change the things you can (your own work, your own team, your own
>   agency)
> And the wisdom to know the difference

So how do you get started? To begin, volunteer at your organization to either start or participate in a positive change process (CQI activity) for a population of concern—such as individuals with CJS involvement and COD, like Mario—that you care about. Talk to your agency leader, stating, for example,

> Hey, I have been reading some stuff about helping, on a population level, people with
> co-occurring mental illnesses who are also involved in the CJS. I want to see if we can
> do some of this cool stuff here. Would it be OK if I pulled together a team of folks to
> look at the issue, and see if we can find some things to improve upon? Don't worry,

we're not looking for ways to spend more money, so much as to use the resources we have more effectively.

Sounds good, right? Scares the bejeezus out of me! But I know that has to be my next step (which I'll discuss more when I talk about Carlo and his family later).

Step four: Don't reinvent the wheel. When your team gets together to implement "COD capability" or "criminal justice capability," try to pay attention to the recommended steps from the literature. Keep it simple. Go slowly. Stay organized. You are learning the "do's" and "don'ts" of population improvement—you *will* make mistakes, as will your team. That's part of the fun, and the process of learning. Keep at it, and ask for help when you need it. Your organization will be able to make progress, and you will steadily improve at being the change agent you want to be as you develop more experience. Your abilities as a clinician, team member, teacher, and change agent can all grow at the same time. This is what is so amazing about community psychiatry: As you get more experience, your ability to reach larger and more complex populations and systems grows dramatically.

Now that I've gotten the go-ahead from my agency leader, I've decided to implement a CQI activity for clients who are involved in the CJS. One of the first steps would involve organizing a team of individuals who are interested in and passionate about this population. Such a team could consist of managers, supervisors, support staff, and even consumers, families, or community members. This step is critical because whatever else may be the case, you can't do it alone, especially in community psychiatry. Having the purchase of other individuals in the organization and community is critical for success. In so doing, you're avoiding the pitfall of reinventing the wheel on two fronts. First, the need for a team is well established in the literature (Engels et al., 2006). Second, the other team members may be able to draw on their own experience, from previous projects, so the overall team doesn't make the mistakes prior efforts have encountered.

After gathering a team of people who are passionate about clients with COD in the CJS, the next step is to engage in a structured CQI process (Minkoff & Cline, 2004). This would involve setting parameters of progress for developing a welcoming organization for this population. One example could be to improve the rate at which clients with CJS involvement return after their first appointment, a potential index of welcoming. Another starting place might be something as basic as identifying how many individuals with co-occurring mental health, substance use disorders, and/or criminal justice needs are currently being served so that an organized and data-driven response for serving them can be developed. From there, your team might choose to improve the identification of stage of change for each individual issue (there is a literature on stage of change identification and treatment for individuals with serious mental illness, criminal justice involvement, and substance use disorders; see DiClemente, Nidecker, & Bellack, 2008; Group for the Advancement of Psychiatry, Committee on Psychiatry and the Community, 2016; Mueser, 2003) as a way of guiding all staff to routinely implement integrated stage-matched interventions with stage-matched outcomes that permit progress in working with individuals who have complex needs in a hopeful, strength-based way, as clients make small steps of progress over time (just as you are trying to do with your organization). As mentioned previously, keep it simple, go slowly, follow the literature, and capitalize on the wisdom of your mentors. You will make mistakes. In these hypothetical examples, maybe you made the wrong individual the team leader, or perhaps your CQI process was too ambitious. Either way, keep it simple and go slowly, stay committed to the process, and be a change agent who is unafraid to admit fault and give it a second shot.

In the next section, we describe the details of a CQI approach, including implementation of the FOCUS-PDCA process, in thinking about how to help the population represented by Carlo and his family.

Engaging Multiproblem Immigrant Families

The situation Carlo and his family face is arguably even more complex than Mario's situation. What's more, the number of families facing similarly complex issues continues to grow. Many (although not all) immigrant families suffer from high rates of poverty, unsteady housing, and unstable employment; many live in fear at the prospect of deportation; and of course, most have language barriers. Clearly, immigrants—especially refugees—are the type of underserved and at-risk population that community psychiatrists seek out and embrace.

Much like in Mario's case, there are both clinical and organizational challenges that have to be addressed. But how does this take place? The answer lies in focusing on what you *can* do to help this population in need—specifically, by applying the previously discussed four steps in the CQI process to aid in the design and implementation of best practice approaches that fit the needs of the target population or community (in this case, multiproblem families with significant cultural/linguistic challenges) rather than trying to fit the challenging population to what you currently offer.

How do I begin this process? First, as mentioned previously, I can safely assume that there are approaches out there that have been effective for immigrant families such Carlo and his family; my job is to review the literature and speak with others in the field to identify them. In my review of the literature on engaging multiproblem immigrant families, I come to understand that there are established "best practices" for meeting the considerable needs of refugee children and their families in resettlement (such as Carlo).

For example, the National Child Traumatic Stress Network (NCTSN) identifies several components of comprehensive services for refugee children, including trauma-informed treatments, school-based cognitive–behavioral therapy (CBT) interventions, psychoeducation, parenting interventions for mothers, and art and expressive therapy (Birman et al., 2005). The NCTSN also notes a number of critical strategies to be employed across interventions, including certain approaches to cultural competence, enhancing cultural awareness and sensitivity of mainstream providers, and identifying ethnically matched professionals and paraprofessionals.

The second step, now that I have worked toward identifying some practices that appear to have been successfully employed by other organizations, is to familiarize myself with the techniques of organizational change. Specifically, I have to develop experience with the practices and principles of COCQI, mentioned previously, in order to be equipped with strategies to deal with the challenges that I'm bound to encounter in designing and implementing services to help the kinds of clients represented by Carlo and his family. The FOCUS-PDCA process, also discussed previously, is ideally suited to the situation we are facing with Carlo and his family. You'll remember that the FOCUS process calls for *finding* something to improve; *organizing* a team to improve the process; *collecting* information on the process to identify a baseline; *understanding* the contributors to the current results at a level of detail; and then *selecting* some things to improve.

Starting with "F," finding a process to improve, I think hard about the many problems Carlo and his family are facing. Clearly, they are in need of—and deserve—access to all of the previously discussed components recommended by the NCTSN, and they are all critical. But given that I want to choose one actionable thing that I can improve, I decide to focus on the delivery of trauma-informed care in our organization. School-based CBT interventions, psychoeducation, and parenting interventions for mothers are important as well, but I try to focus on one thing at a time to improve. So I decide to move forward in the FOCUS process with an attempt to improve the delivery of trauma-informed care within our organization—with the full knowledge that this is *just the beginning*.

My next thought is that trauma-informed care sounds great, but what *is* trauma-informed care exactly? Essentially, trauma-informed care (TIC) is a manner of approaching families such as Carlo's in a way that is safe and sensitive to their histories. The impact of trauma is deep and life-shaping—touching virtually every aspect of one's existence—and great care needs to be taken by providers when working with these clients. Families affected by trauma are in high need, indeed!

Next, my goal is to organize a team to work on the initiative. As discussed in the CJS and COD example presented previously, teams should consist of individuals from all levels of the organization and also include families, consumers, and community members.

So I reach out to the receptionist Bob, the social worker James, my fellow psychiatrist Carol, a community member and neighbor Tom, and a client of the center, Jose, who is also an immigrant and refugee. All of these individuals are passionate about the delivery of TIC and excited about the prospect of working as a team to improve the organization's efforts on this front.

At this point, I consider the (sadly, apocryphal) Gandhi quote about being the change you wish to see in the world and try to "be the change agent I want to see in the world." Of course, any change agent that wants to avoid burnout will, at times, need to keep the aforementioned Serenity Prayer of System Change, but the point remains: It's time to get to work! I arrange a meeting with my agency leader to discuss my interest, passion, and even devotion to this cause. I tell her—or even better, show her—how much I care about the well-being of immigrant refugees and their families. Perhaps most important, I make sure to convey that I'm knowledgeable about the subject. In this case, I have to know more about the plight of immigrant children and importance of TIC than simply what *The New York Times* front page states. If I'm not informed, I run the risk of coming across as naive, ill-prepared, or worse. I let her know that I would volunteer to lead the efforts and have identified five other individuals interested in the project. I reassure her that I'm not trying to change the world overnight, and I am most certainly not asking for more money. Rather, I'm seeking to understand how our organization can serve this population better and to identify a way to use our current resources more effectively. Having received her stamp of approval (hopefully), it's time to act.

So, how to begin? Perhaps an example of where *not* to begin will be instructive. Say, for example, that when the team discusses the issue of improving the experience of families such as Carlo's, an immediate idea is that we want to increase access to Spanish-speaking staff. Indeed, the literature suggests that bilingual health care providers and/or medical interpreter services are critical for meeting the needs of non-native speakers (Flores, 2005). The problem, however, is that this measure may be impossible to implement at this point, given the budgetary limitations the organization faces and the lack of immediate availability of bilingual clinicians in our community. Remember, we only have one staff member who speaks Spanish, and she can't see every Spanish-speaking patient who walks through the door. In addition, we can't just hire more; it's not like our organization is swimming in money. And we can't just magically train several employees to speak Spanish overnight. Everyone knows it takes months, and more likely years, to become even conversational. So what do we do?

Unfortunately, some community psychiatrists at this step will get "stuck." And indeed, we feel like we're stuck and want to give up. What can we possibly do to address this critical problem, if not hire more Spanish speakers? "But soft, what light, through yonder window breaks. It is the east, and . . . and the FOCUS process is our sun." Forgive the Romeo and Juliet reference, but the FOCUS process is our Juliet, and it *will* save us as long as we remain committed to using it! The whole point of a structured CQI process such as FOCUS-PDCA is to *avoid* having everyone on the team think of a "good idea" and then get stuck trying to fund it (which increasing access to Spanish-speaking providers will most certainly require). You must examine all the processes that impact the population you are serving and identify the ones that you *can* improve, prioritizing based on what is both relevant and feasible. Then, you keep going—that's what makes it "continuous" improvement.

Returning to the FOCUS process model: We have found a process to improve (improving organization delivery of trauma-informed care) and organized a team, so the next step would be to learn something about our current baseline of delivering trauma-informed care. This is the "C" in the FOCUS process—collect information on the process to establish a baseline. After all, CQI should always start with some sort of measurement of a baseline. This is a critical step because without baseline information, one cannot be assured that a given initiative had any effect.

How do you collect baseline information about delivery of TIC? If you don't have a good understanding of your agency's ability and capacity to deliver TIC (which is likely), tools have been created to help a program improvement team—and programs themselves—measure TIC baseline. For example, consider the Creating Cultures of Trauma-Informed Care (CCTIC) assessment, which helps agencies assess their readiness to design, implement, evaluate, and monitor trauma-informed programs (Fallot & Harris, 2009; Harris & Fallot, 2001). This self-assessment evaluates the organization on the basis of six domains: program procedures and settings; formal services policies; trauma screening, assessment, service planning, and trauma-specific services; administrative support for program-wide trauma-informed services; staff training and education; and human resources practices. Fortunately, there are other self-assessment tools as well, including the five-component assessment from the Trauma Informed Care Project (http://traumainformedcareproject.org). In any case, whether you use a tool such as CCTIC or the Trauma-Informed Care Project tool, the goal of this step, of course, is to collect information about the organization baseline.

We elect to use the CCTIC and administer it to staff. Meanwhile, we work as a team to involve our colleagues in being excited about the concept of improving our TIC and in joining us in finding ways to improve. It is important for us as a "change team" to work to find partners and allies in the staff, not to imply that the staff members are "deficient" in some way. After all, we all share a passion for trying to find ways within our available resources to improve the experiences and outcomes of the most challenging individuals and families we serve. Taking time to engage program leaders and staff in sharing the goal of improving our ability to be sensitive to the trauma of these complex families, and work hard to make sure we don't re-traumatize them unintentionally, allows more of the staff to get excited about using the CCTIC to collect baseline information. In that process, we discover, unsurprisingly, that although we do well in many areas, there are also many areas in which each program, team, or clinician can improve.

Given the many domains of the CCTIC self-assessment, my next thought (which I share with the TIC change team) is that implementing proper TIC will be a herculean task! How are we ever going to improve our organization's care across all of these domains? But together we remember that the FOCUS-PDCA approach will give us a round of applause for helping each program or team start with one or two small changes they can make, among the many ways in which the organization could improve its efforts to deliver TIC. As a change team, we can gather up many ideas and possibilities and then identify a few to start with. Our role is not to create the change so much as to provide resources, support, and encouragement for our colleagues to take steps forward. For example, we could start by increasing the expectation that all staff are trauma-informed, equipped with the specific knowledge of how to help refugee families feel safe. Alternatively, we could start by implementing welcoming policies and procedures for immigrant refugee children and families who come in the door so that all staff understand there is an expectation that these individuals will be welcomed. In either case, the goal is to start by aspiring to make one or two small changes that can be measured and monitored as our organization makes progress in small steps over time (so that there can be an organized data-driven response for implementation and opportunities to celebrate successes).

To guide our efforts at making one or two small changes, we turn to the results from the CCTIC self-assessment. We notice that the results from Domain 5, Staff Training and Trauma Education, show that there is an impressive knowledge deficit within the organization about what TIC means. Many—if not most—respondents indicated through their responses that they did not have an adequate understanding of many core principles of trauma-informed care, including the relationship between traumatic stress and physical health, the relationship between traumatic stress and mental health, how trauma affects child development, and the relationship between childhood trauma and adult re-victimization.

Given this baseline understanding of our TIC knowledge deficit, our next goal in FOCUS-PDCA is to understand the various contributors to the results we've found in the baseline assessment (namely that the staff is not well-versed in trauma-informed care). In the course of the self-assessment, we learned that 10% of respondents had never received any formal education on trauma-informed treatment. Clearly, not having received education on TIC will get in the way of delivering gold-standard, trauma-informed treatments! Armed with this information, we now understand a little bit more about one of the reasons the staff is not well-versed enough in trauma-informed care: They've never received any education on it.

Given this information, the FOCUS model's last stage tells us to select some things to improve. In this situation, we want to start with things that do *not* require extra hiring or money. The goal is to find the small steps that the organization can and will do. In the case of trauma-informed treatment delivery, our actionable item could be increasing the agency expectation that all staff are trauma-informed, with a specific understanding of how to help refugee families feel safe. Having learned that many respondents lacked knowledge in the basic principles of trauma-informed care, we decide to act by leading an education effort aimed at increasing staff knowledge about the subject.

Now that an activity is selected, the task is to engage in plan–do–check–act cycles with the team to make step-by-step progress. We begin by establishing a "plan." The team decides that a good first step may be to educate the staff about what TIC means. We decide that several 30-minute staff meetings/lectures during lunch, in which the basics of TIC are presented and discussed, might be a good place to begin. On behalf of the team, we ask the leader of the agency if she would have an issue with such a series of presentations, and fortunately she agrees without reservation.

Next, we "do": The team crafts a presentation, schedules the staff meetings many weeks in advance, and advertises it throughout the organization. We deliver the presentation and think it went well. To confirm, we re-administer Doman 5 of the self-assessment and find that three times as many respondents demonstrated adequate knowledge about the basics of trauma-informed care. Then, we "check" the data and results, comparing them to our expected outcomes. For example, we want to be assured that we administered the same test before and after the presentation (we did) and that no mistakes were made in analysis of the data (none were made). At this point, the "check" phase showed that the "plan" phase was put in place and carried out in the "do" phase to good effect (i.e., three times as many people demonstrated sufficient adequate knowledge about TIC). The next step is to act on the basis of these data. We decide as a team that a reasonable expectation for staff members is that 100% of them—not just most of them—should be trauma-informed. We speak with our agency leader, and all agree that this is an appropriate new standard for the organization. Because the PDCA process is iterative, our next goal is to go back to P, and plan a way to help the staff meet this new standard.

But if (and when) we eventually achieve 100% compliance in terms of TIC knowledge, the work is not done, by any means! Because CQI is continuous (by definition), our team is motivated to look forward to potential next steps, even as we continue the education initiative. In the course of the self-assessment, in addition to noticing knowledge deficits, we also came to realize how utterly incomprehensible and unnavigable the various individual service systems (mental health, substance use, intellectual disability services, etc.) must be for Carlo and his family, especially in light of their language limitations. Putting ourselves in their shoes, we wonder if we would be able to navigate the various systems ourselves, even *with* benefits that Carlo and his family *don't* have (being in our country of origin and not having a language barrier). We conclude, naturally, that we would struggle mightily. Given the many different services the family requires—Carlo has mental health service needs, his father has significant substance use disorder needs, and his sister has intellectual disabilities—we decide to begin a second pilot CQI activity that involves a family-based, wrap-around, culturally appropriate approach to serving families such as Carlo's (like the kind discussed in Palmer et al., 2011). What do we do next? Well of course we return to the FOCUS-PDCA process model—and begin anew.

This, then, represents one approach to developing a welcoming and customer service-oriented approach to helping a population in need. Three acronyms—CQI, FOCUS, and PDCA—can guide you in your approach to developing welcoming and customer service-oriented care. It is not the only way, but it is most certainly one good way. It is not going to be easy, but it will most certainly be rewarding. Most important, it will be fun—if you let it be. Do your best not to be so hard on yourself; let yourself fail, or else you'll never have the chance to succeed. Lean on others, and let others lean on you. But especially, trust in your mentors. After all, the chapter is called "Back to the Future," right?

CASE STUDIES: CONCLUSION

Let's return to the beginning of the chapter for the moment. The image that appears in the opening pages depicts Maitreya, who is considered to be the next Buddha in most Buddhist cosmological systems. Like all Buddhas, Maitreya is also considered to be a Bodhisattva, or one who has dedicated himself to helping all sentient beings attain enlightenment, or nirvana. These individuals vow to never rest until all beings have been liberated from suffering and the causes of suffering. According to such world views, once the teachings of the current historical Buddha have dissipated—an indeterminate number of years from now, perhaps thousands or more—Maitreya will be reborn to spread Buddhist teachings once again.

Living in Nepal among Tibetan refugees in a small village outside the capital of Kathmandu, I encountered the image of Maitreya time and again. In writing this chapter, and thinking about the future of community psychiatry, Maitreya is no less present to me. You see, in these Buddhist world views, Maitreya is part of an infinitely long lineage of Buddhas, all of whom are dedicated to liberating sentient beings from suffering. When Maitreya is reborn, sometime in the future, I can't help but think that he will be going Back to the Future as well—back to the principles, ideals, and values of the Buddhas who have served the world in previous lifetimes.

Similarly, the present historical moment in community psychiatry is witnessing a rebirth of the values of the founders of the field, as early career psychiatrists seek to carry their mantle into the future. In the case studies presented, we discussed two values in particular: working with persons who are most in need (i.e., the difficult patients) and working with challenging and at-risk populations. Although the patients in these cases, and the clinicians caring for them, experienced a number of forces colluding to make such work difficult—including a narrowing definition of whom we would serve and a focus on billing rather than caring for communities—aspiring community psychiatrists are electing to travel Back to the Future, tapping into the foundational wisdom of the community psychiatry movement. The cases presented prioritize two strategies for countering the forces that oppose Back to the Future values: welcoming difficult patients and meeting the needs of at-risk populations, rather than fitting their needs to our system. In other words, we're doing our best imitation of Maitreya, trying to invoke the wisdom of our forebears for the benefit of those we serve.

Community psychiatrists are not Buddhas or Bodhisattvas, and I certainly don't mean to equate the two. Nor should early career community psychiatrists hold out hope of becoming Maitreya, as we struggle to serve the needs of patients such as Mario and Carlo. But the notion of a *future* someone who is dedicated to alleviating the suffering of others resonates well with the subject of the chapter. Sometime in the future, in these Buddhist cosmologies, Maitreya will offer teachings for the benefit of people who are suffering, drawing on the wisdom of those Buddhas who came before him. Somehow, this doesn't sound all that dissimilar from the world of future community psychiatrists, who one day will embody and implement the values and principles of community psychiatrists who came before them, so as to benefit those suffering from mental illness.

REFERENCES

Birman, D., Ho, J., Pulley, E., Batia, K., Lynn Everson, M., Ellis, H., . . . Tsai, J. (2005). *Mental health interventions for refugee children in resettlement.* Los Angeles, CA: National Child Traumatic Stress Network.

Buswell, R. E. (Ed.). (2004). *Encyclopedia of Buddhism.* New York, NY: Macmillan.

Cline, C. A., & Minkoff, K. (2012). Inspiring a welcoming, hopeful culture. In H. L. McQuistion, W. E. Sowers, J. M. Ranz, & J. M. Feldman (Eds.), *Handbook of community psychiatry* (pp. 93–102). New York, NY: Springer-Verlag. https://doi.org/10.1007/978-1-4614-3149-7

DiClemente, C. C., Nidecker, M., & Bellack, A. S. (2008). Motivation and the stages of change among individuals with severe mental illness and substance abuse disorders. *Journal of Substance Abuse Treatment, 34*(1), 25–35. https://doi.org/10.1016/j.jsat.2006.12.034

Engels, Y., van den Hombergh, P., Mokkink, H., van den Hoogen, H., van den Bosch, W., & Grol, R. (2006). The effects of a team-based continuous quality improvement intervention on the management of primary care: A randomised controlled trial. *British Journal of General Practice, 56*(531), 781–787.

Fallot, R., & Harris, M. (2009). *Creating Cultures of Trauma-Informed Care (CCTIC): A self-assessment and planning protocol.* Washington, DC: Community Connections 2.2.

Flores, G. (2005). The impact of medical interpreter services on the quality of health care: A systematic review. *Medical Care Research and Review, 62*(3), 255–299. https://doi.org/10.1177/1077558705275416

Group for the Advancement of Psychiatry, Committee on Psychiatry and the Community. (2016). *People with mental illness in the criminal justice system: Answering a cry for help.* Arlington, VA: American Psychiatric Association Publishing.

Harris, M., & Fallot, R. (Eds.). (2001). *Using trauma theory to design service systems: New directions for mental health services.* San Francisco, CA: Jossey-Bass.

Minkoff, K., & Cline, C. A. (2004). Changing the world: The design and implementation of comprehensive continuous integrated systems of care for individuals with co-occurring disorders. *Psychiatric Clin North Am, 27*(4), 727–743. https://doi.org/10.1016/j.psc.2004.07.003

Minkoff, K., & Cline, C. A. (2005). Developing welcoming systems for individuals with co-occurring disorders. *J Dual Diagn, 1*(1), 65–89. https://doi.org/10.1300/J374v01n01_06

Minkoff, K., & Cline, C. A. (2016). *Compass-ez 2.0.* San Rafael, CA: ZiaPartners.

Mueser, K. T. (2003). *Integrated treatment for dual disorders: A guide to effective practice.* New York, NY: Guilford.

Palmer, S., Vang, T. J., Bess, G., Baize, H., Moore, K., De La Torre, A., . . . Gonzalez, J. (2011). Implementing culture-based wraparound. In E. J. Bruns & J. S. Walker (Eds.), *The resource guide to wraparound.* Portland, OR: National Wraparound Initiative, Research and Training Center for Family Support and Children's Mental Health.

Substance Abuse and Mental Health Services Administration. (2002). *Report to Congress on the prevention and treatment of co-occurring substance abuse disorders and mental health disorders.* Washington, DC: US Department of Health and Human Services.

ZiaPartners. (2016). *Overview of the Zia tools.* Retrieved December 11, 2018, from http://www.ziapartners.com/tools

INDEX

Note: *For the benefit of digital users, indexed terms that span two pages (e.g., 52–53) may, on occasion, appear on only one of those pages.*
Tables, figures and boxes are indicated by *t*, *f* and *b* following the page number

ACA (Affordable Care Act), 24–25
academic accreditation requirements, community
    psychiatry, 152–53
academic–community partnership
  academic accreditation requirements, 152–53
  case study, 150, 153, 156–57, 163
  community psychiatry rotation, 157–65
    advocacy, 163
    attending physicians, 159
    community case management, 161
    didactics, 164
    evaluation, 164
    forensic populations, 163
    homelessness, 162
    objectives, 157
    rotation sites and experiences, 160
    severe and persistent mental illness in
      community, 160
  contract negotiations, 154
  contracts, 154
  exploratory discussions, 154
  fellowships, 165–66
  financing, 155–57
  fostering empathy, 153
  fourth-year electives, 166
  leadership, 154–55
  Milestones Project, 158
  monitoring and evaluation, 154
  overview, 151
  partnerships, 154
  principles for formation of, 154
  public psychiatry tracks, 165
  public sector workforce development, 152

access to care
  caseload capacity, 35
  quality of care versus, 34–41
    access to optimal services, 34, 37
    front-door access, 34, 35
    use of services, 34, 38
  queuing theory, 35, 37
  triage process, 36
ACGME (Accreditation Council for Graduate
    Medical Education), 152–53, 211, 215*b*
ACT (assertive community treatment), 63, 173–74
  assertive care teams, 20–21
  Cochrane systematic review, 174
  Dartmouth dual diagnosis study, 174
  REACT, 174
  UK700 study, 174
adherence to treatment
  challenges to, 38
  psychoeducation programs and, 39–40
admission process, asylum model of care, 10–11
advanced practice nurses (APNs), 45–46, 48
advocacy, 25–26
  ACGME core competencies, 215*b*
  advocacy education, 211
  advocacy pearls, 212*t*
  case study, 194, 200, 209, 210, 216
  Clifford Beers, 14–15, 22
  community psychiatry rotation and, 163
  defined, 196
  defining mental health, 196
  defining mental illness, 195
  disparities advocacy, 201*b*, 201
  engaging populations in need

advocacy (*cont.*)
    multiproblem immigrant families, 244
    people with mental illness in criminal justice
        system, 240
    historical context, 197–200
    milestones highlighting importance of, 215*b*
    National Committee for Mental Hygiene, 15,
        142, 199–200
    overview, 195
    potential vulnerable populations, 202*b*, 202
    recovery-oriented model of care, 21–24
    resources, 209–16
        national and regional organizations, 209,
            211*t*, 214*b*
        online, 210
    role in community awareness, 206*b*, 206
    role in prevention, 203*b*, 203
    role in social justice/ legislative advocacy,
        207–8*b*, 207
Affordable Care Act (ACA), 24–25
agoraphobia, 57
almshouse concept, 9
Alzheimer's Disease Neuroimaging Initiative, 178
AMA (American Medical Association), 197
American Academic of Medical Colleges, 153
American Board of Psychiatry and Neurology, 14
American Medical Association (AMA), 197
American Psychiatric Association. *See* APA
Anatomical Expression of Rage painting (Bell),
        127*f*, 128
Anatomy of the Human Body, The (Bell), 128
Angelman syndrome, 80*t*
anticholinergics, 90–91
Anti-Insane Asylum Society, 13*b*
antipsychotics
    for ASD, 87
    caps on access to, 43
    CATIE trial, 43–44, 171–72, 176, 185–86, 188–89
    intellectual disability behaviors, 94
    side effects, 90–91
anxiety disorders, 57
    dual diagnosis with intellectual disability, 86
    GAD-7, 108, 113
    interventions for, 205*t*
APA (American Psychiatric Association)
    defining mental illness, 196
    mental health advocacy, 209–10
    resource document, 211
APNs (advanced practice nurses), 45–46, 48
aripiprazole, 87
Aristotle, 195–96

art therapy, 7
ASD (autism spectrum disorder), 86
assertive community treatment. *See* ACT
assisted outpatient treatment, 172
asylum model of care, 9
    admission process, 10–11
    alternatives to, 12
    Benjamin Rush, 9
    dual purpose of, 10
    moral treatment, 11–12
    New York Retreat, 10
    Public Hospital of Williamsburg, 9
    role superintendent, 11
    social isolation, 11
    Thomas Kirkbride, 11
autism spectrum disorder (ASD), 86

Back to the Future vision of community psychiatry
    case studies, 227–29, 250–51
    challenges facing, 223–25
    contributing forces and ideologies, 225–26
    customer service, 229
    defined, 225
    engaging populations in need
        multiproblem immigrant families, 244
        people with mental illness in criminal justice
            system, 240
    managing guilt, 230
    Triple Aim, 226
    "welcoming," 229, 234
Barye, Antoine-Louis, 75*f*
Beard, John, 22–23
Beers, Clifford, 14–15, 22, 142, 199–200
Beggar Woman with Rosary (Callot) (etching), 31*f*
Behavioral Consultation and Primary Care
        (Robinson and Reiter), 110
behavioral/functional models, ID, 92, 93*b*
behavioral health consultants, role in integrated
        care, 114–15
behavioral phenotype models, ID, 91, 92*b*
behavioral therapy
    CBT, 118, 244–45
    intellectual disability with comorbid mental illness, 88
Bell, Charles, 127*f*, 128
Besnard, Paul-Albert, 3*f*, 4
Bini, Luigi, 15–16
bipolar disorder
    dual diagnosis with intellectual disability, 85
    psychoeducation and, 113
bloodletting, 11, 198
Blue Cross/Blue Shield, 112

Bodhisattva Maitreya (The Buddha of the Future), 221*f*, 222
Boerhaave, Herman, 6–7
Braslow, J. T., 10–11, 18
Brigham, Amariah, 12
Bureau of Justice Statistics National Inmate Survey, 66
burnout, physician, 138–39

Cade, John, 17
Callot, Jacques, 31*f*, 32
camphor shock therapy, 15–16
caregiver burden, 206–7
Cartesian dualism (dualistic categorizations), 6
caseload capacity
    defined, 35
    jail-based care, 36*b*
case managers
    on clinical multidisciplinary teams, 58
    role in integrated care, 115
cathartics, 11
CATIE (Clinical Antipsychotic Trials of
        Intervention Effectiveness) trial, 43–44,
        171–72, 176, 185–86, 188–89
CBPR (community-based participatory research), 188
CBT (cognitive-behavioral therapy), 118, 244–45
CCISC (Comprehensive, Continuous Integrated
        System of Care), 241
CCM (collaborative care model), 107–9
    components of, 107
    drawbacks to, 109
    IMPACT studies, 108–9
    variations on, 109
CCTIC (Creating Cultures of Trauma-Informed
        Care) assessment, 247–48
Cerletti, Ugo, 15–16
challenging behaviors, associated with ID, 88–94
    behavioral/functional models, 92, 93*b*
    behavioral phenotype models, 91, 92*b*
    interventions, 94
    lack of skills, 93*b*, 93
    medical illness, 89, 90*b*
    medication side effect, 90, 91*b*
    mental illness, 89*b*, 89
Cherokee Health Systems, 111, 112, 123–24
Children, The (Halberstam), 142
chlorpromazine, 16
chromosome 15q11.2-13.1 duplication, 80*t*
Cicero, 195–96
CITI Program (Collaborative Institutional Training
        Initiative), 188

Civil Rights Act of 1964, 13*b*
Clare, John, 32–33, 34
Cline, C. A., 231, 242
Clinical Antipsychotic Trials of Intervention
        Effectiveness (CATIE) trial, 43–44, 171–72,
        176, 185–86, 188–89
clinical care
    case study, 32, 42, 48–49
    collaborating with other medical providers, 45–46
    controlling medication costs, 43–45
    overview, 33–34
    quality of care versus access to care, 34–41
        access to optimal services, 34, 37
        front-door access, 34, 35
        use of services, 34, 38
    quality of care versus productivity, 41–42
    in rural practice, 46–49
clinical multidisciplinary teams, 55
    barriers to effective teamwork, 60, 61
    case study, 56, 62, 69–70
    clinical models, 61
    conflict management, 60–61, 61*b*, 62
    leadership, 60
    models of care, 62–67
        Assertive Community Treatment, 63
        co-occurring substance use disorders, 65
        crisis services, 63
        hospital transition teams, 67
        jail-based care, 66
    role of psychiatrist on, 58, 59
        benefits of teams, 58
        engaging with team, 60
        fostering high-functioning teams, 61
    team members, 58–59
    treatment planning, 67–70
clinical pharmacist, role in integrated care, 115
clubhouse model, 22–23
CMHCs (community mental health
        centers), 172–73
Coalition Against Major Diseases, 178
COCQI (customer-oriented continuous quality
        improvement), 242, 245
COD (co-occurring disorders), 240–44
cognitive-behavioral therapy (CBT), 118, 244–45
cohort studies, 180–81
collaborative care model. *See* CCM
Collaborative Institutional Training Initiative
        (CITI Program), 188
Colonial America, mental illness in, 8
Columbia University's academic–community
        partnership, 165

community awareness, role of advocacy in, 206b, 206
community-based participatory research (CBPR), 188
community-based research
    assertive community treatment, 173–74
    case study, 170, 188–89
    CATIE trial, 176
    cohort studies, 181
    design of, 178
    effectiveness research, 171–72
    effect size, 182
    evidence-based medicine, 180–81
    finding opportunities for, 177
    health services, 183b, 183
    health technology, 187
    historical context, 172–73
    IMPACT model, 176
    interpreting results of, 180
    NAVIGATE intervention, 177
    obtaining approval for, 180
    odds ratio, 182
    overview, 171–72
    PACE, 175
    pharmaceutical industry, 182
    RAISE Early Treatment Program trial, 177
    randomization, 181–82
    relative risk, 182
    STAR-D study, 171–72, 175, 188–89
    substance use disorders, 186
    violence and mental illness, 171–72, 185
community case management, 161
Community Mental Health Act of 1963, 18–19, 172–73
community mental health centers (CMHCs), 172–73
Community Mental Health Centers Act of 1963, 200
community mental health system, 19
community psychiatry movement
    Back to the Future vision of
        case studies, 227–29, 250–51
        challenges facing, 223–25
        contributing forces and ideologies, 225–26
        customer service, 229
        defined, 225
        engaging multiproblem immigrant families, 244
        engaging people with mental illness in criminal justice system, 240
        managing guilt, 230
        Triple Aim, 226
        "welcoming," 229, 234
    defined, 1
    foundation of, 222–23
    recent developments in, 224
community psychiatry rotation, 157–65
    advocacy, 163
    attending physicians, 159
    community case management, 161
    didactics, 164
    evaluation, 164
    forensic populations, 163
    homelessness, 162
    objectives, 157
    rotation sites and experiences, 160
    severe and persistent mental illness in community, 160
Comprehensive, Continuous Integrated System of Care (CCISC), 241
Connecticut Society for Mental Hygiene, 199–200
consumer/survivor/ex-patient movement, 22
co-occurring disorders (COD), 240–44
Cow Tipping Press, 76
CQI (continuous quality improvement), 241, 243–44, 247, 249–50
Creating Cultures of Trauma-Informed Care (CCTIC) assessment, 247–48
criminal justice system
    engaging people with mental illness in, 240
    mental health care for prisoners, 20b
crisis services, 63
    law enforcement as first response, 64–65
    medical emergency departments, 64
    mobile services, 64–65
    residential services, 64
Critical Path Institute Consortia, 178
culture
    engaging multiproblem immigrant families, 244
    influence on understandings of mental illness, 17b
    treatment planning, 68b, 68
customer-oriented continuous quality improvement (COCQI), 242, 245
customer service, 229

Dartmouth dual diagnosis study, 174
DD (developmental disability)
    defined, 77–78
    intellectual disability
        barriers to health care, 77
        case study, 76–77, 80, 94–95, 97–99

clinical assessment, 83, 83t
comorbid mental illness, 84–88
defined, 77–78
diagnosis, 78, 79t
etiologies, 78, 80t
etiologies of challenging behavior, 88–94
legal Issues, 96
prevalence of, 77, 78
transition from pediatric to adult-based
services, 97
deinstitutionalization, 18
Delay, Jean, 16
delusional disorder. See also psychotic disorders
Deniker, Pierre, 16
depression
caregiver burden, 206–7
DIAMOND, 109–10
imipramine, 16–17
interventions for, 205t
RESPECT-Mil, 109, 110
STAR-D study, 171–72, 175, 188–89
Depression Initiative Across Minnesota, Offering a
New Direction (DIAMOND), 109–10
developmental disability. See DD
Diagnostic and Statistical Manual of Mental Disorders
(DSM-5), 77–78
Diagnostic Manual-Intellectual Disability
(DM-ID), 84
DIAMOND (Depression Initiative Across
Minnesota, Offering a New
Direction), 109–10
Dickinson, Emily, 56–57, 106, 122
didactics, community psychiatry rotation, 164
"disease theory of race," 198–99
disparities advocacy, 201b, 201
dissociative identity disorder, 171
distributed leadership, 60
Dix, Dorothea, 5, 13b, 194–95, 199
DSM-5 (Diagnostic and Statistical Manual of Mental
Disorders), 77–78
dualistic categorizations (Cartesian dualism), 6

Earle, Piney, 11–12
early intensive behavioral intervention (EIBI), 87
Eastern Lunatic Asylum/ Eastern State Hospital
(Public Hospital of Williamsburg), 9
eating disorders, 205t
EBM (evidence-based medicine), 180–81
ECA (Epidemiologic Catchment Area) study, 185
ECT (electroconvulsive therapy), 7–8, 15–16, 88

education. See also academic–community
partnership
ACGME, 152–53, 211, 215b
advocacy education, 211
psychoeducation, 39–40, 113
effectiveness research, 171–72
effect size, community-based research, 182
EIBI (early intensive behavioral intervention), 87
Eisenhower, D., 18–19
electroconvulsive therapy (ECT), 7–8, 15–16, 88
Eliot, T. S., 128–29
empathy, 39, 153, 198, 238–39
engaging populations in need
multiproblem immigrant families, 244
people with mental illness in criminal justice
system, 240
potential vulnerable populations, 202b, 202
Epidemiologic Catchment Area (ECA)
study, 185
equipoise stratified randomization, 175–76
ethics
ethical basis for randomization, 175–76
leadership, 143–46, 144–45b
evaluation
community psychiatry rotation, 164
PACE, 175
REACT, 174
Everdingen, Allart van, 169f, 170
evidence-based decision-making, 44–45
evidence-based interventions, mental
disorders, 205t
evidence-based medicine (EBM), 180–81

FaceTime, 47
fail-first policies, formulary restrictions, 43
Faulkner, L. R., 154
Fauquier, Francis, 9
fetal alcohol spectrum disorder, 80t
financing/funding, 18–19
CMHCs, 172–73
in-home support services, 95
integrated care, 138
public psychiatrists as educators, 155–57
Fiorilli, Vince, 76
Fitbits, 187
FOCUS-PDCA process, 242, 245, 246–47, 248–49
forensic populations
community psychiatry rotation and, 163
engaging people with mental illness in criminal
justice system, 240
jail-based care, 36b, 39, 66

formulary restrictions (medication), 43–45
    CATIE trial, 43–44
    evidence-based decision-making, 44–45
    fail-first policies, 43
    medical algorithms, 44
    patient assistance programs, 44
    pharmaceutical benefit management companies, 43
    tiered formularies, 43
    treatment-decision tools, 43–44
fragile X syndrome (FXS), 78, 80t, 87
front-door access to care, 34, 35
functional behavior assessment, 92–93

GAD-7 (General Anxiety Disorder 7-item scale),
        108, 113
Galen, 195–96
gender. See race and gender
Gibran, Kahlil, 150–51
Grob, Gerald, 8
guardianship, for intellectually-disabled patients, 96

Halberstam, David, 142
Harvard University's academic–community
        partnership, 162
health services research, 183b, 183
health technology research, 187
HEDIS (Health Plan Employer Data and
        Information System), 135
Herrman, H., 60
Hippocrates, 195–96
Hogarth, William, 193f
Home and Community Based Services waivers, 95
homelessness, 19, 65, 162
hospital/clinic medical director, public psychiatrists
        as, 131, 133b
    establishing medical policy, 131–32
    fiscal health of organization, 132
    human resource responsibilities, 131, 133
    interpersonal literacy, 133–34
    systems literacy, 132
hospital transition teams, 67
housing-first programs, 65–66b, 65
human resource responsibilities, 131, 133
"hysteria," 171

I Am! poem (Clare), 32–33, 34
ID (intellectual disability)
    barriers to health care, 77
    case study, 76–77, 80, 94–95, 97–99
    clinical assessment, 83, 83t
    comorbid mental illness, 84–88

    anxiety disorders, 86
    autism spectrum disorder, 86
    mood disorders, 84
    obsessive-compulsive disorders, 86
    prevalence of dual diagnosis, 84
    psychotic disorders, 85
    treatment considerations, 88
defined, 77–78
diagnosis, 78, 79t
etiologies, 78, 80t
etiologies of challenging behavior, 88–94
    behavioral/functional models, 92, 93b
    behavioral phenotype models, 91, 92b
    interventions, 94
    lack of skills, 93b, 93
    medical illness, 89, 90b
    medication side effect, 90, 91b
    mental illness, 89b, 89
legal issues, 96
    guardianship, 96
    interactions with law enforcement, 96
prevalence of, 77, 78
transition from pediatric to adult-based
        services, 97
I Felt a Funeral, in My Brain (Dickinson), 56–57
If I Can Stop One Heart from Breaking
        (Dickinson), 106
imipramine, 16
IMPACT (Improving Mood-Promoting Access to
        Collaborative Treatment), 107, 108–9, 176
Insel, Thomas R., 170
institutional review board (IRB), 180
insulin shock therapy, 7–8, 15–16
integrated care, 107–8b, 110–11b, 112b
    career considerations, 122–23b, 122–25, 124b
    case study, 124–25
    legal issues, 119
    models for, 107–14
        choosing and adapting, 112
        collaborative care model, 107–9
        primary care behavioral health, 110
        reverse integrated care, 113
    role of psychiatrist in, 115–19, 117b, 118b, 136
        as consultant, 115–16
        as educator, 116
        as supervisor, 115–16
    serious mental illness, 121
    specialty care, 119
    team member roles, 114–15
    telepsychiatry, 120
Integrated Care (Raney), 107

intellectual disability. *See* ID
interpersonal literacy, 133–34
interventions
  for anxiety disorders, 205*t*
  for challenging behavior with ID, 93
  EIBI, 87
  evidence-based interventions, 205*t*
  NAVIGATE intervention, 177
  for psychotic disorders, 205*t*
  for substance use disorders, 205*t*
involuntary outpatient commitment, 183
IRB (institutional review board), 180

jail-based care, 36*b*, 39, 66. *See also* forensic
  populations
Johnson-Powell, Gloria, 142
Joint Commission on Mental Illness and
  Health, 18–19

Kendra's Law, 183–84
Kennedy, John, 19
Kennedy, Rosemary, 19
Kevin's Law, 183–84
Khatri, Parinda, 123–24
Kirkbride, Thomas, 11, 13*b*
Kraepelin, Emil, 12–14, 142
Kuhn, Roland, 16

lack of skills, ID, 93*b*, 93
La Femme (Besnard) (etchings), 4
Lauriks, S., 135
law enforcement. *See also* forensic populations
  as first response in crisis, 64–65
  interactions with intellectually-disabled
    patients, 96
  jail-based care, 36*b*, 39, 66
leaders, public psychiatrists as
  addressing physician well-being, 138
  Adolf Meyer, 141
  Benjamin Rush, 140
  case study, 128, 145–46
  educators, 154–55
  Gloria Johnson-Powell, 142
  hospital/clinic medical director, 131, 133*b*
  importance of, 129
  integrated care, 136
  leadership ethics, 143–46, 144–45*b*
  quality management, 135, 136*b*
  state-level medical director, 134*b*, 134
  training for, 139
  unit medical director, 129, 130*b*

legal issues
  integrated care, 119
  intellectual disability, 96
Legros, Alphonse, 55*f*, 56, 150
Lentz, Amanda, 123–24
lithium, 17
Lokko, Hermioni, 153
Lowdermilk, E., 121

MacArthur Violence Risk Assessment
  Study, 185
Maryland Plan, 152
mass incarceration, 20*b*
MAT (medication-assisted treatment), 186
  alcohol use disorder, 186
  opiate replacement therapies, 186–87
Meal Time etching (Strang), 149*f*
Medicaid
  academic–community partnership, 155
  Home and Community Based Services
    waivers, 95
  Mental Health Planning Act of 1986, 172–73
  use of PBMs, 43
Medicaid Act of 1965, 200
medical algorithms, formulary restrictions, 44
*Medical Inquires and Observations Upon the Diseases
  of the Mind* (Rush), 198–99
medical providers, collaborating with, 45–46
  advanced practice nurses, 45–46
  physician assistants, 46, 114
  primary care physicians, 114
Medical Research Council/ AstraZeneca
  Mechanisms of Disease Initiative, 178
Medicare
  academic–community partnership, 155
  use of PBMs, 43
medication-assisted treatment. *See* MAT
Meduna, Ladislas, 15
Melancholy (Besnard) (etching), 3*f*
Memoirs on Madness (Pinel), 198
Memorial (Dix), 194–95, 199
Mendota Mental Health Institute, 173–74
mental health, defined, 196
mental health advocacy. *See* advocacy
Mental Health America (National Committee for
  Mental Hygiene), 15, 142, 199–200
mental health nurses (psychiatric nurses), 59
mental health parity legislation, 24
Mental Health Planning Act of 1986, 172–73
Mental Health Study Act, 18–19
Mental Hygiene Movement, 199–200

mental illness
  defined, 195
  serious mental illness in integrated care, 121
  severe and persistent mental illness in
    community, 160
Metzl, J., 17b
Meyer, Adolf, 12–14, 15, 141
Mind That Found Itself, A (Beers), 14–15, 199–200
Minkoff, K., 231, 242
mood disorders, 57, 84
moral treatment, 7, 11–12, 25

naltrexone, 186–87
NAMI (National Alliance on Mental Illness),
    22, 196
National Alliance on Mental Illness (NAMI),
    22, 196
National Center on Minority Health
    Disparities, 142–43
National Child Traumatic Stress Network
    (NCTSN), 244–45
National Committee for Mental Hygiene (Mental
    Health America), 15, 142, 199–200
National Institute of Mental Health (NIMH)-
    funded clinical trials, 171–72
National Institutes of Health, 142–43, 177–78, 188
NAVIGATE intervention, 177
NCTSN (National Child Traumatic Stress
    Network), 244–45
New Freedom Commission on Mental Health of
    2003, 23
New York Retreat, 10
NIMH (National Institute of Mental Health)-
    funded clinical trials, 171–72
Norfleet, K. R., 122

Obolensky, Michael, 22–23
obsessive-compulsive disorders, 86
odds ratio, community-based research, 182
Oliver, Mary, 222, 229
Olmstead Supreme Court decision, 95
One Mind for Research partnership, 178
On Teaching (Gibran), 150–51
opium, 11
optimal services, access to, 34, 37
outpatient settings, 12–14. See also community-
    based research; community psychiatry
    movement
  involuntary outpatient commitment, 183
  outpatient commitment studies, 172
  PGY- 2 experience, 162

PACE (Personal Assessment and Crisis
    Evaluation), 175
Packard, Elizabeth, 13b
partnerships. See also academic–community
    partnership
PAs (physician assistants), 46, 48
patient assistance programs (PAPs), 44
patient-directed care
  intellectually-disabled patients, 95
  treatment planning, 67–68
patient navigators, role in integrated care, 115
PBMs (pharmaceutical benefit management
    companies), 43
PCBH (primary care behavioral health), 110
Peasant in a Round Hat etching (Legros), 55f
peer support services, 23–24
peer support specialists, 59
Personal Assessment and Crisis Evaluation
    (PACE), 175
person-centered treatment
    planning, 40b, 40–41
person-directed care
  intellectually-disabled patients, 95
  treatment planning, 67–68
pharmaceutical benefit management companies
    (PBMs), 43
pharmaceutical industry, 182
phenylketonuria, 80t
Phipps, Henry, 142
PHQ-2 assessment tool, 114
PHQ-9 assessment tool, 108, 110, 113
physician assistants (PAs), 46, 48
physicians
  on clinical multidisciplinary teams, 57–58
  community psychiatry rotation, 159
  physician burnout, 138–39
  role in integrated care, 114
Pinel, Philippe, 7, 198
Plato, 195–96
polypharmacy, 88, 90–91, 94
post-traumatic stress disorder, 7
practice facilitation, 137–38
Prader-Willi syndrome, 80t
President's New Freedom Commission on Mental
    Health, 67
prevention, role of advocacy in, 203
  primary prevention, 204, 205t
  secondary prevention, 203b, 204
  tertiary prevention, 204
primary care behavioral health (PCBH), 110
primary care physicians. See physicians

prisons. *See* criminal justice system; forensic populations
Pritchard, Thomas Octavius, 34
productivity, quality of care versus, 41–42
Project ECHO, 121
Prophet, The (Gibran), 151
psychiatric nurses (mental health nurses), 59
Psychiatry Genomics Consortium, 178
psychoanalysis, 7
psychopharmacology, 7–8
  chlorpromazine, 16
  imipramine, 16
  lithium, 17
psychotic disorders
  dual diagnosis with intellectual disability, 85
  interventions for, 205*t*
  schizophrenia, 17*b*, 38
Public Hospital of Williamsburg (Eastern State Hospital; Eastern Lunatic Asylum), 9
public psychiatrists
  as clinical team members, 55
    case study, 56, 62, 69–70
    role of psychiatrist on, 58–61
    service array, 62–66
    treatment planning, 67–70
  as clinicians
    case study, 32, 42, 48–49
    collaborating with other medical providers, 45–46
    controlling medication costs, 43–45
    overview, 33–34
    quality of care versus access to care, 34–41
    quality of care versus productivity, 41–42
    in rural practice, 46–49
  history of, 3
    Affordable Care Act, 24–25
    asylum alternatives, 12
    asylum model of care, 9
    chlorpromazine, 16
    Colonial America, 8
    community mental health system, 19
    deinstitutionalization, 18
    Dorothea Dix, 5
    imipramine, 16
    influence of culture on understandings of mental illness, 17*b*
    lithium, 17
    mass incarceration, 20*b*
    mental health parity legislation, 24
    race and gender in early public psychiatry, 13*b*
    recovery paradigm, 22

    shifting paradigms in psychiatry, 6–8
    shock therapy, 15
    somatic treatments, 15
  multiple roles of, 2
public psychiatry
  case study, 4, 18, 21, 25–26
  defined, 1
  tenets of, 1–2

quality of care
  access to care versus, 34–41
    access to optimal services, 34, 37
    front-door access, 34, 35
    use of services, 34, 38
  productivity versus, 41–42, 42*b*
  role of public psychiatrists in, 135, 136*b*
queuing theory, 35, 37

race and gender
  culturally competent care, 38–39
  disparity in access to care, 38
  in early public psychiatry, 13*b*
  schizophrenia diagnosis, 17*b*
  treatment of women and African Americans in early public psychiatry, 13*b*
  treatment planning, 68
RAISE (Recovery After an Initial Schizophrenia Episode), 171–72, 188–89
RAISE Early Treatment Program trial, 177
Rake's Progress, A painting (Hogarth), 193*f*
Randomised Evaluation of Assertive Community Treatment (REACT), 174
randomization, 179–80, 181–82
  CATIE trial, 43–44, 171–72, 176–77, 185–86, 188–89
  equipoise stratified randomization, 175–76
  IMPACT model, 107, 108–9, 176
Raney, L. E., 107, 115–16
REACT (Randomised Evaluation of Assertive Community Treatment), 174
Read, R., 61
Recovery After an Initial Schizophrenia Episode (RAISE), 171–72, 188–89
recovery-oriented model of care, 21–24
  academic–community partnership and, 157
  assertive community treatment, 63
  person-directed treatment planning, 67–68, 69
  recovery paradigm, 22
Re-Engineering Systems of Primary Care Treatment of PTSD and Depression in the Military (RESPECT-Mil), 109, 110

Reiter, J. T., 110
relative risk, community-based research, 182
research. *See* community-based research
resources, advocacy, 209–16
    national and regional organizations, 209,
        211*t*, 214*b*
    online, 210
RESPECT-Mil (Re-Engineering Systems of
        Primary Care Treatment of PTSD and
        Depression in the Military), 109, 110
Rett syndrome, 87
reverse integrated care, 113
risperidone, 87
Robinson, P. J., 110
Rockland State Hospital, 22–23
Rothman, D. J., 8, 10
Rubinstein-Taybi syndrome, 80*t*
rural practice, 21
    asylum model of care, 10, 11
    boundary issues with patients, 47
    clinical care, 46–49
    in colonial America, 8
    professional isolation, 47
    telemedicine, 48
    telepsychiatry, 120
    work–life balance for psychiatrist in, 47*b*
Rush, Benjamin, 9, 13*b*, 140, 198–99

Sakel, Manfred, 15
SAMHSA (Substance Abuse and Mental Health
        Services Administration), 18–19, 203–4
Santos, A., 159
Schermerhorn, Elizabeth, 22–23
schizoaffective disorder. *See also* psychotic disorders
schizophrenia, 17*b*, 38. *See also* psychotic disorders
Schreiber, Flora Rheta, 171
Seascape with Three Figures to the Right etching
        (Everdingen), 169*f*
selective serotonin reuptake inhibitors
    autism spectrum disorder, 87
    intellectual disability behaviors, 94
Sequenced Treatment Alternatives to Relieve
        Depression (STAR-D) study, 171–72,
        175, 188–89
sequential intercept model, 66
Sequeyra, John de, 10, 25
"Serenity Prayer of System Change" (Minkoff and
        Cline), 242
service-utilization. *See* use of services
shock therapy, 15
Silveira, Nise da, 7

Skype, 47
Slagle, Eleanor Clark, 141
smartphone applications, 187
Smith-Magenis syndrome, 80*t*
social isolation, as part asylum model of care, 11
social justice/legislative advocacy, 207–8*b*, 207
social workers, on clinical multidisciplinary
        teams, 59
somatic treatments/therapies, 15, 25
    chlorpromazine, 16
    electroconvulsive therapy, 7–8
    imipramine, 16
    insulin shock therapy, 7–8
    lithium, 17
    shock therapy, 15
specialty care, 119
STAR-D (Sequenced Treatment Alternatives
        to Relieve Depression) study, 171–72,
        175, 188–89
state-level medical directors, 134*b*, 134
Strang, William, 150
Stribling, Francis T., 13*b*
Student Nonviolent Coordinating Committee, 142
suboxone, 186–87
Substance Abuse and Mental Health Services
        Administration (SAMHSA), 18–19, 203–4
substance abuse counselor, role in integrated
        care, 115
substance use disorders
    clinical multidisciplinary teams, 65
    community-based research, 186
    incarceration, 66
    interventions for, 205*t*
    supported housing, 65–66*b*, 65
suicide, 203–4, 205*t*
Sybil (Schreiber), 171
systems literacy, 132

Talbott, J., 154, 155
talk therapy, 7
team member roles, integrated care
    behavioral health consultants, 114–15
    case managers, 115
    clinical pharmacist, 115
    primary care physician, 114
    substance abuse counselor, 115
telemedicine, 48
telepsychiatry, 120
TIC (trauma-informed care), 245, 247–50
tiered formularies, formulary restrictions, 43
Tiger Approaching Pool (Barye) (watercolor), 75*f*

training
  CITI Program, 188
  leadership training, 139
  "training in community living model," 173–74
trans-institutionalization phenomenon, 172–73
transition from pediatric to adult-based services, 97
trauma-informed care (TIC), 245, 247–50
Trauma-Informed Care Project tool, 247
treatment-decision tools, formulary
      restrictions, 43–44
trephination, 198
triage process, 36
Triple Aim, 226
Trisomy 21 and Down syndrome, 78, 80*t*
tuberous sclerosis, 80*t*, 87
Tuke, William, 10
22q11.2 deletion syndrome, 80*t*

UK700 study, 174
unit medical directors, public psychiatrists as,
      129, 130*b*
University of Florida's academic–community
      partnership, 162
University of Texas Southwestern Medical Center's
      academic–community partnership,
      161, 162
urban practice
  almshouse concept, 9
  asylum model of care, 9–10
  in colonial America, 8–9
  jail-based care, 36*b*, 39
  telemedicine, 48

use of services, 34, 38
  adherence to treatment, 38, 39–40
  case management, 39
  clinician empathy and, 39
  culturally competent care, 38–39
  disparity in access to care, 38
  obstacles to, 38
  patient/clinician communication, 39–40
  person-centered treatment planning, 40*b*, 40
  psychoeducation programs and, 39–40
  self-directed care, 40–41

Vallas, Rebecca, 20*b*
violence and mental illness, 171–72
  community-based research, 185
  MacArthur Violence Risk Assessment Study, 185
Vittoz, Roger, 129

Waste Land, The (Eliot), 128–29
"welcoming," 229–34
What a Tiger Can Do (Fiorilli), 76
When Death Comes (Oliver), 222
WHO (World Health Organization)
  defining mental health, 196
  defining mental health advocacy, 197
  port on quality improvement for mental
      health, 135
Williams syndrome, 80*t*
World Health Organization. *See* WHO
World War II, influence on psychiatry, 18–19

Yale University, 163